THE skinnytaste COOKBOOK

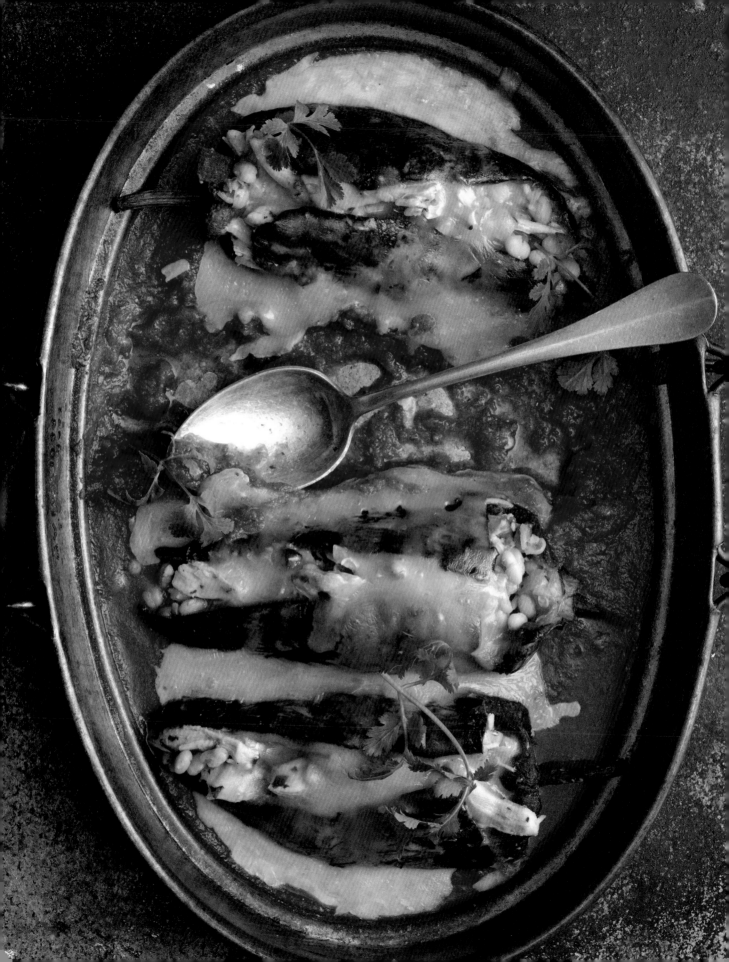

THE skinnytaste COOK BOOK

light on calories, big on flavour

GINA HOMOLKA

with Heather K. Jones, R.D.

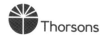 Thorsons

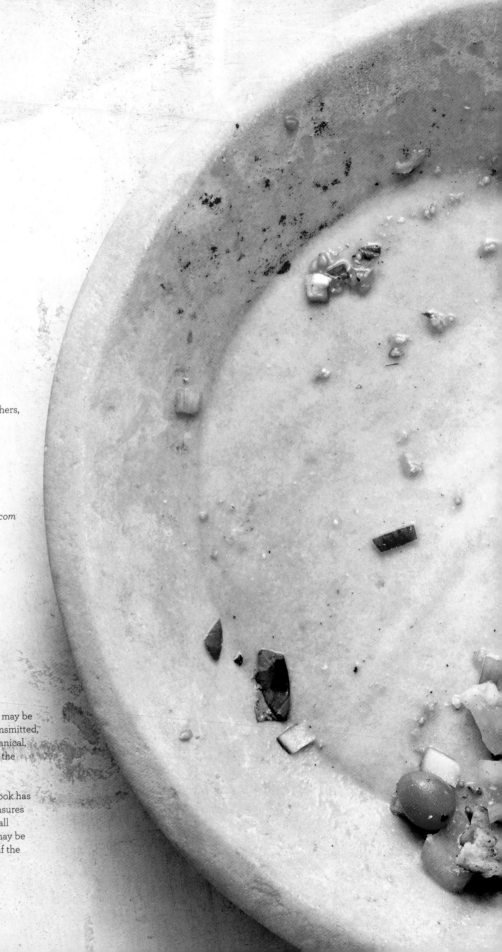

Thorsons
An imprint of HarperCollins*Publishers*
1 London Bridge Street
London SE1 9GF

www.harpercollins.co.uk

Published in the US by Clarkson Potter/Publishers,
a Penguin Random House Company 2014
First published in the UK by Thorsons 2015

10 9 8 7 6 5 4 3 2 1

A catalogue record of this book is
available from the British Library

ISBN 978-0-00-812805-0

Book design by Stephanie Huntwork

Printed and bound in Poland

The nutritional information included in this book has
been calculated using the original US cup measures
and ingredients. The publisher has converted all
measures as accurately as possible but there may be
a degree of variation in the nutritional values if the
UK metric measures are followed.

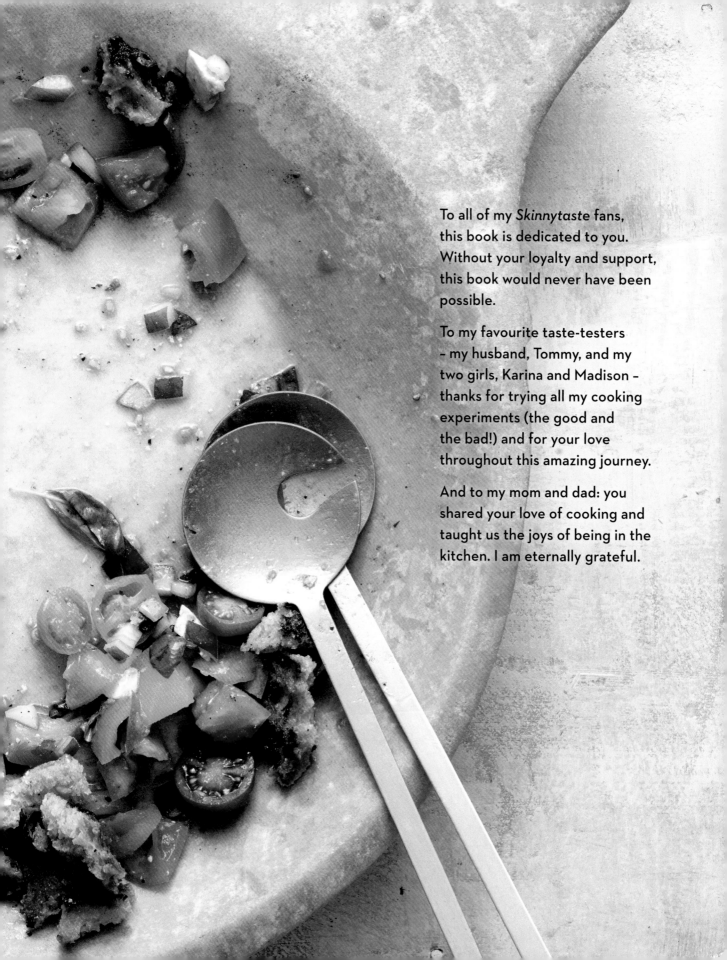

To all of my *Skinnytaste* fans,
this book is dedicated to you.
Without your loyalty and support,
this book would never have been
possible.

To my favourite taste-testers
– my husband, Tommy, and my
two girls, Karina and Madison –
thanks for trying all my cooking
experiments (the good and
the bad!) and for your love
throughout this amazing journey.

And to my mom and dad: you
shared your love of cooking and
taught us the joys of being in the
kitchen. I am eternally grateful.

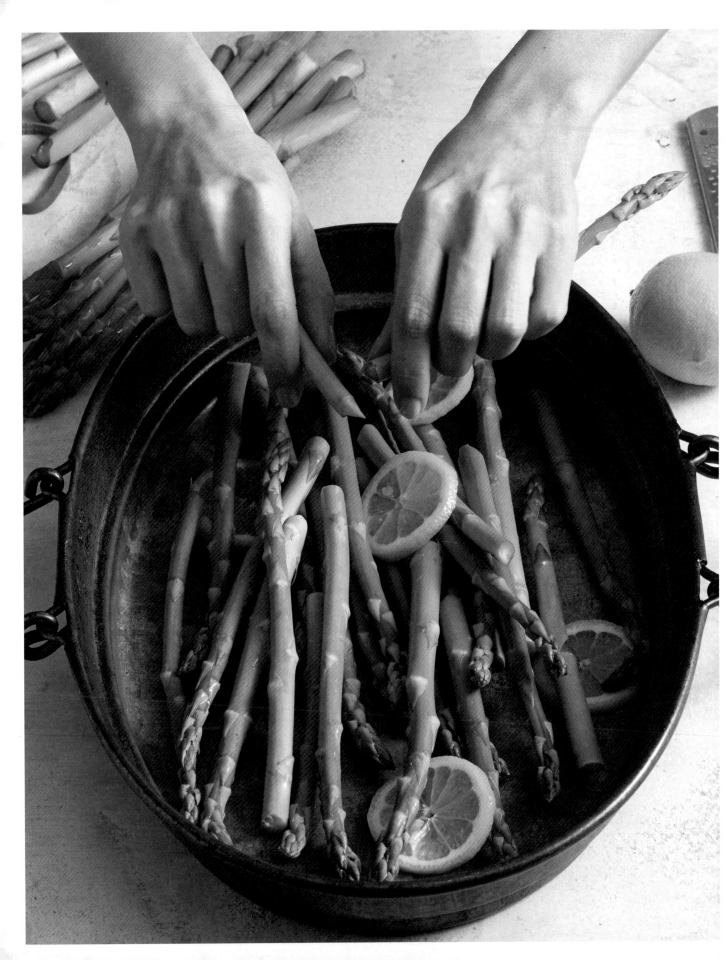

CONTENTS

INTRODUCTION

Struggling to shed some pounds while still eating healthfully and feeding your family meals that they will love? Considering that about 64 per cent of adults in the UK are overweight or obese, and families are looking for meals they can all enjoy together, the answer for most is yes. The problem is that too many people get sucked into the 'diet' trap, buying processed, so-called 'weight loss' food that is nothing more than junk (some of it isn't even *food*) loaded with artificial ingredients that can actually make you sick. Well, I'd like to offer a better suggestion: head to the kitchen and get cooking!

Okay, I know what you're thinking. You're running through a list of reasons you just can't do it. Maybe you don't have time, or it's too expensive, or it takes too much effort. Perhaps you have no idea what you're doing in the kitchen or you believe healthy food tastes bland. I'm sure you have a tonne of reasons – and I've heard most of them.

I'm going to bust all the excuses that keep you out of your kitchen, and show you that cooking – even cooking healthy, nutritious food – is quick, easy and, dare I say it, painless. It's not nearly as pricey as buying processed, packaged junk food, or, down the line, treating the diseases caused by obesity, including cancer, heart disease and diabetes. Cooking at home is both delicious and satisfying – and it can encourage healthy habits in your family, too.

Still sceptical? Doubt I can change your mind about healthy cooking? If you don't believe me, just take it from the millions of readers of my recipe and healthy-eating blog, *skinnytaste.com*. Since 2008, I've been converting the most reluctant eaters, and I'm hoping you'll be next on my list! I'm thrilled (and so humbled) by the incredible number of Skinnytaste success stories – people who have turned to my site for inspiration, advice and help in creating delicious meals that enable them to lose weight and keep it off. Speaking of success stories, I consider myself one, too.

THE ORIGINAL SKINNYTASTE SUCCESS STORY

I was one of those skinny teens who could eat whatever I wanted and never gain a pound (I actually used to try to *put on* weight). But like all good things, it didn't last. Once I was in my twenties, those days of eating whatever I wanted without worrying about weight gain soon came to an end, as pregnancy, children, a slower metabolism and a love for eating out led to weight gain. Like many, I turned to lots of fad diets, which inevitably didn't stick. My turning point was trying Weight Watchers, which is really more of a lifestyle than a diet. The programme gave me the tools to learn how to eat right, which helped me form a healthy relationship with food.

But still I found myself faced with a huge hurdle: I couldn't find any healthy and tasty recipes that supported my lifestyle. Sure, there were plenty of so-called 'diet' recipes out there, but many of them used processed foods or they tasted, well, diet-y. I realized that Weight Watchers – or any other diet plan, for that matter – wouldn't work for me unless I found a way to love the food I was eating.

I've always loved to cook, and I love a challenge, so I set my mind to figuring out how to make some of my favourite meals lighter.

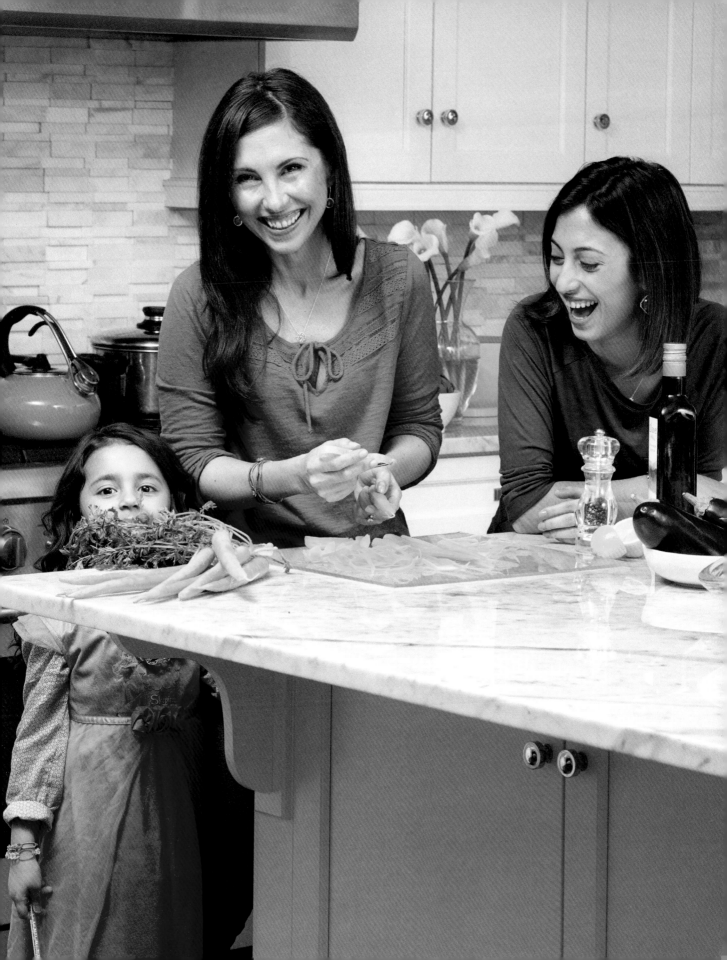

I was thrilled when I discovered that many of my favourite dishes could easily be tweaked to lower the fat and calorie content. But here's the thing: it wasn't enough that the dishes tasted good and were good for me – they also had to appeal to my family. After all, having to make a meal for myself and then a separate meal for the rest of the family was not an option. Really, who has the time for that?

Happily, my kitchen experiments worked. I uncovered the secret formula to kitchen and waistline success: if you skinny-fy (that is, put a healthy spin on) dishes you already love, you'll feel satisfied as you slim down – no sacrificing or deprivation necessary. And a big bonus, my family loved the meals I prepared.

Needing a place to house all of my skinny creations, I started *skinnytaste.com* purely for fun. As a graphic designer, my blog allowed me to marry several of my passions: creating fabulous skinny meals, design and photography. As my blog grew more popular, the feedback started pouring in. It was incredibly gratifying to read weight-loss stories from *Skinnytaste* fans and receive heartfelt letters from people who were slimming down cooking my recipes (and loving them!). I was touched by their praise, and this motivated me to keep my pots in action! *Skinnytaste.com* is now my full-time job – one that I love. (Can someone please pinch me?)

SO, WHAT'S YOUR EXCUSE?

Now that you know a little about me, let's talk about you. What is keeping you from whipping up healthy, homemade meals? If you're not sure, take a quick look at some of the following reasons people struggle to embrace cooking. Do any sound familiar? This book is going to help you get beyond those excuses.

you don't have the time

I hear you – really, I do. For those who just can't seem to find the time, I've created loads of recipes that you can pull together in 30 minutes or less – those recipes are all labelled with a **Q** symbol for quick. I've also cooked up a bunch of slow-cooker meals, so you can throw everything together in the morning and then forget about it until it's time to eat that night. Those recipes are all marked with the **SC** symbol. In addition, you'll find recipes you can double up on and freeze for future use; look for the **FF** for freezer-friendly.

it's too much work

The little effort I put into prepping and cooking my meals is nothing compared with the rewards. Nothing makes me happier than having my family and friends sitting around my dinner table, laughing, eating and enjoying my food. I want you to get to a point where you're comfortable enough in the kitchen that cooking becomes not only easy but also enjoyable. You can get there, and I'm here to help.

Recipe Key

Look for these helpful icons throughout the book:

V – Vegetarian

GF – Gluten-Free

Q – Quick (ready in 30 minutes or less)

FF – Freezer-Friendly

SC – Slow Cooker

it costs too much

At first glance, the meal deal at your local fast-food joint seems to be the better buy. But fresh ingredients go beyond one meal – you can stretch them out over the course of several days or more in a variety of meals. Another problem: many people buy fresh ingredients, only to throw them out because they go bad too fast. If that happens to you, I can see why you think it's more expensive to eat healthfully. I'll show you how to buy the right things and plan ahead so you use it all without wasting.

you don't know the difference between grilling and braising

Not a kitchen pro? Don't sweat it. You'll find a number of simple dishes with easy-to-follow, step-by-step directions for cooks of all levels. And don't be afraid to make mistakes – they provide some of the best lessons.

healthy food sounds about as appetizing as eating paper

I don't know about you, but crispy Buttermilk Oven 'Fried' Chicken (page 151), creamy Too-Good-to-Be-True Baked Potato Soup topped with bacon (page 58) and cheesy Loaded 'Nacho' Potato Skins (page 105) don't sound like diet food at all. Lucky for you, I'm completely obsessed with figuring out ways to make the dishes I just can't live without skinnier and healthier, and yet unbelievably tasty. I also stay away from artificial ingredients and fake sweeteners and, instead, use what the earth has provided: quality ingredients, fresh herbs, spices and seasonal produce that will tantalize your taste buds.

my family won't eat healthy stuff

Can't get anything green past your two-year-old? Have a meat-and-potatoes husband who won't even entertain the idea of chicken, or, gasp, fish? Or maybe your family eats pretty healthfully but doesn't need to lose any weight? There is something for everyone in this book, from picky kids to those with upscale palates. And I haven't forgotten those with food allergies or eating limitations. Gluten-free recipes are marked (GF); I've also given suggestions on how to adapt various recipes. Vegetarian options are marked with a (V).

But it's not all about the recipes. This book is filled with easy-to-understand advice that simplifies healthy eating and cooking. And as a special bonus, I've partnered with registered dietitian Heather K. Jones to provide healthy food facts and useful nutritional information, so you can feel good about enjoying the recipes you love.

So step into my kitchen and cook yourself skinny with me!

A Note About This Edition

The nutritional information included in this book has been calculated using the original US cup measures and ingredients. For this UK edition the cup measures have been converted as accurately as possible, but there may be a degree of variation in the nutritional values if the UK metric measures are followed. In some cases an alternative ingredient has been suggested. If these ingredients are used, the nutritional values included will no longer be valid.

THE SKINNY BASICS

create a good-for-you kitchen and lifestyle

Be honest with yourself: aren't you over all the excuses? What have they done for you, besides keep you from achieving your goals and creating a better life for yourself? By picking up this book, you've already taken the first step to end the excuses. Congratulations! You are now officially on the path towards your goals and a healthier life.

I can assure you that every single recipe in this book will help you on your road to a leaner lifestyle. How do I know this? I've tested and retested every recipe for accuracy in the Skinnytaste test kitchen, which has a staff of just two, my aunt and me. My aunt is a baker, so she's accustomed to following a recipe precisely as written. She catches any blunders and she doesn't overlook small details, so we make the perfect team. (Plus, she lives only minutes away from me.) As you can imagine, testing recipes for a book while also creating new recipes for my blog every day left me with A LOT of extra food at the end of the day. Each afternoon, my aunt and I had a Skinnytaste lunch together, and I would send her home with more food to eat for dinner each night. All this food, and yet there was not a single pound gained. In fact, as the months passed, my aunt dropped over 2 stone and went from a size 14 to a size 6. At first, she thought there might be something wrong, so she went to her doctor to get a full checkup. The good news: her doctor said she was in the best shape of her life, her cholesterol was great, and she had more energy than ever. Her doctor asked her secret, and she happily told him to visit *skinnytaste.com*. I can't even tell you how great it makes me feel that she is another Skinnytaste success story!

The pages that follow will hopefully make you one, too. I will show you that cooking – even cooking healthy, nutritious food – is quick, easy, and even FUN. It's time to get back into the kitchen, where you can start improving and refining your healthy cooking skills while you simultaneously make your way back into your skinny jeans. And guess what? It's not as hard as you think. Here's how to whittle your waist without skimping on taste, Skinnytaste style.

PLAN AHEAD AND EAT HEALTHY ALL WEEK

Whipping up a week's worth of light, filling and family-friendly meals is as easy as one, two, three:

1 **Plan your menu for the week.**

2 **Make a shopping list.**

3 **Head to the supermarket or shops to get all the ingredients you need.** You can choose one or two freezer-friendly recipes to make on your day off; these will serve as more than one meal so you can have leftovers for lunch or dinner later in the month.

TAKE CHARGE OF YOUR KITCHEN

The bottom line: when *you're* in charge of the cooking, you can control what you eat and what you put into your food. The benefits of home cooking are too many to list, but one that's worth repeating is the fact that making your own meals and snacks is the easiest way to control the types of ingredients and the amount of calories you consume.

Don't be intimidated! You don't have to put together elaborate four-course meals, you don't have to spend hours in front of the stove, and you don't have to use recipes that feature ingredients you can't even pronounce. Just get in the kitchen and start cooking. No matter what your comfort level, these recipes will work for you. And if you make a mistake, it's okay! That's the best way to learn. Cut yourself some slack and enjoy the process (and the results)!

DUMP THE JUNK

The road to Skinny isn't paved with processed food. And yet, supermarket shelves are jam-packed with them. What's the draw? They may help save a little time and effort, but try to read the label – there will be a long list of ingredients you've never even heard of or can't pronounce. Even the so-called 'healthy' foods can be loaded with sodium, calories, sugar and fat. If that's what's in your fridge, freezer or pantry, the road to Skinny will be a bumpy one.

Having a properly stocked kitchen, on the other hand, can help set you up for weight loss success. (See A Skinny Kitchen Makeover, page 17.) Whenever a snack attack strikes, you'll be fully prepared with healthy snacks.

FALL IN LOVE WITH REAL FOOD

My eating philosophy is built on utilizing in-season, whole foods – those that are in their unprocessed and natural state. Whole foods are healthier and there's no doubt they taste better. Not only that, when you cook with whole foods, you know exactly what you're putting into your body. Head to your local farmers' market, check out the organic and produce sections of your neighbourhood supermarket or visit a health food shop to stock up on the freshest, tastiest, most nutritious ingredients. Another option is vegetable box schemes. When you join one, you'll get a weekly box of fresh produce and other foods delivered. It's a win-win: you'll be supporting farmers and you'll get the opportunity to experiment with new foods. It's time to reconnect with real food.

KEEP IT SIMPLE

If you're intimidated by healthy eating, you're not alone. But there's no need to stress, because I like to keep things simple. I base my meals largely on nutrient-packed, energy-boosting vegetables, fruits, beans, whole grains and healthy fats. You'll eat fish and only modest amounts (if you choose to) of lean meat and dairy products. You'll also cut back on salt, refined sugars, white flour and partially hydrogenated oils. That's it!

FORGET THE FADS

Here's a Skinny secret: typical fast-fix diets don't work. I've tried several diets that either required me to eat the same bland, tasteless food every day or that required me to cut out carbs completely. Sure, those diets may help you lose weight in the short-term, but they very rarely keep the pounds away for good. In fact, more often than not, they lead to dangerous yo-yo dieting, which could permanently damage your relationship with food. To really shrink your waistline – and keep it that way – you must alter your eating habits and lifestyle in a way that's easy to stick with in the long run.

SERVE UP PERFECT PORTIONS

If you stick to the recipes in this book, your portions will automatically be controlled. Of course, that's not the case if you're making a different recipe or you're dining out.

A good guideline that always helps me at home: picture a plate divided in half. Fill one half with salad and veggies, one quarter with whole grains and the last quarter with lean protein. You can mix up your food options at each meal to maximize your nutrient intake and shake things up for your taste buds. Another trick to use at home is to eat on smaller plates; studies show you'll eat less but you will still feel full.

When you eat out, try to use a few tricks to keep portion sizes under control. For instance, pass on the bread basket (it's too easy to lose track of slices), order a starter as your full meal, split a main with a dining companion, or take half the meal home for lunch the next day.

Make Your Calories Count

While all food contains calories, some are better than others at helping your body look and feel its best. In other words, the quality of your calories counts as much as the quantity. These 'high-quality calories' come from healthy fats, lean protein and high-fibre carbohydrates.

While exact calorie needs depend upon a variety of factors (height, weight, activity levels, etc.), an intake of around 1,500 to 1,600 calories per day will lead to a healthy weight loss of about two pounds per week for most women. (For extra help keeping track, use a free calorie counter app, such as myfitnesspal.com.)

An ideal meal combines at least two of these three groups to help you feel full, maintain normal blood sugar levels, stop you from overeating and promote a healthy glow from the inside out. Create your own meals and snacks by picking foods from at least two of these three categories:

healthy fats

Monounsaturated and polyunsaturated fats help improve blood cholesterol levels, which reduces your risk of heart disease. Plus, they're filling, so they contribute to weight control.

TRY: olives, avocados, hummus, peanut butter, hazelnuts, almonds, cashews, pumpkin seeds, sesame seeds and olive oil

lean protein

Lean protein is super-satisfying and low in saturated fat, which is a huge help for weight loss and heart health. Protein also provides building material for muscles, and muscles are your friends. In addition to making your body look sexy and sculpted, they burn calories **ALL THE TIME**, even when you're asleep.

TRY: eggs, beans, tofu, edamame, turkey, roast beef, pork fillet, fat-free Greek yoghurt, low-fat milk, nuts and nut butters, seeds and fish

high-fibre carbohydrates

Fibre is a type of indigestible carbohydrate that slows carbohydrate digestion, blunting the rise in blood sugar and keeping hunger at bay. It's also linked to reduced risk of heart disease and diabetes.

TRY: oatmeal, nuts and seeds, fruit, beans, peas, wholemeal bread, whole wheat pasta, whole grains (like brown rice, quinoa and popcorn) and vegetables

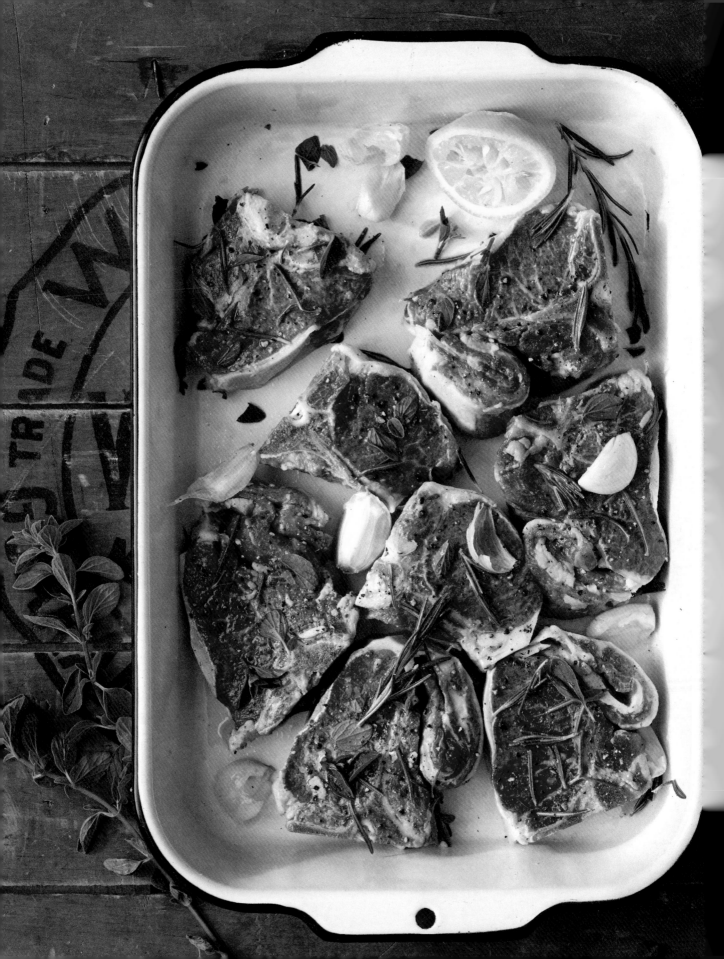

PASS ON PERFECTION

Theodore Roosevelt said it best: 'Comparison is the thief of joy.' This is my favourite quote, and it can apply to so many facets of life. In this case, I mean the idea of that perfect body. We all come in different shapes and sizes, so try to be the best version of yourself and stop comparing yourself to those perfect magazine models. By the way, I worked for years in photo retouching, where we'd spend hours retouching the models to get that 'perfect' look. You would be surprised if you saw the before and after photos. Even the prettiest of models and celebrities have flaws just like you and me.

GIVE YOURSELF A BREAK

Food is my life. I test recipes, write about food, attend food blog conferences and go on lots of awesome food trips hosted by large brands where I get fed some pretty darn good food. If you think I'm passing up any of these delightful dishes because I'm watching my weight, you're wrong. I make good choices all week so I can still enjoy a great meal out here and there. Going out to dinner with my husband or enjoying a night out with the girls is one of my favourite things to do. I learn about new flavours and foods and I get inspiration from those meals. But I still maintain my healthy weight because I factor that in to my life.

So shed that all-or-nothing attitude. Perfection does not equal success when it comes to losing weight or becoming comfortable in the kitchen. Allow yourself some wiggle room and be patient. Remember, you didn't put on the extra weight overnight.

Also keep in mind that no food is considered off-limits or 'bad' when eating the Skinnytaste way. The more you deprive yourself of certain foods, the more you're going to crave them. Enjoy your favourite foods in moderation from time to time, be it a planned indulgence once in a while or a spontaneous bite of a favourite dessert. This is a realistic way of eating that you can keep up for the rest of your life.

EXERCISE, STRESS LESS AND GET PLENTY OF SLEEP

As irresistible as my healthy recipes are, eating a nutritious diet alone is not enough to get your best body – you have to consider the big picture. It involves all the components of a healthy life: a healthy balance of exercise, plenty of sleep, stress relief and fun.

Exercise is an important part of life, as staying fit and being active on a regular basis will not only help you lose weight and decrease your risk for a variety of diseases, but it will also boost your energy levels and improve your mood. It is also a great way to relieve stress. High levels of stress can wreak havoc on your body, so it's also important to manage your stress levels. Unwind by doing some yoga, treating yourself to a massage or other spa treatment, playing with your kids or even just listening to music. And don't forget sleep!

Don't Forget to Hydrate

Even mild dehydration can bring on fatigue and snack attacks. Aim for a daily goal of at least eight 225ml glasses of fluid, with most of that coming from water. Be wary of calorie-dense, high-sugar energy drinks and juice. It takes just a few minutes to drink a few hundred calories, and you'll still feel hungry when you're done because your body doesn't feel as full from drinking liquid as it does from eating food.

I function best after seven to nine hours a night, though everyone is different. When I'm well rested, I'm alert and ready to take on the new day. Figure out the amount of sleep you need to function at your best, and then make sure you get that amount each night.

Lastly, don't forget about the fun factor. You're creating this amazing, healthy Skinny life for yourself – make sure you take full advantage of it. Take some time to think about what you enjoy, and then make a point to do one or more of those things each day.

A SKINNY KITCHEN MAKEOVER

Ready to get on the path to a healthier, leaner new you? Your first step is to give your fridge, freezer and cupboards a healthy makeover. Some of you might think you already have this all figured out, but I'm sure if I sneaked a peek at your kitchen, I'd find at least a few hidden obstacles just waiting to trip you up. Use the strategies below to set up your kitchen for healthy eating success.

THE FRIDGE

keep it real

Your focus should be on health before weight. To accomplish this goal, stock your fridge with real ingredients – that means whole, unprocessed foods. A little real and flavourful food goes a long way, so I keep it in moderation.

be choosy with cheese

Cheese is a stellar source of calcium and protein. For certain varieties – like mozzarella, Swiss or cheddar – I don't mind opting for reduced-fat. But for stronger flavoured cheeses, such as mature cheddar or Gorgonzola, I stick

with the real thing because I can use smaller quantities to get the same flavour hit. And I always have naturally lower-in-fat cheeses, such as Pecorino Romano or Parmesan, in my fridge to boost the flavour in a variety of dishes.

lose light butters and vegetable spreads

You're better off going for a dab of real butter instead of those highly processed spreads. I usually cook with healthy oils, but once in a while, butter is necessary. Cookies, pastry and scones, for instance, often require butter; and for those occasions, I go for the real thing and simply use smaller amounts.

replace artificially sweetened yoghurt

Stock up instead on plain, fat-free or low-fat yoghurt or Greek yoghurt. You'd be surprised by how many low-calorie yoghurts use artificial sweeteners to keep the calories down. Plain Greek yoghurt doesn't have any added sweeteners and it's higher in protein. Sweeten it yourself with fresh fruit or a drizzle of honey.

dispose of shop-bought salad dressings

Lose those bottled salad dressings (yes, even the low-fat ones) and make your own from scratch. It's easy, tastes better, will save you money and will put you in control over what you add to your recipe. (See Fabulous Main-Dish Salads on page 123 for dressing recipes.)

ditch the fizzy drinks

Don't drink your calories away! You can save hundreds of calories by simply swapping fizzy drinks and other sugar-sweetened beverages for still or sparkling water. Need a little flavour? Toss in some fruit, such as watermelon slices, berries or lemon, lime or orange wedges; or add some slices of cucumbers or fresh mint.

THE FREEZER

forgo frozen mains

How about real home cooking instead of all those preservatives? Sure, it takes some extra time to prepare, but the health benefits are worth the effort – look for all my recipes with the **FF** tag and make your own healthier, freezer-friendly meals!

stock up on frozen fruits and vegetables

The problem with tinned vegetables is that they tend to lose a lot of nutrients during the preservation process (a notable exception is tomatoes). Frozen vegetables, on the other hand, may be even more healthy than some of the fresh produce sold in supermarkets because they are flash-frozen when they're at their peak.

opt for better ice cream alternatives

Don't break the calorie bank on full-fat ice creams. Instead, opt for nonfat frozen yoghurt or sorbet. Or you can make your own healthier frozen treats: try freezing ripe bananas to make a quick and healthy one-ingredient frozen treat in your food processor or make your own ice lollies with fresh fruit purées or create a granita (see recipe on page 310).

THE CUPBOARDS

replace white with whole grains

This one simple swap – replacing refined white bread, pasta and rice with whole grains – will increase the amount of fibre and antioxidants you get each day. Plus, whole grains take longer to digest so they keep you feeling fuller, longer. Experiment with different varieties of rice and pastas or try some new grains, such as quinoa, farro, barley, bulgur, wheatberries, spelt and more.

opt for healthy oils

Say hello to a variety of heart-healthy oils: rapeseed, olive and groundnut oils are high in monounsaturated fats, while sunflower and sesame oils are high in healthy polyunsaturated fats.

stock up on whole-grain cereals

Skip the sugary cereals and instead load up on a variety of fibre-rich whole-grain cereals. Go for oats and granola, or try using quinoa in place of your porridge.

buy beans and legumes

Dried or canned beans and legumes are not only economical, they're also a perfect store cupboard staple because they keep for a while and can be used in a variety of dishes. They're a smart buy for health: they're high in fibre and protein as well as B vitamins and iron.

sweeten smartly

Less refined sweeteners, like raw sugar, raw honey and pure maple syrup, contain more antioxidants and give your blood sugar a gentler rise. Still, you'll want to sweeten smartly because these more natural sweeteners are high in calories, so use them sparingly.

be prepared for a snack attack

Toss all those salty fried snacks and instead opt for raw or dry-roasted nuts, like almonds, peanuts, cashews and walnuts. A handful of nuts is a fibre-rich snack that's high in healthy fats. Combine them with dried fruit and whole-grain cereal to make your own trail mix. You can also stock up on nut butters, baked tortilla chips, whole-grain crackers, air-popped popcorn, dark chocolate and fresh fruit (on the counter or in the fridge) so you always have healthier snack alternatives on hand.

Bottom line: having a properly stocked kitchen can help set you up for success. In fact, when your cupboards, fridge and freezer are loaded with the right ingredients and products, healthy eating becomes a breeze.

Stay Motivated

Everyone gets in a slump once in a while, and sometimes it's hard to find your way out. But don't throw in the towel! Instead, find a way to get back in control. Here are some tricks:

- **SURROUND YOURSELF WITH PEOPLE WHO INSPIRE YOU.** I like to be around fit people because they inspire me to work out more. Finding a workout buddy can also help give you that push to keep you on track.

- **PENCIL YOURSELF IN.** We are all busy, and finding time for exercise can be hard. I schedule my workouts in my calendar, as I would a business meeting or doctor's appointment.

- **GO PUBLIC.** Committing yourself publicly, whether it's to friends in person or on social media or even via a blog, can help you stay on track. We don't like to let others down, so this public proclamation can keep us from breaking our commitment to ourselves.

- **THINK SMALL.** Sure, you may want to lose 20, 30 or 40 pounds, or maybe even more. But think of it this way: Every pound lost brings you a pound closer to your goal. So celebrate every small accomplishment, whether it's simply hitting the gym instead of the snooze button or passing on seconds of your favorite dessert.

- **MAKE A LIST AND CHECK IT OFTEN.** Jot down a list of all the reasons you want to eat healthfully, get in better shape and lose weight. Maybe it's for your family or an upcoming holiday; maybe you're sick and tired of feeling sick and tired. Keep the list handy and refer to it whenever your motivation starts to flag.

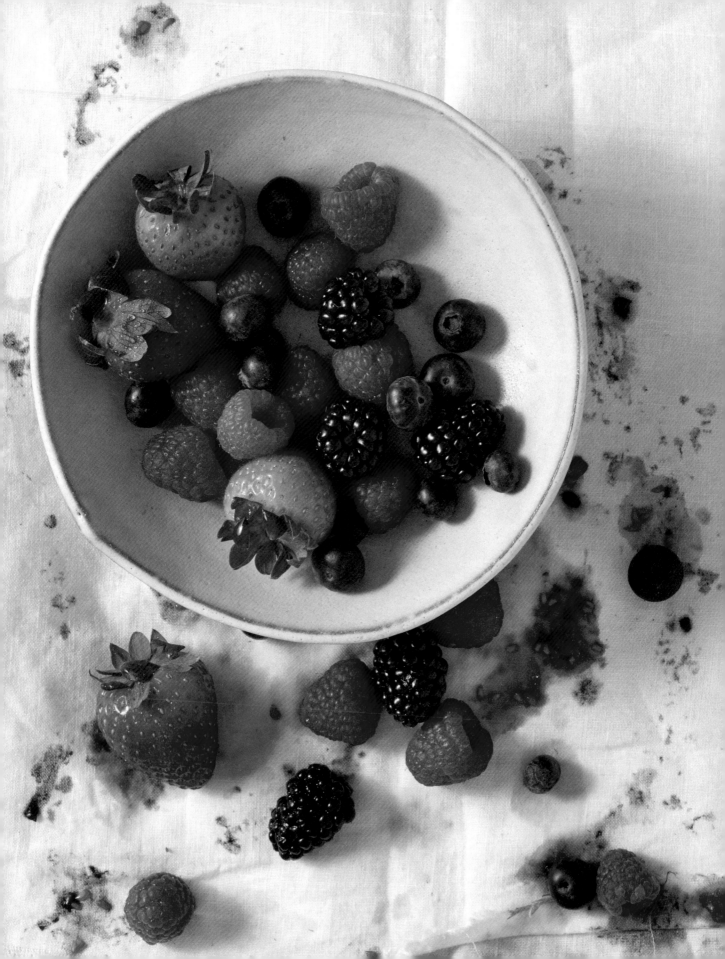

SUNNY MORNINGS

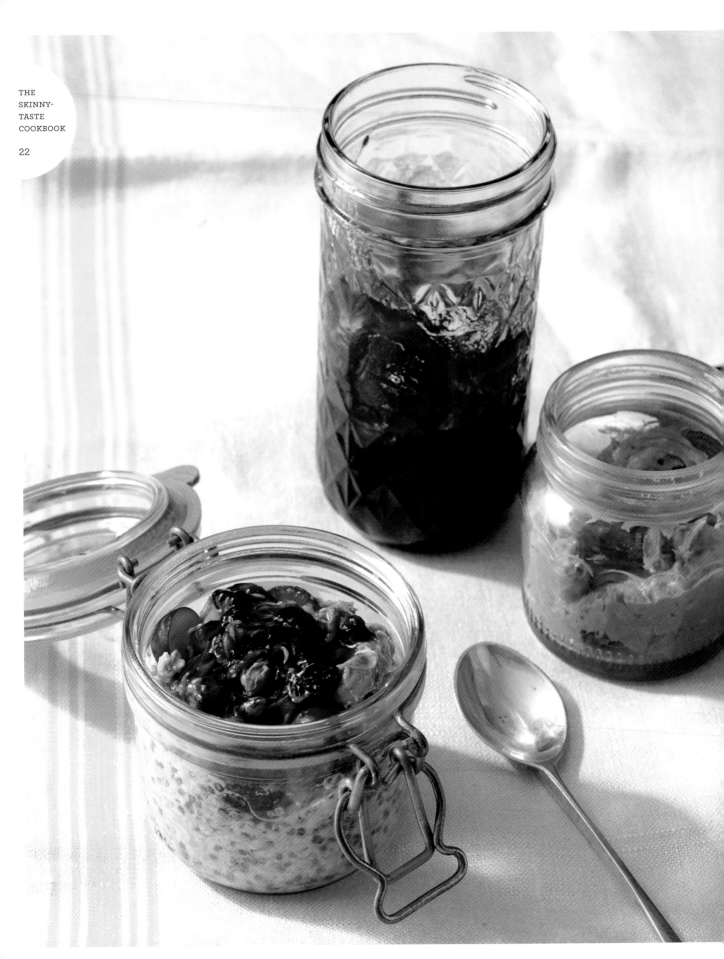

PB & J Overnight Oats in a Jar

SERVES 1

I always found comfort in those mornings when my mom made us porridge for breakfast. I've never liked the instant stuff, and so I've always made my porridge from scratch, just like my mom did. But recently, I discovered overnight oats, which makes a made-from-scratch version, to be eaten cold, possible on those busy weekdays. Plus, it's packed with protein, fibre, vitamins and nutrients – score!

OATS

½ cup (120ml) unsweetened almond milk (or skimmed or soy)

¼ cup (25g) rolled oats*

¼ cup (45g) red seedless grapes, halved

½ tablespoon chia seeds

1 teaspoon sugar (I prefer raw cane sugar)

TOPPINGS

1 tablespoon crunchy peanut butter

1 tablespoon reduced-sugar grape jelly or strawberry jam

Read the label to be sure this product is gluten-free.

For the oats: In a 225ml mason jar, combine the milk, oats, grapes, chia seeds and sugar. Close the jar with the lid, shake the mixture and refrigerate overnight.

For the toppings: The next day, take the jar out of the refrigerator, stir in the peanut butter and jelly or jam and serve.

FOOD FACTS fill up with oats
If you're looking for an easy and satisfying morning meal that can keep hunger in check until lunchtime, oats are the answer. Oats are loaded with soluble fibre, which slows digestion and can keep you feeling fuller longer. They also contain a good amount of protein, which is more satiating than fat or carbs. And studies show the soluble fibre in oats can help reduce LDL ('bad') cholesterol, which can cut your risk for heart disease.

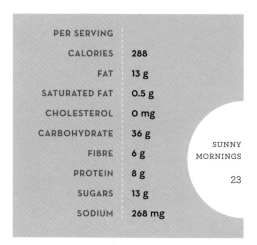

PER SERVING	
CALORIES	288
FAT	13 g
SATURATED FAT	0.5 g
CHOLESTEROL	0 mg
CARBOHYDRATE	36 g
FIBRE	6 g
PROTEIN	8 g
SUGARS	13 g
SODIUM	268 mg

SUNNY MORNINGS

23

Coco-Loco Mango Green Smoothie

SERVES 1

The first time I made a green smoothie, I was a little scared to taste it. But after my first sip, I was hooked. In fact, I start my morning with a green smoothie three or four days each week. Even my toddler loves them, and I like knowing that she's getting a healthy serving of greens. You can use any combination of fruit you like, but I'm wild about the pairing of coconut and sweet ripe mango. I like adding chia seeds to my smoothies, but I also play around with other superfoods, such as flaxseed, hemp seeds and berries. And I also experiment with different greens, like baby kale and baby chard.

1 cup (225ml) coconut milk drink

½ cup (160g) chopped ripe mango

1 cup (45g) baby spinach

1 tablespoon sweetened coconut flakes*

1 teaspoon chia seeds

1 medium dried stoned date (or 1 teaspoon sugar)

1 cup (135g) ice

*Read the label to be sure this product is gluten-free.

In a blender, combine the coconut milk, mango, spinach, coconut flakes, chia seeds and the date and blend until smooth. Add the ice and blend again until smooth.

FOOD FACTS **little seed, big nutrition**
Indigenous to Central America, chia seeds have been a staple energy source for centuries and are high in omega-3 fatty acids, which have been shown to improve cardiovascular health. They have incredible satiating effects, a high fibre content and a good amount of healthy fats and antioxidants.

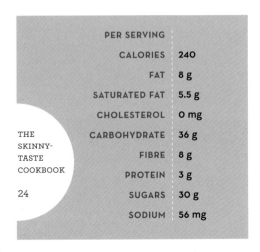

PER SERVING	
CALORIES	240
FAT	8 g
SATURATED FAT	5.5 g
CHOLESTEROL	0 mg
CARBOHYDRATE	36 g
FIBRE	8 g
PROTEIN	3 g
SUGARS	30 g
SODIUM	56 mg

THE SKINNY-TASTE COOKBOOK

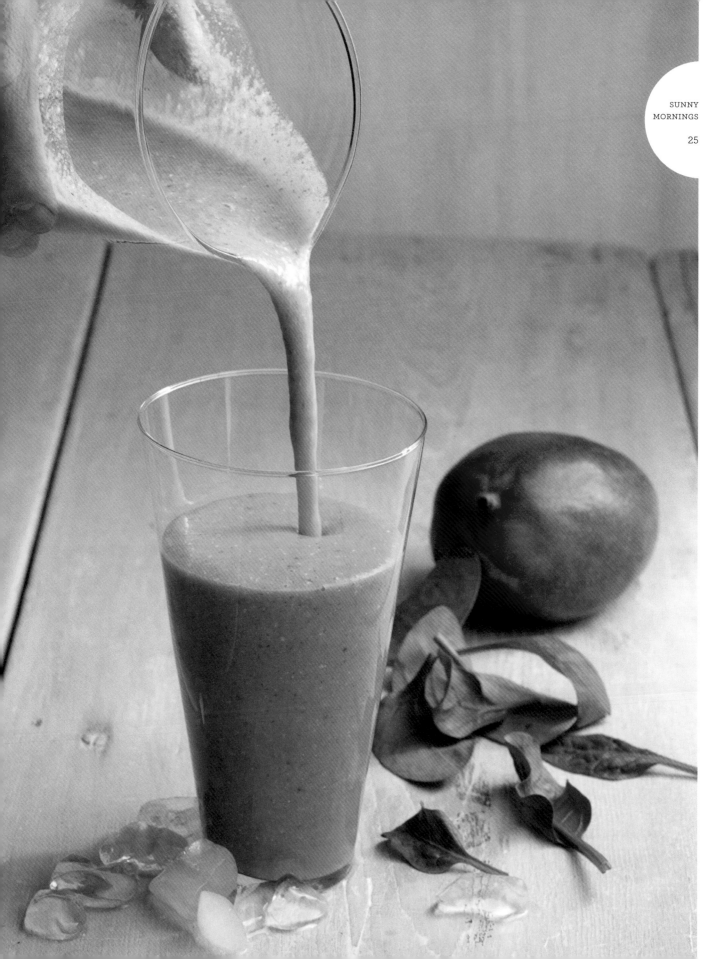

Good-for-You Granola

SERVES 11

Here's how I like my cereal: fill a bowl with a cup of whatever fruit is to hand, top it with some homemade granola and pour in some unsweetened almond milk. This is my basic granola recipe – you can add any combination of dried fruit, nuts or other ingredients that you like. Whatever you use, you'll feel good knowing that this recipe is lower in fat than shop-bought granola.

¼ cup (50g) quinoa

1½ cups (150g) rolled oats*

¼ cup (15g) sweetened coconut flakes

¼ cup (30g) ground flaxseeds

¼ cup (30g) slivered or flaked almonds

¼ cup (30g) chopped walnuts

¼ cup (40g) dried blueberries

¼ cup (40g) dried cherries

¼ cup (90g) honey

1 teaspoon virgin coconut oil (or rapeseed)

½ teaspoon pure vanilla extract

¼ teaspoon ground cinnamon

Sea salt

Read the label to be sure this product is gluten-free.

skinny**scoop**

I make a batch of granola on weekends when I have free time. Kept in an airtight jar, it can last a month or longer.

Preheat the oven to 160°C/140°C fan/Gas 3. Line a baking sheet with baking parchment.

Rinse the quinoa thoroughly under cold water in a fine-mesh sieve. Drain well and pat dry with kitchen paper.

Spread the quinoa, oats and coconut out on the baking sheet. Toast in the oven, stirring once, until golden, about 10 minutes. Transfer the oat mixture to a medium bowl and add the ground flaxseeds, almonds, walnuts and dried fruit. (Leave the oven on.)

In a separate medium bowl, combine the honey, oil, vanilla, cinnamon and a pinch of salt. Pour the mixture over the oats and stir together with a spatula.

Spread the mixture out on the lined baking sheet. Bake until golden brown, 10 to 12 minutes.

PER SERVING	
CALORIES	173
FAT	6.5 g
SATURATED FAT	2 g
CHOLESTEROL	0 mg
CARBOHYDRATE	27 g
FIBRE	3.5 g
PROTEIN	4 g
SUGARS	13 g
SODIUM	8 mg

Paradise Sundae

SERVES 2

When I make a sundae, there are no rules – I use whatever I have to hand. However, the one guideline I try to follow is to make it as colourful as possible. We eat with our eyes, so I often consider how something will look when I make it. Layering is one way to make a dish more visually appealing. The mango and coconut give it a tropical flair and offer up one-and-a-half fruit servings, as well as protein and fibre.

1½ cups (350g) fat-free plain Greek yoghurt

½ cup (90g) chopped strawberries

½ cup (80g) chopped pineapple

½ cup (95g) chopped mango

¼ cup (15g) sweetened coconut flakes*

2 teaspoons honey

Read the label to be sure this product is gluten-free.

Layer the yoghurt, strawberries, pineapple and mango in clear sundae or champagne glasses. Top with coconut flakes, drizzle with honey and serve.

A DIY Sundae Party Bar

Start with fat-free Greek yoghurt and let your guests pick their favourite mix-ins. Choose a variety for maximum flavour, colour and crunch:

FRUITY: fresh berries, cherries, bananas, peaches, kiwi, pomegranate seeds, pineapple, mango, fresh figs, dried fruit

CRUNCHY: granola, toasted nuts (chopped pecans, walnuts, pistachios and almonds), coconut flakes (toasted, optional)

SWEET: cocoa nibs, dark chocolate, honey, peanut butter, maple syrup

'SPICE-Y': cinnamon, cocoa powder, nutmeg

NUTRITION BOOSTERS: chia seeds, hemp seeds, ground flaxseeds, goji berries, toasted quinoa

PER SERVING	
CALORIES	220
FAT	3 g
SATURATED FAT	3 g
CHOLESTEROL	0 mg
CARBOHYDRATE	32 g
FIBRE	3 g
PROTEIN	18 g
SUGARS	26 g
SODIUM	85 mg

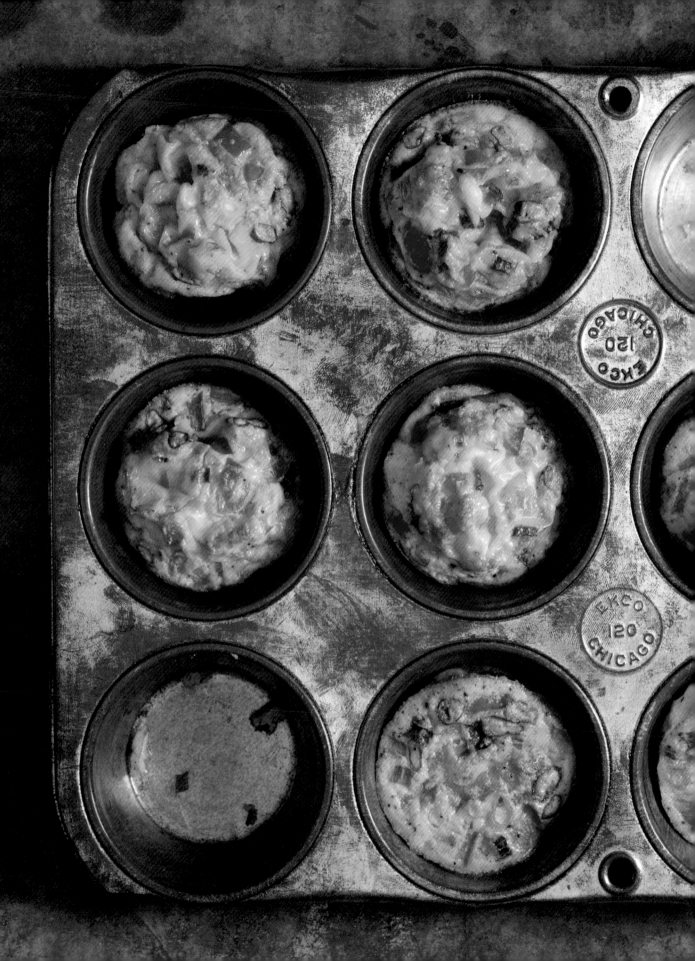

Make-Ahead Ham, Onion and Pepper Omelette 'Muffins'

MAKES 12 MUFFIN-SIZE OMELETTES • SERVES 6

These make-ahead muffin-size omelettes are the perfect solution for breakfasts on the run. Bake them up and you'll have breakfast ready for the next few days. Just keep them refrigerated and portioned in ziplock plastic bags. Simply reheat right before heading to work or the gym, or getting your kids off to school. To make these light, I swap half the egg yolks with egg whites. That way, you still get the nutrients of the egg yolk, but with half the fat.

Olive oil cooking spray or oil mister

6 large eggs

6 large egg whites

¼ teaspoon sea salt

Freshly ground black pepper

75g sliced ham (about 4 slices), finely chopped

50g lighter Swiss cheese, chopped

½ cup (90g) finely chopped red or orange pepper

¼ cup (30g) chopped spring onions

Preheat the oven to 180°C/160°C fan/Gas 4. Lightly spray a standard 12-cup nonstick or silicone muffin tin with oil.

In a medium bowl, beat the whole eggs and egg whites with a fork. Season them with the salt and a pinch of black pepper. Mix in the ham, Swiss cheese, pepper and spring onions. Pour the egg mixture into each muffin cup and carefully place the tin in the oven.

Bake until the eggs set, 20 to 24 minutes.

skinnyscoop

You can freeze leftovers or make a double batch. To freeze, wrap cooled egg muffins in clingfilm. To reheat, unwrap frozen egg muffins and microwave for about 1 minute or place on a baking sheet and bake at 180°C/160°C fan/Gas 4 until heated through, about 25 minutes.

PER SERVING	
CALORIES	119
FAT	6 g
SATURATED FAT	2 g
CHOLESTEROL	195 mg
CARBOHYDRATE	2 g
FIBRE	0.5 g
PROTEIN	14 g
SUGARS	1 g
SODIUM	329 mg

Apple 'n' Spice Baked Oatmeal

SERVES 6

Apples and spice and everything nice! I love baked oatmeal. It's almost like having dessert for breakfast – without the guilt. Whenever I make it, I can trick my toddler, Madison, into eating it cold because she thinks it's cake. I personally prefer eating it warm, right out of the oven, and I make this anytime I need something delish for brunch.

APPLE FILLING

2 tablespoons honey

2 cups (200g) peeled and chopped Gala apples

¾ cup (90g) sultanas

1 tablespoon cornflour

¾ teaspoon ground cinnamon

¼ teaspoon ground nutmeg

Cooking spray or oil mister

OATMEAL

1 cup (100g) rolled oats*

⅓ cup (40g) chopped walnuts or pecans

½ teaspoon baking powder

Sea salt

1 cup (225ml) skimmed milk

1 large egg

2 tablespoons raw honey

1 teaspoon pure vanilla extract

FOOD FACTS fill up on fibre! Studies show that people lose more weight when they fill up on high-fibre foods, such as fruit, oats and other whole grains. Your goal: at least 25 grams of fibre a day for women, 38 grams for men.

Read the label to be sure this product is gluten-free.

For the apple filling: In a large heavy pot, combine ⅓ cup (75ml) water, the honey, apples, sultanas, cornflour, cinnamon and nutmeg. Bring to a simmer over low heat and cook, stirring occasionally, until the apples are soft, about 25 minutes.

Preheat the oven to 190°C/170°C fan/Gas 5. Lightly spray a 20 x 20cm or 23 x 23cm ceramic baking dish with oil. Put the apples into the bottom of the prepared baking dish.

For the oatmeal: In a bowl, combine the oats, half of the walnuts, baking powder and a pinch of salt. Pour over the apples.

In a separate bowl, whisk together the milk, egg, honey and vanilla. Pour the milk mixture over the oats, making sure to distribute the mixture as evenly as possible.

Sprinkle the remaining walnuts over the top. Bake until the top is golden brown and the oatmeal is set, about 30 minutes. Cut into 6 rectangles and serve warm from the oven.

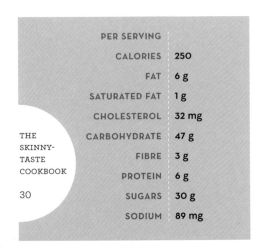

PER SERVING	
CALORIES	250
FAT	6 g
SATURATED FAT	1 g
CHOLESTEROL	32 mg
CARBOHYDRATE	47 g
FIBRE	3 g
PROTEIN	6 g
SUGARS	30 g
SODIUM	89 mg

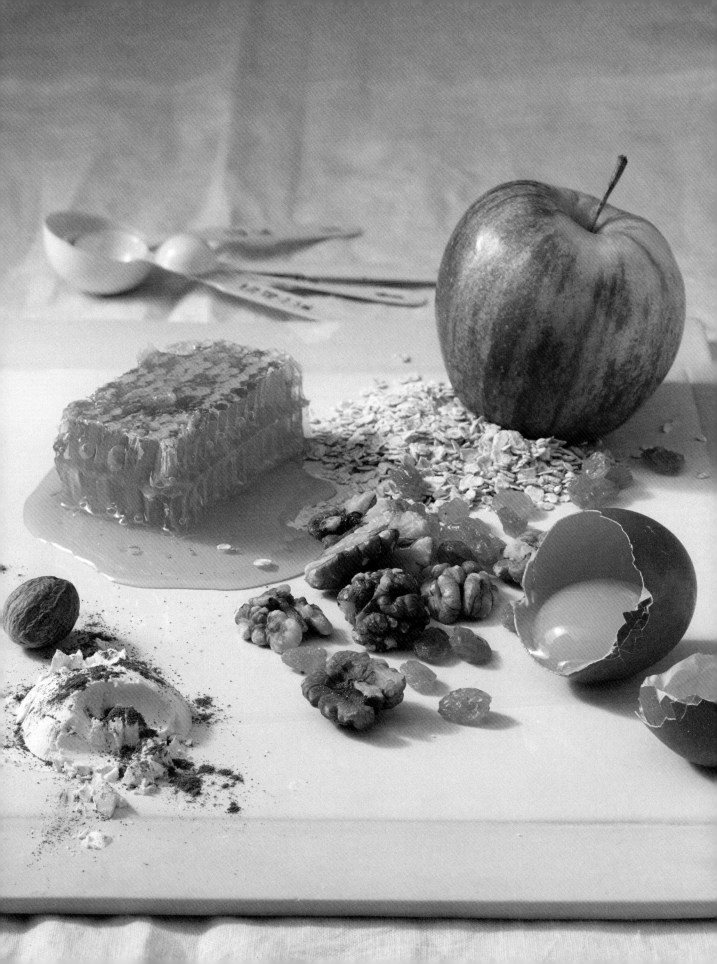

Naked Eggs Benedict

SERVES 4

When I was a teenager, my mom owned a café eponymously named Marlene's Kitchen. She worked behind the counter cooking breakfast for all her customers and I helped out, working as a waitress on weekends. It was a quaint little place, where everyone knew one another and felt at home. Of all the breakfast options there, poached eggs topped with cheese were my favourite. I'm also fond of another popular poached pick: Eggs Benedict. But the Hollandaise sauce is all butter, and just a few tablespoons contain a whopping 200 calories. No thanks! My 'skinny' solution is simple: use wholemeal muffins, add some greens and skip the Hollandaise sauce. Then I don't feel bad splurging with a little light Havarti cheese on top.

4 slices back bacon

4 large eggs

2 multigrain or wholemeal muffins, split and toasted

1 cup (45g) loosely packed baby spinach

Sea salt and freshly ground black pepper

50g light Havarti cheese, grated†

1 tablespoon finely chopped fresh chives, for garnish

Heat a large frying pan over medium-high heat. Add the bacon and cook until lightly browned on each side, about 1 minute.

Fill a large deep frying pan with about 5cm of water and bring to a boil. Reduce the heat to low to maintain a simmer. Crack the eggs into individual bowls. Gently slide the eggs one at a time into the simmering water. Using a spoon, gently nudge the egg whites in towards the yolk. Cook for 2 to 3 minutes for a semi-soft yolk or 3 to 4 minutes for a firmer-set yolk. Using a slotted spoon or spatula, transfer the eggs one at a time to a plate lined with kitchen paper to drain.

Divide the toasted muffin halves among 4 serving plates. Top each muffin half with a piece of bacon, a quarter of the baby spinach and a poached egg. Season each with a pinch of salt and black pepper to taste. Sprinkle with grated cheese and finely chopped chives and serve hot.

† If you can't find light Havarti cheese, you can use standard Havarti or Tilsit instead.

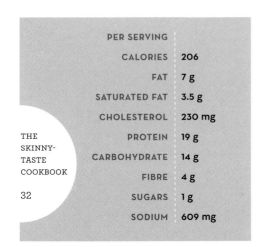

PER SERVING	
CALORIES	206
FAT	7 g
SATURATED FAT	3.5 g
CHOLESTEROL	230 mg
PROTEIN	19 g
CARBOHYDRATE	14 g
FIBRE	4 g
SUGARS	1 g
SODIUM	609 mg

Greek-a-licious Egg White Omelette

SERVES 4

Egg white omelettes can be boring, but not when you fill them with flavour! This savoury omelette is packed with spinach, tomatoes, feta and dill, reminiscent of the popular Greek pie *spanakopita*. Greek food holds a special place in my heart because I was born in Astoria, New York, which has a large Greek population. Years later, I landed one of my first jobs there, and I used to eat at a little Greek hole-in-the-wall that made the best spanakopita – I ordered it nearly every day. This dish has a lot fewer calories than the original since it skips the flaky pastry, calls for egg whites and uses light feta cheese.

1 tablespoon extra-virgin olive oil

½ cup (60g) finely chopped spring onions

1 garlic clove, crushed

2 vine-ripened tomatoes, finely chopped

275g frozen chopped spinach, thawed and excess liquid squeezed out

1 tablespoon chopped fresh dill

2 tablespoons chopped fresh parsley

Sea salt

½ cup (70g) crumbled light feta cheese

2 tablespoons grated Parmesan cheese

12 large egg whites

Freshly ground black pepper

Cooking spray or oil mister

In a medium frying pan, heat the oil over medium heat. Add the spring onions and garlic and cook until soft, about 2 minutes. Add the tomatoes, spinach, dill, parsley and a pinch of salt. Cook until the tomatoes soften and everything is heated through, 3 to 5 minutes. Season with ¼ teaspoon salt and cook for 1 more minute. Remove the pan from the heat, stir in the feta and Parmesan, and cover the pan to keep warm.

In a medium bowl, whisk the egg whites with 2 tablespoons water, ⅛ teaspoon salt and a pinch of black pepper. Lightly spray a large nonstick frying pan with oil and heat the pan over medium-low heat. When hot add a quarter of the egg mixture (about ½ cup), swirling to evenly cover the bottom of the pan. Cook until set, about 2 minutes. Spoon a quarter of the spinach mixture (about ½ cup) onto half of the omelette, fold the omelette over and slide it onto a serving plate. Repeat with the remaining ingredients.

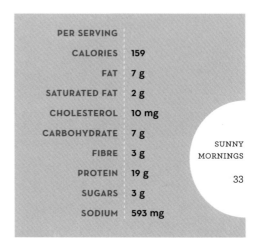

PER SERVING	
CALORIES	159
FAT	7 g
SATURATED FAT	2 g
CHOLESTEROL	10 mg
CARBOHYDRATE	7 g
FIBRE	3 g
PROTEIN	19 g
SUGARS	3 g
SODIUM	593 mg

SUNNY MORNINGS

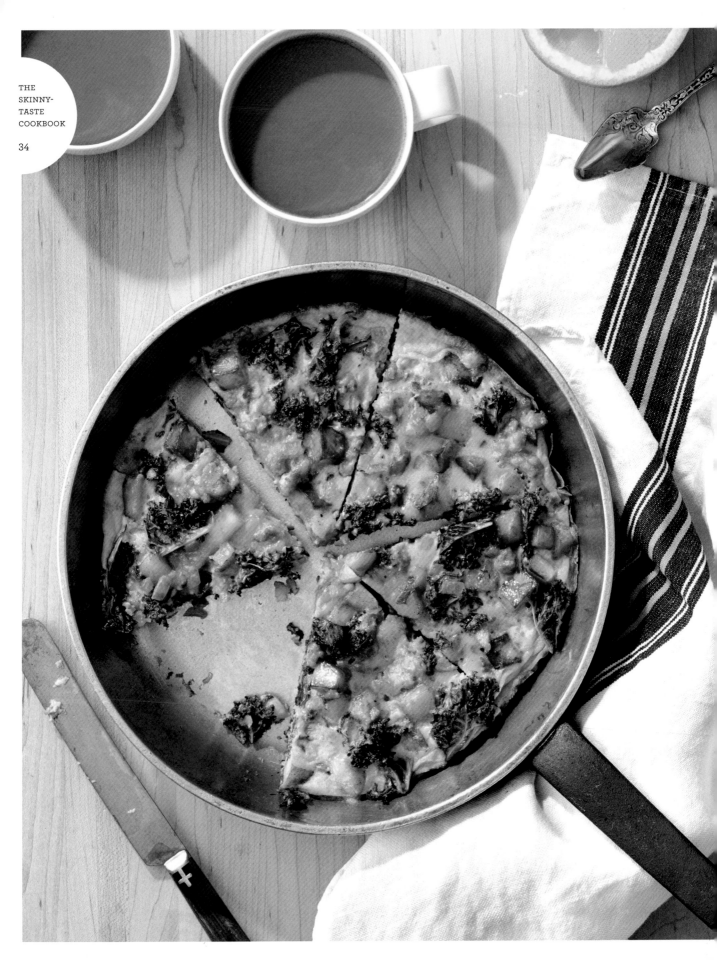

Winter Potato, Kale and Sausage Frittata

SERVES 6

With sausage, potatoes, eggs and kale, this frittata is a meal in one! Frittatas are so versatile, both in what you can put in them and for the fact that they're delicious for breakfast, lunch *or* dinner. You can literally clean out your refrigerator to come up with countless ways to whip one up. This dish starts out on the hob and finishes in the oven, so you'll need to use an ovenproof frying pan. If you don't own one, you can also slide the half-cooked frittata onto a large plate, then carefully flip it back into the pan and finish cooking the other side over low heat on the hob.

5 large eggs

3 large egg whites

2 tablespoons grated Pecorino Romano cheese

Sea salt

Freshly ground black pepper

2 teaspoons olive oil

170g fresh sweet Italian chicken sausages, casings removed*†

1 small onion, chopped

2 medium (350g) peeled all-purpose potatoes, diced into 1cm pieces

⅛ teaspoon garlic powder

⅛ teaspoon paprika

1 cup (70g) chopped kale, stems and ribs removed

*Read the label to be sure this product is gluten-free.

Preheat the oven to 200°C/180°C fan/Gas 6.

Crack the eggs and egg whites into a large bowl. Add grated Pecorino Romano, ⅛ teaspoon of the salt and a pinch of black pepper and beat until blended.

Heat a 25cm nonstick ovenproof frying pan over medium heat. Add 1 teaspoon of the oil, the sausage meat and the onions to the pan and cook, breaking the meat up with a wooden spoon, until it's cooked through and the onions are golden, 5 to 6 minutes. Transfer the sausage and onions to a plate.

Add the remaining 1 teaspoon of oil to the pan, then add the potatoes. Season with ½ teaspoon salt, garlic powder, paprika and a pinch of black pepper. Cover and cook the potatoes over medium-low heat, stirring occasionally, until crisp and tender,

(recipe continues)

PER SERVING	
CALORIES	184
FAT	8.5 g
SATURATED FAT	2.5 g
CHOLESTEROL	178 mg
CARBOHYDRATE	13 g
FIBRE	2 g
PROTEIN	14 g
SUGARS	1 g
SODIUM	383 mg

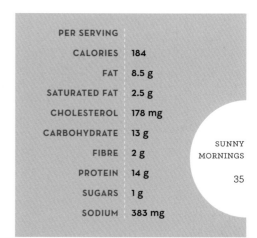

SUNNY MORNINGS

35

Any dark leafy green can be swapped for the kale – try spinach or Swiss chard. You can freeze leftovers to reheat for another day. To freeze, cut the cooked, cooled frittata in wedges, wrap each wedge in clingfilm, wrap in foil and freeze until hard. To reheat, unwrap frozen frittata and microwave it, or bake at 180°C/160°C fan/ Gas 4 until heated through, about 35 minutes.

10 to 12 minutes. Add the kale, cover, and cook until wilted, 2 to 3 minutes.

Add the cooked sausage and onions to the pan and stir to combine. Pour the egg mixture into the pan. Reduce the heat to low and cook until the edges are set, 6 to 8 minutes.

Transfer the pan to the oven and bake until the frittata is completely set and cooked through, 8 to 10 minutes. Remove from the oven, place a plate over the pan, and turn the frittata out onto the plate. Cut into 6 wedges and serve.

† If you can't find Italian chicken sausages, another kind of chicken sausage or reduced-fat pork sausages will work well.

Breakfast Excuse Buster

Research shows that skipping meals – breakfast in particular – can lead to weight gain. The fact is breakfast should be a morning must! But it doesn't have to be time-consuming – it could be something as simple as a slice of wholemeal toast with nut butter and bananas (five minutes, tops!), yoghurt or some hard-boiled eggs with fruit.

For an egg-streamly easy breakfast, I boil a dozen eggs in advance and keep them in the refrigerator for a handy, hunger-busting breakfast. A piece of fruit plus one large egg are only 200 calories, and the mix of protein, fat and fibre will keep you satisfied until lunch. For a more substantial start to the day, you can whip up my favourite Egg, Tomato and Spring Onion Sandwich (page 90) in minutes, because the eggs are already cooked. (Bonus: no sticky frying pan to clean!)

Cali Avocado Egg Sandwich

SERVES 4

I'm always impressed with how health-conscious people in California are, and it excites me to see that they put avocados on everything. (If you haven't noticed yet, I'm a bit avocado-obsessed myself. I always have three or four avocados in my kitchen at any given time.) You can find healthy food options everywhere in the Golden State – even the airport, which is where I actually got the inspiration for this sandwich.

8 large egg whites

Sea salt

Freshly ground black pepper

Cooking spray or oil mister

¼ cup (30g) chopped spring onions

¼ cup (50g) seeded and chopped tomatoes

¼ cup (45g) chopped red pepper

8 slices wholemeal bread, toasted

1 medium (110g) avocado, thinly sliced

In a medium bowl, beat together the egg whites, ¼ teaspoon salt and black pepper to taste.

Heat a 23cm nonstick frying pan over medium heat. When hot, lightly spray the pan with oil. Add 1 tablespoon each of the spring onions, tomatoes and pepper, and season with a pinch of salt. Cook, stirring, for 1 minute. Pour in a quarter of the egg whites and rotate the pan. Reduce the heat to medium-low and cook until the eggs are set, 1 to 1½ minutes. Fold the eggs in half so they look like a half moon and cook for 30 more seconds. Fold the eggs in half again.

Transfer the eggs to a piece of toasted bread. Top each with one-quarter of the avocado, a pinch more of salt and black pepper and a second slice of bread. Cut in half and serve. Repeat with the remaining ingredients to make 3 more sandwiches.

skinny**scoop**

After I get back from shopping, I leave one avocado out on the counter to ripen, and put the rest in the refrigerator so they last longer. If I don't use a whole avocado, I keep the stone in the remaining avocado, cover it tightly with clingfilm and refrigerate it.

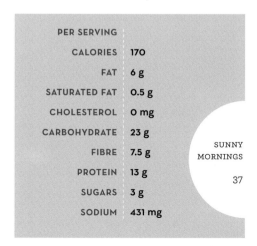

PER SERVING	
CALORIES	170
FAT	6 g
SATURATED FAT	0.5 g
CHOLESTEROL	0 mg
CARBOHYDRATE	23 g
FIBRE	7.5 g
PROTEIN	13 g
SUGARS	3 g
SODIUM	431 mg

SUNNY MORNINGS

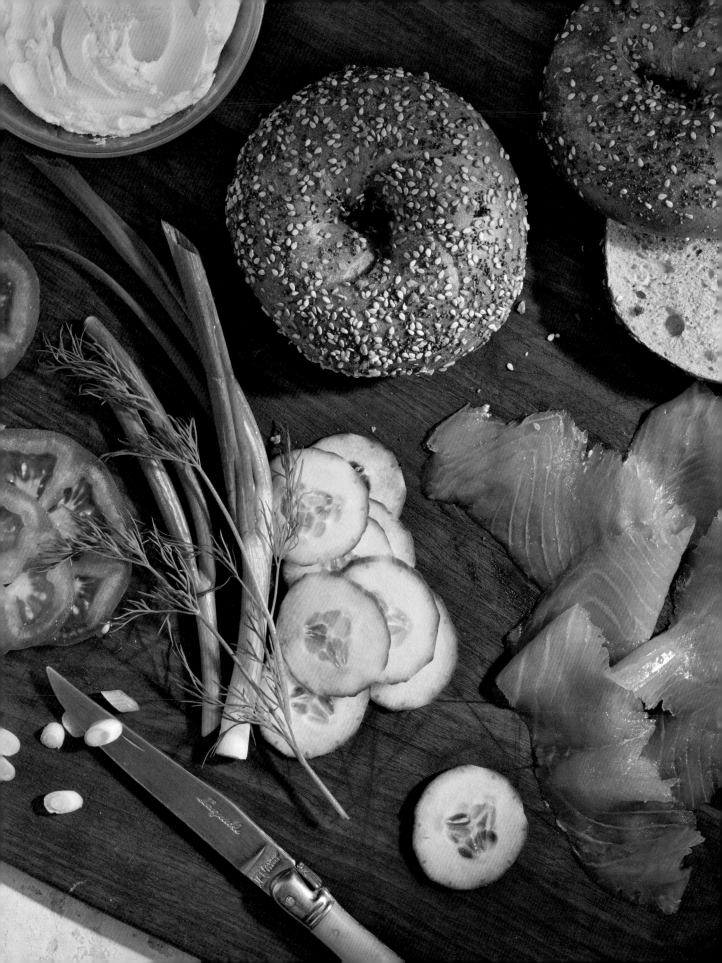

Open-Face Bagels
with Spring Onion-Lox Cream Cheese

SERVES 4

Bagels and lox is a New York City classic. The dish – which is perfect for breakfast, lunch or brunch – takes just minutes to whip up and is delicious, especially when topped with a few slices of fresh tomatoes and cucumbers. The bagels they sell here in New York are pretty large, so I find half a bagel, which is roughly 60 grams, to be the perfect size. My favourite bagel is wholemeal, but any whole-grain type is a great option.

110g light cream cheese, at room temperature

50g smoked salmon or lox, finely chopped

¼ cup (30g) finely chopped spring onions

1 tablespoon finely chopped fresh dill

2 large wholemeal bagels, sliced in half, or 4 small bagels

1 medium tomato, thinly sliced

½ medium cucumber, thinly sliced

Sea salt

Freshly ground black pepper

In a medium bowl, combine the cream cheese, salmon, spring onions and dill. Spread 3 tablespoons of the cream cheese mixture onto each bagel half. Top each half with tomatoes and cucumber slices, and finish with a pinch of salt and black pepper.

skinny**scoop**

Although smoked salmon and lox can be refrigerated for about a week (make sure they're tightly wrapped), they're best eaten as soon as possible because the intensity of flavour and firmness of texture will diminish as the days go by.

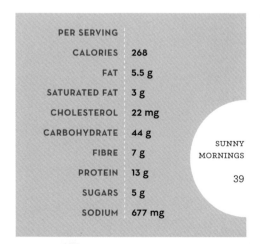

PER SERVING	
CALORIES	268
FAT	5.5 g
SATURATED FAT	3 g
CHOLESTEROL	22 mg
CARBOHYDRATE	44 g
FIBRE	7 g
PROTEIN	13 g
SUGARS	5 g
SODIUM	677 mg

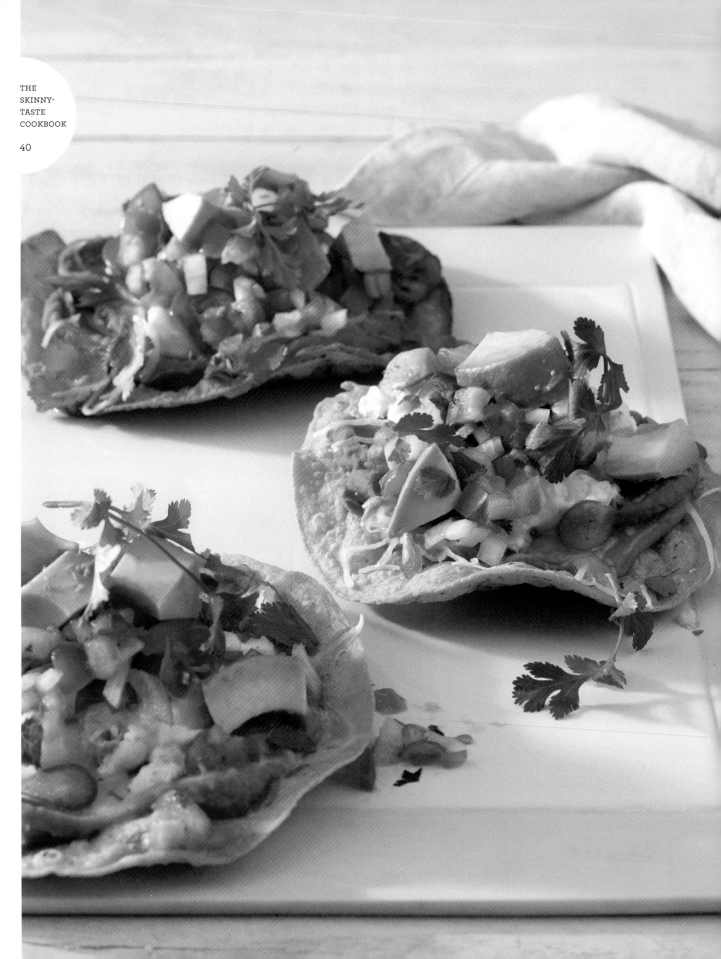

'Que Rico' Breakfast Tostada

SERVES 4

Scrambled egg whites with spring onions piled high on a crispy tostada with refried beans, melted cheese, salsa, jalapeño and diced avocado – can I get an 'Olé!' Whenever I'm craving a bit of spice to start my day, I love making these Mexican-inspired breakfast tostadas. (No worries if you don't care for spicy food – you can easily leave out the jalapeño.)

8 large egg whites

Sea salt

Freshly ground black pepper

3 tablespoons chopped spring onions

Cooking spray or oil mister

1 cup (230g) refried beans*

1 teaspoon ground cumin

4 corn tostadas*†

1 cup (125g) grated reduced-fat Mexican cheese blend‡

1 jalapeño or other green chilli, thinly sliced

¼ cup (50g) pico de gallo, homemade (page 120) or shop-bought fresh salsa

½ medium (50g) avocado, cut into 1cm chunks

4 sprigs of fresh coriander, for garnish (optional)

*Read the label to be sure this product is gluten-free.

Preheat the oven to 180°C/160°C fan/Gas 4.

In a medium bowl, beat together the egg whites, ¼ teaspoon salt and a pinch of black pepper. Add the spring onions and mix well.

Heat a medium nonstick frying pan over medium heat. When hot, lightly spray the pan with oil and add the eggs. Cook, stirring occasionally, until set, about 3 minutes. Remove the pan from the heat.

In a medium bowl, combine the refried beans, cumin and ⅛ teaspoon salt. Arrange the tostadas on a baking sheet and spread a quarter of the bean mixture over each tostada. Top each with a quarter of the scrambled egg whites, a quarter of the cheese and a few slices of jalapeño.

Bake the tostadas until the cheese melts, 4 to 5 minutes. Transfer the tostadas to plates. Top with pico de gallo or salsa and avocado and garnish with coriander, if desired.

† If you can't find corn tostados, you can use corn tortillas instead – just brush with a little oil and bake in the oven at 190°C/170°C fan/Gas 5 for 5 to 10 minutes until crisp and lightly golden before adding the topping.

‡ If you can't find Mexican cheese, lighter cheddar will work well.

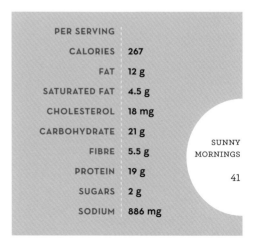

PER SERVING	
CALORIES	267
FAT	12 g
SATURATED FAT	4.5 g
CHOLESTEROL	18 mg
CARBOHYDRATE	21 g
FIBRE	5.5 g
PROTEIN	19 g
SUGARS	2 g
SODIUM	886 mg

Pumpkin-Obsessed Vanilla-Glazed Scones

MAKES 12 SCONES

These light and fluffy buttermilk scones – made with pumpkin purée, autumn spices and a vanilla pod glaze – will warm up your home and fill it with an intoxicating scent that no fancy candle can come close to replicating. I've lightened these up substantially by using buttermilk instead of cream and replacing some butter with pumpkin purée. They taste just as good as any scone you would buy in a fancy coffee shop with half the calories.

SCONES

Cooking spray or oil mister

½ cup (120ml) cold buttermilk

1 large egg

1 teaspoon pure vanilla extract

5 tablespoons tinned unsweetened pumpkin purée

¼ cup packed (55g) dark brown sugar

1 vanilla pod

1 cup (130g) wholemeal flour

1 cup (150g) plain flour, plus more for the work surface

1 tablespoon baking powder

2 teaspoons pumpkin pie spice†

¼ teaspoon ground nutmeg

¼ teaspoon ground cinnamon

½ teaspoon sea salt

3 tablespoons very cold butter, cut into small pieces

GLAZE

2 tablespoons cold skimmed milk

1 cup (125g) icing sugar, sifted

Preheat the oven to 190°C/170°C fan/Gas 5. Spray a baking sheet with oil.

For the scones: In a medium bowl, whisk together the buttermilk, egg, vanilla, pumpkin purée and brown sugar. Using the tip of a sharp knife, cut along the length of the vanilla pod to split it open. Scrape half of the seeds into the bowl and whisk well; reserve the remaining seeds for the glaze.

In a large bowl, whisk together the flours, baking powder, pumpkin pie spice, nutmeg, cinnamon and salt. Using a pastry blender or 2 knives, cut in the chilled butter until the mixture resembles coarse breadcrumbs. Add the buttermilk mixture and stir until just moist.

† If you can't get hold of pumpkin pie spice, you can blend your own – just combine 1 teaspoon ground cinnamon, ½ teaspoon ground ginger, ¼ teaspoon ground cloves and ⅛ teaspoon ground nutmeg.

(recipe continues)

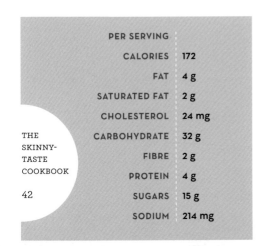

PER SERVING	
CALORIES	172
FAT	4 g
SATURATED FAT	2 g
CHOLESTEROL	24 mg
CARBOHYDRATE	32 g
FIBRE	2 g
PROTEIN	4 g
SUGARS	15 g
SODIUM	214 mg

skinnyscoop

For perfect scones, be
careful not to overwork
the dough and be sure
your butter is well chilled.
I always keep a packet of
butter in the freezer just
for making scones.

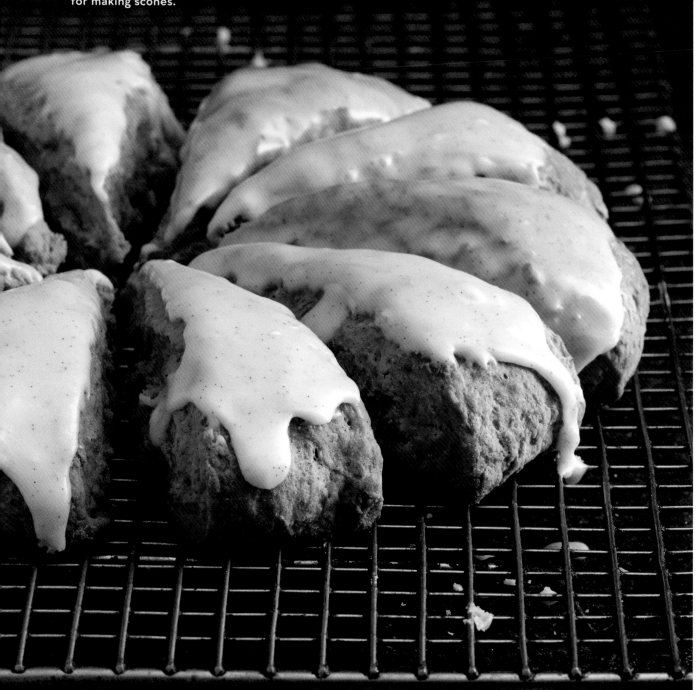

Turn the dough out onto a floured work surface and knead lightly four times with floured hands. Transfer the dough to the baking sheet and shape it into a 23cm round about 2cm thick. Using a knife, cut the dough all the way through into 12 wedges.

Bake until golden brown, 18 to 20 minutes. Transfer to a wire rack and let cool for about 10 minutes before glazing.

For the glaze: Meanwhile, in a medium bowl, whisk together the remaining seeds from the vanilla pod and the milk. In another bowl add the icing sugar. Using a spatula mix in the milk and combine well until it is mixed through and forms a thick glaze.

Put the scones on baking parchment and drizzle the vanilla glaze over the scones using a spoon. Alternatively you can dip the tops of the scones into the glaze, and then let them sit on the paper to harden.

Serve warm. Leftovers can be stored in airtight containers for up to 2 days.

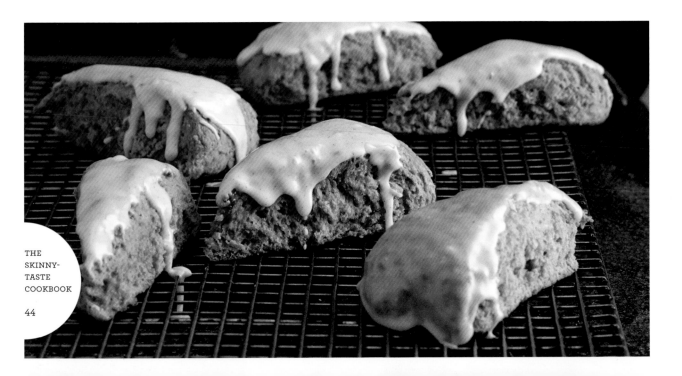

Heavenly Banana-Nut Oat Muffins

MAKES 12 MUFFINS

This recipe is like a cross between banana bread and baked oatmeal – two of my favourite breakfast foods! They are so delicious, you won't believe that the recipe calls for just a single tablespoon of oil. They get their moisture instead from very ripe mashed bananas, which also add a natural sweetness, allowing you to use less sugar. Aside from the fact that these just taste pretty darn good, you'll also score some filling fibre and satiating protein from the oats.

Cooking spray or oil mister

1½ cups (150g) rolled oats

1¼ cups (300ml) unsweetened almond milk

½ cup packed (115g) dark brown sugar

1 cup (240g) mashed ripe bananas

2 large egg whites

2 tablespoons honey

1 tablespoon rapeseed oil

1 teaspoon pure vanilla extract

½ cup (65g) wholemeal flour

1 teaspoon baking powder

½ teaspoon bicarbonate of soda

½ teaspoon sea salt

¾ cup (90g) chopped walnuts

Preheat the oven to 200°C/180°C fan/Gas 6. Line a standard muffin tin with 12 liners and lightly spray the liners with oil.

Pour the oats into a large bowl, add the almond milk and mix well; soak for about 30 minutes.

Add the brown sugar, mashed bananas, egg whites, honey, oil and vanilla to the oats and mix well.

In a medium bowl, whisk together the flour, baking powder, bicarbonate of soda and salt. Slowly add the flour mixture ingredients to the liquid ingredients and mix with a spatula until just incorporated. Fold in the walnuts. Pour the batter into the prepared muffin tin.

Bake until a toothpick inserted comes out clean, 24 to 28 minutes. Allow to cool before serving.

skinny scoop

Make a batch of these muffins and freeze what you don't eat in a freezer-safe ziplock plastic bag. Pop frozen muffins in the microwave for a few seconds and you'll have a quick breakfast ready for when you're on the go.

PER SERVING	
CALORIES	162
FAT	6.5 g
SATURATED FAT	0.5 g
CHOLESTEROL	0 mg
CARBOHYDRATE	24 g
FIBRE	2.5 g
PROTEIN	4 g
SUGARS	12 g
SODIUM	167 mg

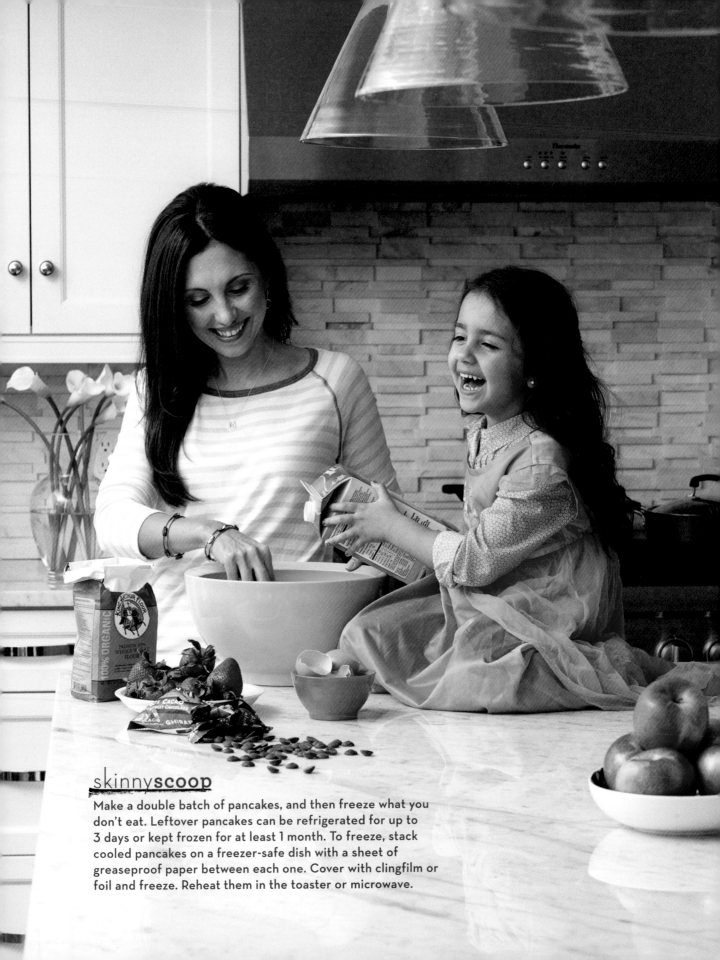

skinnyscoop

Make a double batch of pancakes, and then freeze what you don't eat. Leftover pancakes can be refrigerated for up to 3 days or kept frozen for at least 1 month. To freeze, stack cooled pancakes on a freezer-safe dish with a sheet of greaseproof paper between each one. Cover with clingfilm or foil and freeze. Reheat them in the toaster or microwave.

Guiltless Chocolate Chip Pancakes

MAKES 10 PANCAKES · SERVES 5

These fluffy pancakes are lighter than a standard pancake because I've replaced most of the fat with apple sauce and egg whites – but no one would know. I make these on the weekends for my daughter Madison – she just loves them. Sometimes for fun, I make a smiley face, using fruit for eyes and chocolate chips as the mouth. She usually gets a big chuckle out of that. Personally, I prefer topping my pancakes with fresh strawberries and honey, because they complement the flavour of the chocolate.

½ cup (65g) wholemeal flour

½ cup (75g) plain flour

2 teaspoons baking powder

¼ teaspoon sea salt

½ cup (125g) unsweetened apple sauce†

1 cup (225ml) unsweetened almond milk (or soy or low-fat dairy milk)

3 large egg whites

2 teaspoons rapeseed oil

1 teaspoon pure vanilla extract

Cooking spray or oil mister

¼ cup (45g) chocolate chips

5 large strawberries, sliced

Honey or pure maple syrup, for serving (optional)

In a large bowl, whisk together the flours, baking powder and salt.

In a separate bowl, combine the apple sauce, almond milk, egg whites, oil and vanilla. Stir the flour mixture into the apple sauce mixture until just moist, being careful not to overmix.

Heat a large nonstick frying pan or griddle over medium-low heat. When hot, lightly spray the pan with oil. Scoop out a ladleful of batter for each pancake, then sprinkle 1 teaspoon of chocolate chips on top. Cook until the pancakes start to bubble and the edges begin to set, 1½ minutes. Flip the pancakes over and cook the second side until golden, 1½ minutes. Repeat with the remaining batter.

To serve, put 2 pancakes on each of 5 plates and then top with strawberry slices and honey or maple syrup (if using).

† If you can't get hold of unsweetened apple sauce, use sweetened as an alternative.

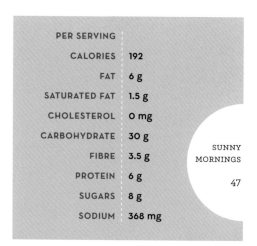

PER SERVING	
CALORIES	192
FAT	6 g
SATURATED FAT	1.5 g
CHOLESTEROL	0 mg
CARBOHYDRATE	30 g
FIBRE	3.5 g
PROTEIN	6 g
SUGARS	8 g
SODIUM	368 mg

Corny Banana-Blueberry Pancakes

MAKES 10 PANCAKES · SERVES 5

I love cornbread and corn muffins, so I thought, why not add some cornmeal to my pancakes? The result: naturally sweet, fluffy, wholemeal pancakes with a corn muffin–like texture. A single serving – 2 pancakes – provides almost 3 grams of fibre, which can help control your appetite until lunch.

¾ cup (90g) wholemeal flour

½ cup (75g) fine cornmeal

2 teaspoons baking powder

¼ teaspoon sea salt

1 large ripe banana, mashed well

1 cup plus 2 tablespoons (255ml) buttermilk

3 large egg whites

2 teaspoons rapeseed oil

1 teaspoon pure vanilla extract

1 cup plus 2 tablespoons (185g) blueberries

Cooking spray or oil mister

5 tablespoons pure maple syrup, for serving

FOOD FACTS beware of maple syrup substitutes
Be careful what you pour over your pancakes. You might be topping your stack with 'pancake syrup', which is a mix of different types of sugar, flavourings and other ingredients. Real maple syrup has just one ingredient: maple syrup. Be sure to check the ingredients list.

In a large bowl, whisk together the flour, cornmeal, baking powder and salt.

In a separate bowl, combine the mashed banana, buttermilk, egg whites, oil and vanilla.

Add the flour mixture to the banana mixture and stir until just moist, making sure not to overmix. Gently fold in the blueberries.

Heat a large nonstick frying pan or griddle over medium-low heat. When hot, lightly spray with oil.

Scoop out a ladleful of batter for each pancake. Cook until it starts to set and the bottom is golden brown, about 3 minutes. Flip the pancake and cook the second side until golden brown, about 2 minutes. Repeat with the remaining batter.

Arrange 2 pancakes on each of 5 plates and serve topped with 1 tablespoon of maple syrup.

PER SERVING	
CALORIES	259
FAT	3 g
SATURATED FAT	0.5 g
CHOLESTEROL	2 mg
CARBOHYDRATE	51 g
FIBRE	3 g
PROTEIN	7 g
SUGARS	22 g
SODIUM	349 mg

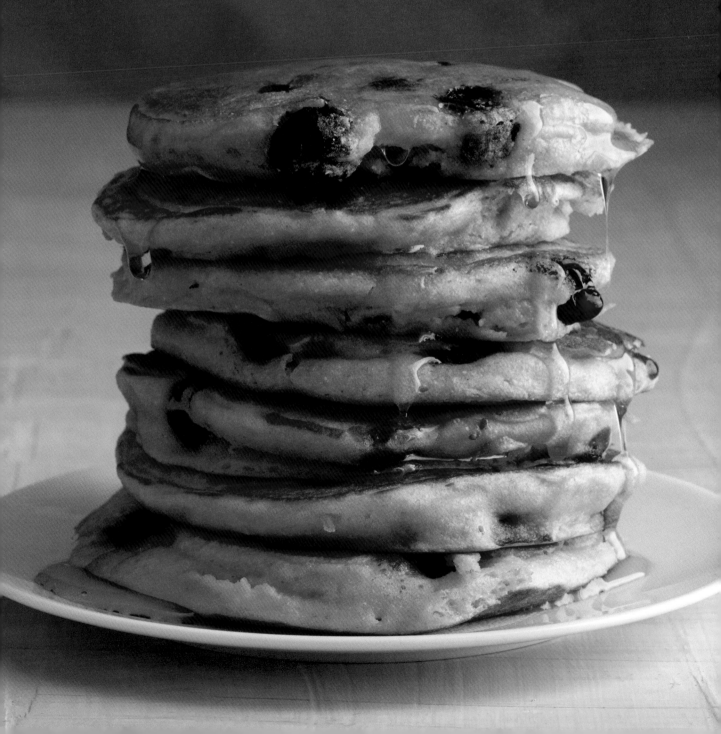

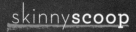

If you have only medium or coarse cornmeal to hand, you can grind it in a clean spice mill until fine.

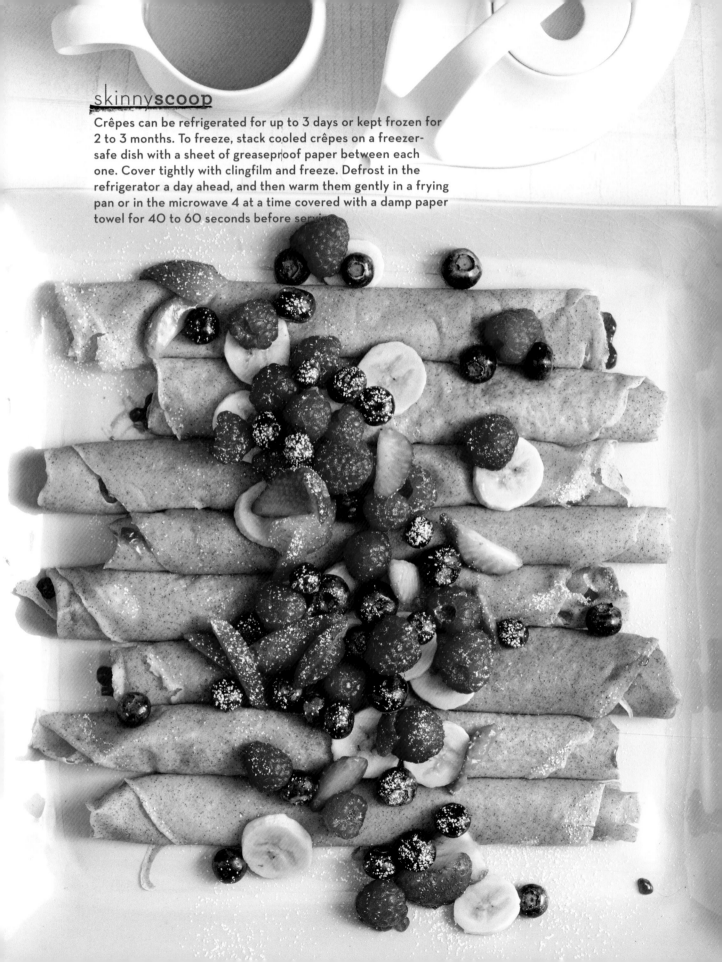

skinnyscoop

Crêpes can be refrigerated for up to 3 days or kept frozen for 2 to 3 months. To freeze, stack cooled crêpes on a freezer-safe dish with a sheet of greaseproof paper between each one. Cover tightly with clingfilm and freeze. Defrost in the refrigerator a day ahead, and then warm them gently in a frying pan or in the microwave 4 at a time covered with a damp paper towel for 40 to 60 seconds before serving.

Dad's Jammin' Crêpes

MAKES 12 CRÊPES · SERVES 6

Crêpes are pretty easy to make once you get the hang of them. My father is originally from the Czech Republic, and crêpes, known there as *palacinky*, were a staple in our home for breakfast or dessert. I've played around with my dad's recipe, swapping the plain flour for wholemeal and the whole milk with skimmed for nearly identical results that would make Dad proud. This is the perfect breakfast when you have guests you want to impress. I buy a variety of fancy fruit jams, set out different bowls of fruit and fillings, and let everyone compose their own.

CRÊPES

1¾ cups (400ml) skimmed milk

2 large egg whites

1 large egg

1 teaspoon rapeseed oil

1 teaspoon pure vanilla extract

1 cup (130g) wholemeal flour

1 teaspoon ground cinnamon

Cooking spray or oil mister

FILLING AND TOPPINGS

¼ cup (80g) of your favourite fruit jams

3 bananas, sliced

¾ cup (110g) sliced strawberries

¾ cup (115g) blueberries

¾ cup (90g) raspberries

1 tablespoon icing sugar, for dusting

For the crêpes: In a blender, combine the milk, egg whites and egg, oil and vanilla. Add the flour and cinnamon and blend until smooth. At this point, the batter may be refrigerated for up to 2 days.

Heat a 25cm nonstick frying pan over medium-low heat. When hot, lightly spray with oil. Pour a ladleful of batter into the pan, swirling the pan slightly to form a thin, even coating on the base. Cook until the bottom of the crêpe sets and is golden in colour, 1 to 2 minutes. Gently flip with a spatula and cook the second side for about 1 minute. Repeat with the remaining batter, stacking the finished crêpes on a plate. You should have 12 crêpes.

For the filling and toppings: To serve, spread 1 teaspoon of the fruit jams in the centre of each crêpe, fold the edge of the crêpe over the filling and roll it into a tube shape. Place the rolled crêpe on a plate, seam side down. Top with fresh fruit, lightly dust with icing sugar and serve immediately.

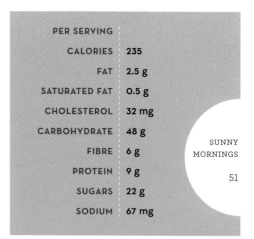

PER SERVING	
CALORIES	235
FAT	2.5 g
SATURATED FAT	0.5 g
CHOLESTEROL	32 mg
CARBOHYDRATE	48 g
FIBRE	6 g
PROTEIN	9 g
SUGARS	22 g
SODIUM	67 mg

SKINNY-LICIOUS SOUPS & CHILLIES

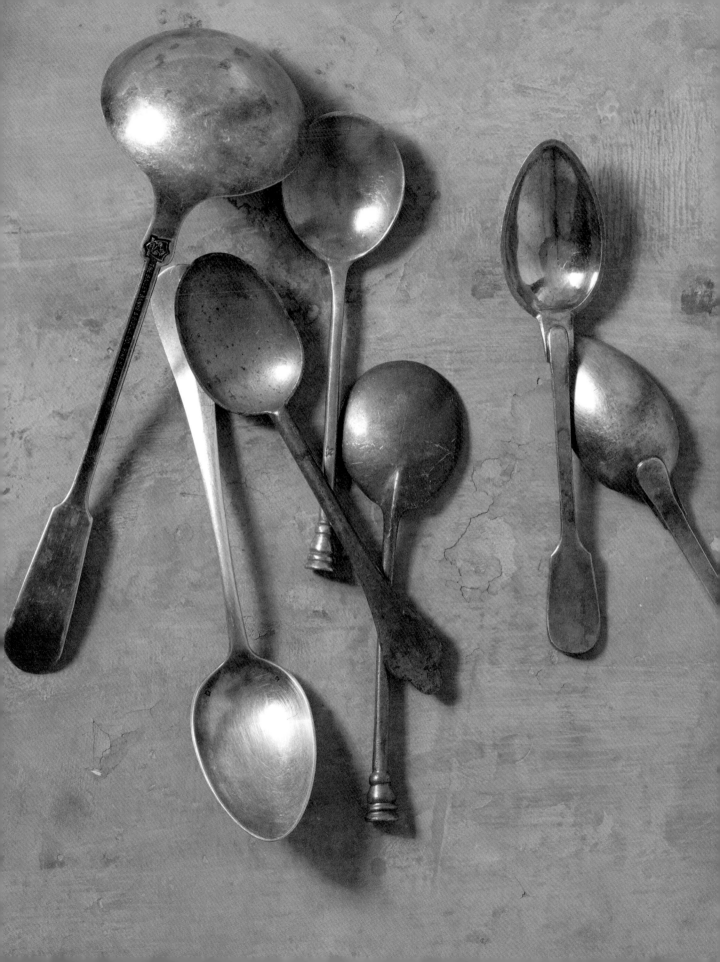

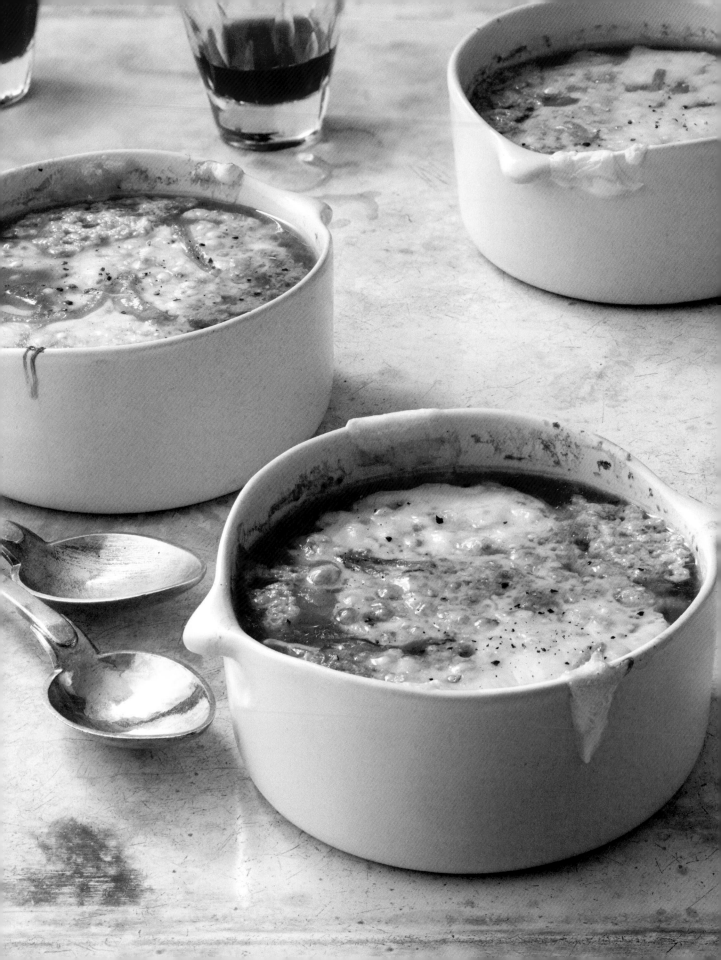

Breadless French Onion Soup with Parmesan-Asiago Crisps

SERVES 6

What's the best part of French onion soup? The melted cheese on top of the savoury broth that's loaded with sweet caramelized onions. Personally, I've never cared for the soggy bread – I'd rather save my carbs for something I really enjoy. So instead I make a cheese crisp to float on top. Not only is it easy, but the combination of the two cheeses is also absolutely heavenly.

SOUP

1 tablespoon olive oil

1 tablespoon unsalted butter

900g sweet brown onions, cut into 2 to 3mm slices

¼ cup (50ml) dry sherry

¼ cup (50ml) dry white or red wine

2 tablespoons plain flour (use glutinous rice flour* for gluten-free)

8 cups (2 litres) good-quality low-salt beef stock

1 sprig of fresh thyme

1 bay leaf

Freshly ground black pepper

6 (25g) slices lighter Swiss cheese

PARMESAN-ASIAGO CRISPS

½ cup (50g) freshly grated Parmesan cheese

¼ cup (25g) freshly grated Asiago cheese†

Read the label to be sure this product is gluten-free.

For the soup: In a Dutch oven or large nonstick pot, heat the oil and butter over medium-low heat until the butter melts. Add the onions and slowly cook until they become soft, stirring from time to time, about 30 minutes. Increase the heat to medium and cook until the onions begin to caramelize, about 20 to 25 minutes, stirring every few minutes. Add the sherry and wine and reduce the heat to low, stirring any brown bits stuck to the pot. Simmer until the liquid cooks down and evaporates, 2 to 3 minutes. Add the flour and cook, stirring, for 3 to 4 minutes. Add the stock, thyme and bay leaf, increase the heat to high and bring to a boil. Cover, reduce the heat to moderately low and simmer until the onions are tender, about 30 minutes. Remove and discard the herbs, and then season with black pepper to taste.

† If you can't find Asiago cheese, either Pecorino Romano or extra Parmesan would work well as an alternative.

(recipe continues)

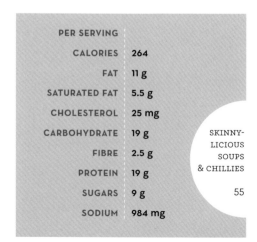

PER SERVING	
CALORIES	264
FAT	11 g
SATURATED FAT	5.5 g
CHOLESTEROL	25 mg
CARBOHYDRATE	19 g
FIBRE	2.5 g
PROTEIN	19 g
SUGARS	9 g
SODIUM	984 mg

SKINNY-LICIOUS SOUPS & CHILLIES

55

For the Parmesan-Asiago crisps: Meanwhile, preheat the oven to 200°C/180°C fan/Gas 6. Line a baking sheet with a silicone baking mat or baking parchment.

In a small bowl, combine the Parmesan and Asiago. Put 2 tablespoons of the cheese mixture onto the baking sheet and lightly pat it with your fingers into a 10cm round. Repeat with the remaining cheese to make 6 rounds, leaving a 1cm space in between each. Bake until golden and crisp, 6 to 8 minutes. Set aside to cool.

When ready to serve, preheat the grill.

Ladle the soup into 6 ovenproof soup bowls, lay one cheese crisp on top of each (it should float), and then lay 1 slice of Swiss cheese over each crisp. Put the bowls on a baking sheet.

Grill until the cheese melts, watching closely so that it doesn't burn, 3 to 4 minutes. Serve hot.

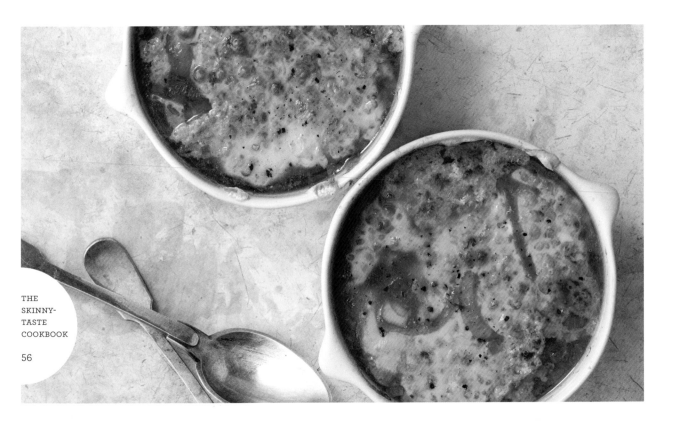

Italian Escarole and White Bean Soup

SERVES 6

  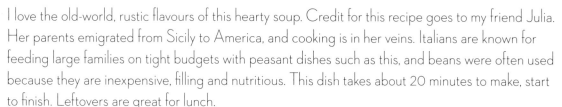

I love the old-world, rustic flavours of this hearty soup. Credit for this recipe goes to my friend Julia. Her parents emigrated from Sicily to America, and cooking is in her veins. Italians are known for feeding large families on tight budgets with peasant dishes such as this, and beans were often used because they are inexpensive, filling and nutritious. This dish takes about 20 minutes to make, start to finish. Leftovers are great for lunch.

275g ditalini pasta (use brown rice pasta for gluten-free)

Sea salt

1 teaspoon olive oil

1 medium onion, chopped

8 cups (2 litres) low-salt chicken or vegetable stock*

1 (400g) tin cannellini beans,* rinsed and drained

Freshly ground black pepper

1 head escarole, leaves washed and torn into a few pieces

Freshly grated Parmesan cheese, for serving (optional)

Read the label to be sure this product is gluten-free.

Cook the pasta to al dente in a pot of salted boiling water according to packet directions. Drain and set aside.

Heat a large nonstick pot over medium heat. When hot, add the oil and onion and cook, stirring, until golden, 3 to 4 minutes. Add the stock and beans and bring to a boil. Season with black pepper to taste, and then add the escarole. Cook until the escarole wilts, about 15 minutes.

To serve, divide the cooked pasta among 6 bowls. Ladle the soup over the pasta and sprinkle with Parmesan, if desired.

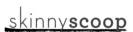

skinnyscoop

Nothing can ruin a dish like mushy pasta. To avoid that situation, cook the pasta in a separate pot. Then, when you're ready to serve, divide the pasta among serving bowls, ladle in the soup and top with cheese.

FOOD FACTS meet escarole
Escarole (pronounced ESS-ka-roll) is a variety of endive whose leaves are broader, paler and less bitter. It contains a number of nutrients, including folate, fibre and vitamins C and K. If you can't find it, you can substitute Swiss chard or any other leafy green vegetable.

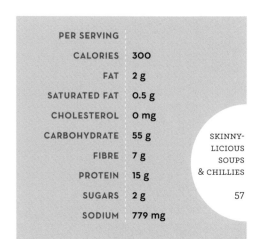

PER SERVING	
CALORIES	300
FAT	2 g
SATURATED FAT	0.5 g
CHOLESTEROL	0 mg
CARBOHYDRATE	55 g
FIBRE	7 g
PROTEIN	15 g
SUGARS	2 g
SODIUM	779 mg

SKINNY-LICIOUS SOUPS & CHILLIES

57

Too-Good-to-Be-True Baked Potato Soup

SERVES 5

This soup is one of my most popular recipes on *Skinnytaste*. It offers everything you love about a baked potato in soup form! In fact, a fan once described it as a 'warm bowl of awesomeness'. You can totally enjoy it without the guilt because it's soooo much lighter than a baked potato. That's because I hide some cauliflower in there, which gives the great taste and texture for fewer calories.

2 medium baking potatoes, about 170g each

3½ cups (450g) cauliflower florets (from 1 small head)

1½ cups (350ml) low-salt chicken stock*

1½ cups (350ml) skimmed milk

½ cup (125g) light soured cream

6 tablespoons chopped fresh chives

¾ teaspoon sea salt

Freshly ground black pepper

10 tablespoons grated lighter mature cheddar cheese

3 slices centre-cut or back bacon, cooked and crumbled

Read the label to be sure this product is gluten-free.

Pierce the potatoes all over with a fork and microwave on high for 5 minutes. Turn them over and microwave until tender, 3 to 5 minutes longer. (Alternatively, bake at 200°C/180°C fan/Gas 6 for 1 hour or until tender.) Allow to cool. When cool enough to handle, peel and coarsely chop the potatoes.

Set a steamer basket in a large pot and fill with about 2.5cm of water. Bring the water to a boil over high heat. Add the cauliflower, cover and steam until tender, 5 to 6 minutes. Drain, remove the steamer basket and return the cauliflower to the pot.

Set the pot over medium heat and add the stock, milk and potatoes. Bring to a boil. Use a hand blender to purée the soup until smooth. Add the soured cream, 3 tablespoons of the chives and season with the salt and black pepper to taste. Reduce the heat to low and cook, stirring occasionally, until thick and creamy, 8 to 10 minutes.

Remove the pot from the heat. Ladle the soup into bowls. Top each with 2 tablespoons of cheese and divide the remaining chives and the bacon among them. Serve hot.

PER SERVING	
CALORIES	200
FAT	7 g
SATURATED FAT	3 g
CHOLESTEROL	17 mg
CARBOHYDRATE	23 g
FIBRE	3.5 g
PROTEIN	14 g
SUGARS	6 g
SODIUM	323 mg

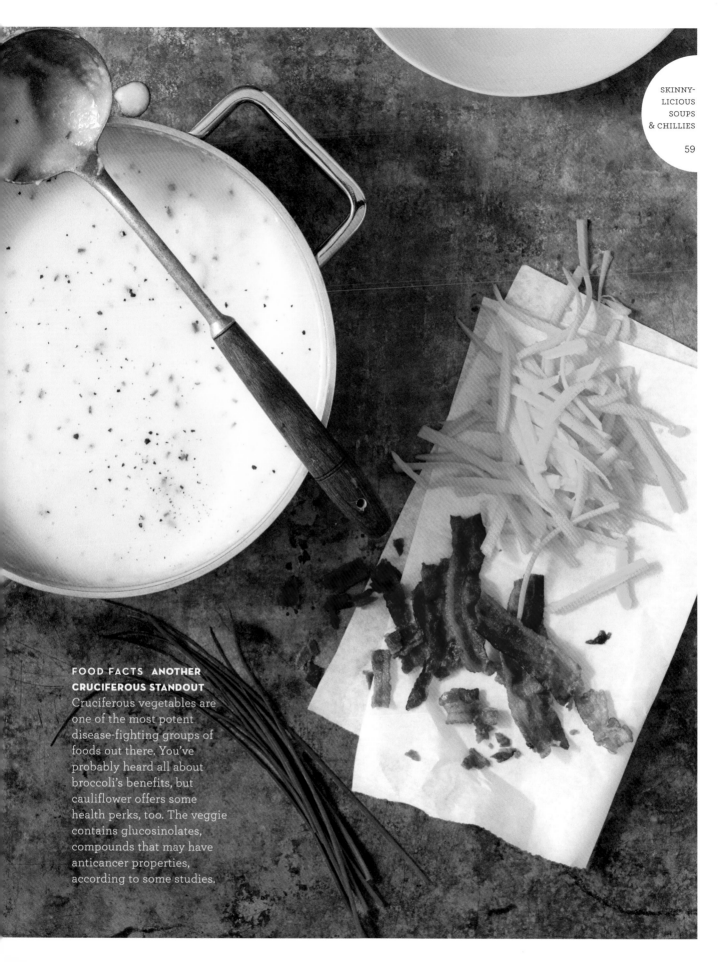

FOOD FACTS ANOTHER CRUCIFEROUS STANDOUT
Cruciferous vegetables are one of the most potent disease-fighting groups of foods out there. You've probably heard all about broccoli's benefits, but cauliflower offers some health perks, too. The veggie contains glucosinolates, compounds that may have anticancer properties, according to some studies.

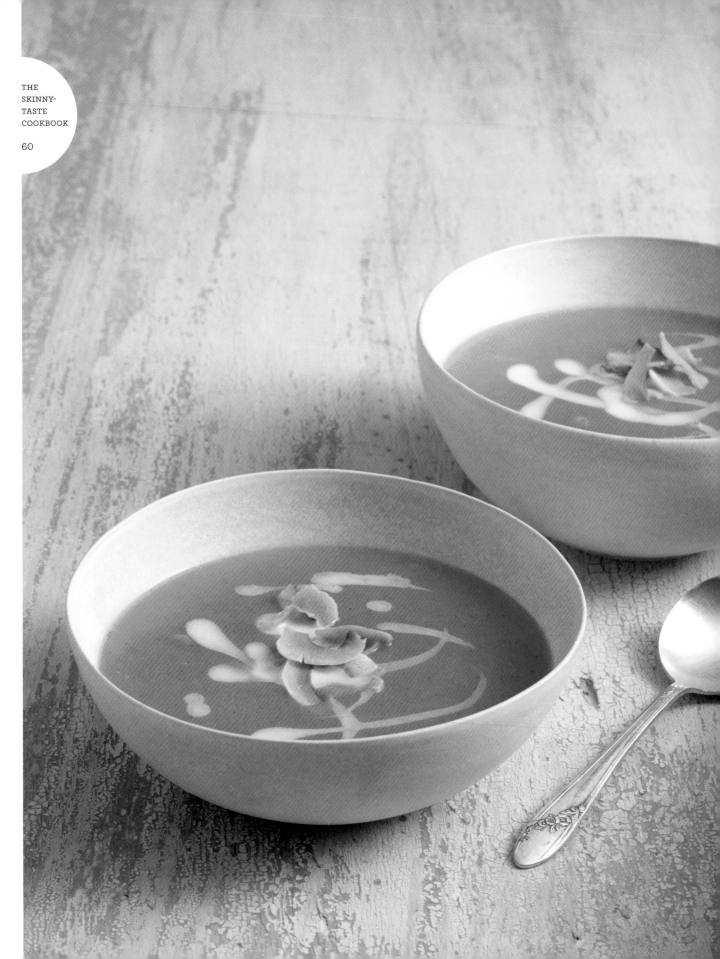

Cinnamon-Roasted Butternut Squash Soup

SERVES 6

I get inspiration for my soups from the fresh produce available as the seasons change. Butternut squash is wonderful when roasted with nutmeg and cinnamon. I then balance out the sweetness with sautéed shallots and purée the whole thing until it's creamy and velvety. I had an 'aha' moment when I was trying to think of a good garnish for the soup. I just happened to be making Coconut Chicken Salad (page 126) for lunch while testing this recipe when it hit me: toasted coconut!

1.2kg peeled and seeded butternut squash, cut into 4cm cubes, from 1 whole

¾ teaspoon ground cinnamon

¼ teaspoon ground nutmeg

6 tablespoons sweetened coconut flakes*

1 tablespoon coconut oil

¼ cup (30g) finely chopped shallots

2¼ cups (500ml) good-quality low-salt vegetable stock,* plus more as needed

1 cup plus 2 tablespoons (275ml) light tinned coconut milk

¾ teaspoon sea salt

Freshly ground black pepper

*Read the label to be sure this product is gluten-free.

Preheat the oven to 190°C/170°C fan/Gas 5.

Put the squash on a large baking sheet. Toss with the cinnamon and nutmeg, cover with foil and roast until tender, 40 to 50 minutes. Allow to cool. (Reduce the oven temperature to 180°C/160°C fan/Gas 4.)

Spread the coconut on a baking sheet and toast in the oven, stirring every 2 minutes, until golden, 6 to 8 minutes. Allow to cool.

Heat a large nonstick pot over medium heat. Add the coconut oil and shallots and cook, stirring, until tender, 5 minutes.

Add the roasted squash to the pot with the shallots. Add the stock and 1 cup of the coconut milk and simmer for about 5 minutes. Using a hand blender or a regular blender in batches, purée the soup until smooth. Add more stock if needed and simmer for 2 to 3 more minutes. Season with salt and pepper.

To serve, ladle the soup into bowls and top each with 1 tablespoon toasted coconut and 1 teaspoon coconut milk.

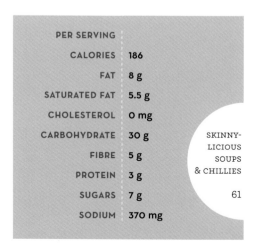

PER SERVING	
CALORIES	186
FAT	8 g
SATURATED FAT	5.5 g
CHOLESTEROL	0 mg
CARBOHYDRATE	30 g
FIBRE	5 g
PROTEIN	3 g
SUGARS	7 g
SODIUM	370 mg

SKINNY-LICIOUS SOUPS & CHILLIES

Silky Edamame Soup

SERVES 4

   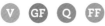

I often get inspiration from great restaurants when I go out to eat, and this soup is the perfect example. While dining with my husband at a new Asian-fusion restaurant in my area, I felt as if the edamame soup on the menu was calling my name. It was a silky soup made of puréed edamame (soya beans), baby spinach, shallots and stock, topped with a dollop of crème fraîche. I loved it so much, I ran straight to the shops afterwards to re-create it myself. Here's the result!

SOUP

1 teaspoon sesame oil

¼ cup (30g) chopped shallots

2 garlic cloves, chopped

4 cups (1 litre) low-salt chicken stock* (or vegetable stock can be used)

1 tablespoon reduced-salt soy sauce (use tamari for gluten-free)

350g fresh or frozen shelled edamame

3 cups (135g) baby spinach

TOPPINGS

Freshly ground black pepper

1 tablespoon sliced spring onions

¼ cup (60g) crème fraîche or light soured cream

Roasted Edamame with Sea Salt (page 107; optional)

PERFECT PAIRINGS

Enjoy this soup as a main course with a salad on the side or as a starter to your own Asian-fusion main. Need a suggestion? Try the **Sweet 'n' Spicy Sriracha-Glazed Salmon (page 215)**.

Read the label to be sure this product is gluten-free.

For the soup: In a medium saucepan, heat the sesame oil over medium heat. Add the shallots and garlic and cook, stirring, until lightly golden and fragrant, 1 to 2 minutes. Add the stock, soy sauce and edamame and bring to a boil. Cover, reduce the heat to medium-low and simmer until the edamame are tender, 15 to 20 minutes. Add the spinach and cook 1 more minute.

Working in batches, purée the soup in a blender. Return it to the saucepan to keep warm.

For the toppings: To serve, ladle the soup into 4 bowls, top each with some black pepper, spring onions and a touch of crème fraîche and roasted edamame.

FOOD FACTS the skinny on soya beans
Soya beans are a super source of protein, with more than 8 grams per ½ cup (30g). In fact, soya beans are considered a complete protein, meaning they contain all of the essential amino acids that our bodies cannot make on their own.

PER SERVING	
CALORIES	173
FAT	10 g
SATURATED FAT	3.5 g
CHOLESTEROL	20 mg
CARBOHYDRATE	11 g
FIBRE	4.5 g
PROTEIN	11 g
SUGARS	3 g
SODIUM	732 mg

'Un'Stuffed Cabbage Soup

SERVES 8

Stuffed cabbage is one of my favourite comfort dishes that my mom used to make, but it can take quite a bit of time to prepare. These days, time is not something I have a lot of with a toddler running around and a full-time career, so when I'm in a rush, I rely on this shortcut: I throw all the ingredients into a big pot and make this soup instead. Most of the cooking time is unattended, so I can spend more time with my family and less time in the kitchen. Bonus: leftovers are even better the next day.

450g lean beef mince

1⅛ teaspoons sea salt

1 large white onion, finely chopped

3 garlic cloves, crushed

1½ teaspoons sweet paprika

½ teaspoon dried thyme

2 (400g) tins chopped tomatoes

225g passata

5 cups (1.25 litres) good-quality low-salt beef stock*

4 cups (300g) chopped green cabbage

Freshly ground black pepper

1 cup (185g) cooked brown rice

Read the label to be sure this product is gluten-free.

In a large pot or Dutch oven set over high heat, season the beef mince with ¼ teaspoon of the salt and cook, using a wooden spoon to break the meat into small pieces as it browns. Drain any fat from the pot and reduce the heat to medium-low. Add the onion, garlic, paprika and thyme and cook until the onions are soft, 5 to 7 minutes. Add the tomatoes, passata, beef stock and cabbage, and season with the remaining salt and black pepper to taste. Bring to a boil, reduce the heat to low, cover and simmer until the cabbage is soft, about 35 minutes.

Add the cooked brown rice and simmer 5 more minutes before ladling the soup into bowls to serve.

skinnyscoop

Soups and stews like this are perfect for freezing. Freeze leftovers in labelled, portion-size containers so you'll have quick meals to reheat when you're pressed for time.

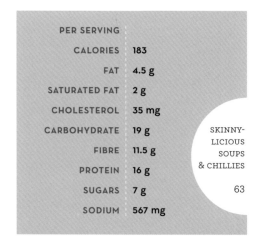

PER SERVING	
CALORIES	183
FAT	4.5 g
SATURATED FAT	2 g
CHOLESTEROL	35 mg
CARBOHYDRATE	19 g
FIBRE	11.5 g
PROTEIN	16 g
SUGARS	7 g
SODIUM	567 mg

SKINNY-LICIOUS SOUPS & CHILLIES

Slow-Cooker Chicken Enchilada Soup

SERVES 6

Call me lazy, but I love a meal that can pretty much cook itself. I also love turning classic meals into a hearty bowl of soup, and the slow cooker allows me to do both. For this dish, I took my standard chicken enchilada recipe and threw the ingredients into a slow cooker. What emerged a few hours later was this delicious chunky soup that I topped with cheese, spring onions, coriander and avocado. If I don't have avocado, I add a touch of light soured cream or crushed tortillas on top. It's everything I love about enchiladas in one neat bowl!

SOUP

2 teaspoons olive oil

½ cup (80g) chopped onion

3 garlic cloves, crushed

3 cups (575ml) low-salt chicken stock*

225g passata

1 to 2 teaspoons chopped chipotle chilli in adobo sauce†

¼ cup (15g) chopped fresh coriander

1 (400g) tin low-salt black beans, rinsed and drained

1 (400g) tin chopped tomatoes

2 cups (300g) frozen sweetcorn kernels

1 teaspoon ground cumin, plus more to taste

½ teaspoon dried oregano

450g boneless, skinless chicken breasts

TOPPINGS

¾ cup (90g) grated lighter cheddar cheese

¼ cup (30g) chopped spring onions

¼ cup (15g) chopped fresh coriander

1 medium (110g) avocado, sliced

6 tablespoons light soured cream (optional)

Read the label to be sure this product is gluten-free.

For the soup: In a medium nonstick frying pan, heat the oil over medium heat. Add the onion and garlic and cook, stirring, until soft, about 3 minutes. Add to the slowcooker along with the stock, passata, chipotle in adobo, coriander, beans, tomatoes, sweetcorn, cumin and oregano. Add the chicken breasts. Cover and cook on low for 4 to 6 hours.

Remove the chicken, shred it with two forks and return it to the slow cooker.

For the toppings: To serve, ladle into bowls and, dividing evenly, top each with 2 tablespoons of cheddar, spring onions, coriander, avocado and soured cream (if using).

† If you can't find chipotle chilli in adobo sauce, chipotle paste would work well as an alternative.

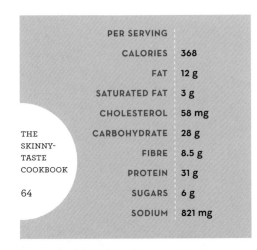

PER SERVING	
CALORIES	368
FAT	12 g
SATURATED FAT	3 g
CHOLESTEROL	58 mg
CARBOHYDRATE	28 g
FIBRE	8.5 g
PROTEIN	31 g
SUGARS	6 g
SODIUM	821 mg

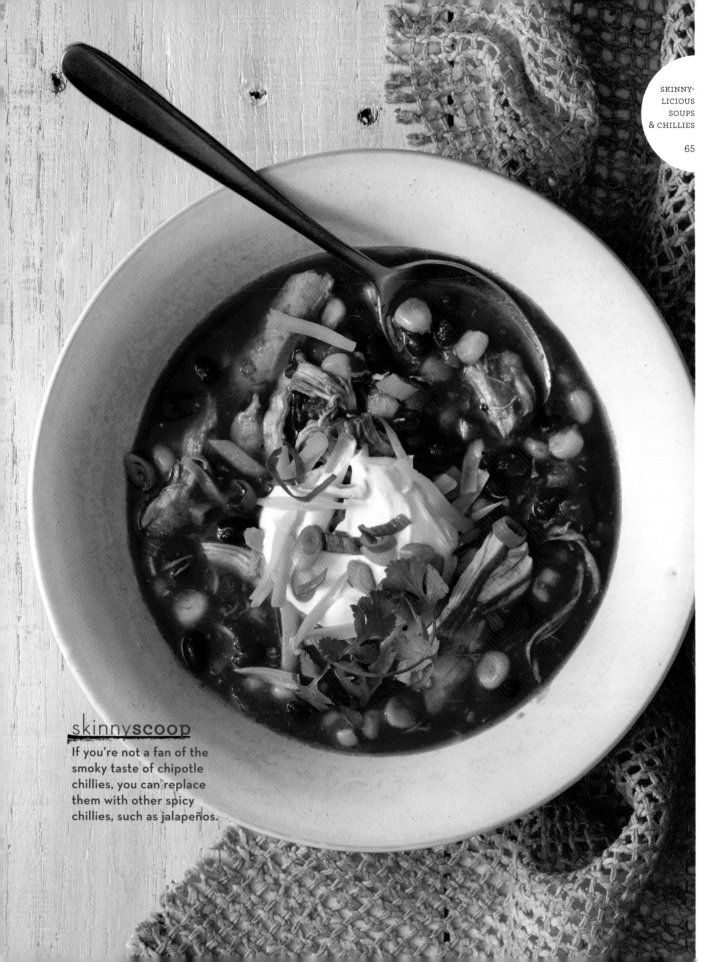

skinny<u>scoop</u>

If you're not a fan of the smoky taste of chipotle chillies, you can replace them with other spicy chillies, such as jalapeños.

Aztec Chicken, Quinoa and Avocado Soup

SERVES 6

Never seen avocado used in soup before? My mom is from Colombia, where it's quite common to add fresh avocado to soup just before eating. It adds a cool, sweet, creamy texture to a warm, hearty bowl of soup. As a kid, I didn't really care for it, but as an adult, I just love it. And luckily, so does my family. To brighten and round out the flavours of this soup, I like to finish it with a squeeze of fresh lime juice just before serving.

2 teaspoons olive oil

7 spring onions, chopped

2 garlic cloves, crushed

1 cup (200g) chopped tomatoes

6 tablespoons chopped fresh coriander

1 teaspoon ground cumin

½ teaspoon sweet paprika or ground annatto

5 cups (1.25 litres) low-salt chicken stock*

1 cup (155g) sliced carrots

½ cup (90g) chopped yellow pepper

Sea salt

Freshly ground black pepper

450g boneless, skinless chicken breasts

1 medium jalapeño or other green chilli, diced (optional)

½ cup (100g) quinoa, rinsed well

1½ cups (300g) fresh or frozen sweetcorn kernels

1 medium (110g) avocado, chopped, for garnish

6 lime wedges, for serving

Read the label to be sure this product is gluten-free.

In a large pot or Dutch oven, heat the oil over medium-low heat. Add the spring onions and garlic and cook, stirring, until soft, about 3 minutes. Add the tomato, 4 tablespoons of the coriander, the cumin and the paprika and cook 2 more minutes. Add the stock, carrots, pepper, ½ teaspoon of salt and black pepper to taste, and bring to a boil. Reduce to a simmer, cover and cook until the vegetables are tender, about 30 minutes.

Add the chicken and jalapeño (if using) and cook until the chicken is cooked through, about 15 to 18 minutes. Remove the chicken, shred it using two forks and set it aside.

Meanwhile, in a medium saucepan, cook the quinoa according to packet directions.

PER SERVING	
CALORIES	230
FAT	8 g
SATURATED FAT	1 g
CHOLESTEROL	48 mg
CARBOHYDRATE	21 g
FIBRE	4.5 g
PROTEIN	21 g
SUGARS	4 g
SODIUM	702 mg

Add the cooked quinoa and sweetcorn to the soup, increase the heat to medium and cook for 5 more minutes. Remove the pot from the heat. Return the shredded chicken to the pot, season with ⅛ teaspoon salt and black pepper to taste and stir in the remaining 2 tablespoons coriander.

Ladle the soup into bowls, garnish with the avocado and serve with lime wedges on the side for squeezing.

FOOD FACTS crazy for quinoa
This grain is a hunger-curbing, power-packed nutritional all-star. Loaded with protein, fibre, calcium, iron and vitamins, this superfood is digested slowly, which keeps blood sugar and insulin levels (and, therefore, energy and appetite) steady.

skinny**scoop**
Annatto is a staple in Latin American cooking, imparting flavour as well as colour. It can be found online. Sweet paprika can be used in its place if annatto is not available.

4 Tips for Making a Better Bowl of Soup

There's nothing better than a one-pot meal (easy cleanup!), and making soup is the easiest way to achieve this. Sure you could pop open a tin, but believe it or not, making soups from scratch is a cinch once you master these simple, basic techniques.

SIMMER SEASONAL
You can capture the essence of each season and come up with endless varieties of soups by simmering seasonal vegetables – it's a smart and healthy way to cook.

START WITH DELICIOUS BROTH
I often make my own homemade stocks when it's time to clean out the refrigerator. But there is no mistaking the convenience of using packaged stock. Adding fresh herbs and aromatics, such as onions, garlic, leeks and shallots, to your shop-bought stock will make them taste like you were simmering them for hours.

SAY CHEESE!
Add a Parmesan rind to your pot – this is simple, but it works like a charm. They are like magic flavour bombs and add a rich, savoury, umami character to your soup. I always save my Parmesan or Pecorino Romano rinds and keep them in my freezer just for this.

BE FRESH
Flavouring your soup at the very end with something fresh and uncooked, such as herbs, avocado or a squeeze of lime juice, will brighten the deep, delicious, melded tastes of the rest of the soup and add a much needed touch of freshness.

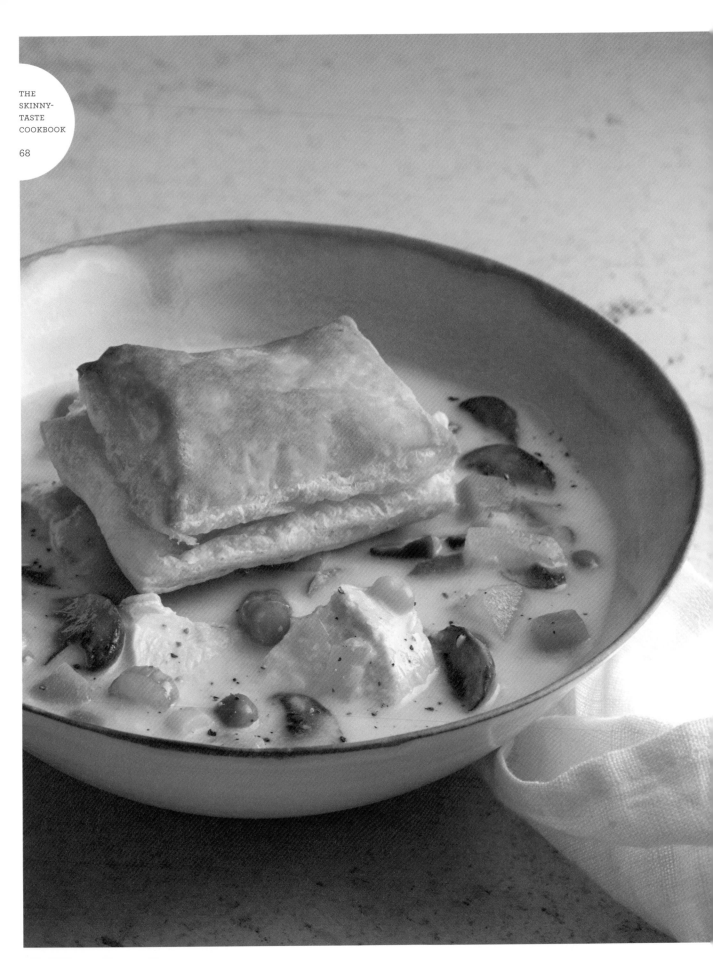

Chicken Pot Pie Soup

SERVES 6

Why not take a classic comfort food and put a new spin on it? Chicken pot pie – one of my childhood favourites – is every bit as delightful when served as a soup. On the nights I want to get extra fancy, I cut out 'croutons' from frozen shortcrust or puff pastry into shapes, bake them until golden and serve on top.

¼ cup (35g) plain flour
(or 2 tablespoons cornflour
for gluten-free)

4 cups (1 litre) skimmed milk

575g boneless, skinless
chicken breasts

275g frozen classic mixed
vegetables (peas, carrots,
green beans, sweetcorn)

1 large celery stalk, chopped

½ medium onion, chopped

225g sliced mini portobello
mushrooms

2 tablespoons good-quality
low-salt chicken stock*

Pinch of dried thyme

Freshly ground black pepper

2 medium all-purpose
potatoes, peeled and diced

Sea salt, if needed

Read the label to be sure this product is gluten-free.

In a small bowl, make a slurry by whisking together ½ cup (120ml) cold water and the flour (or cornflour if making this gluten-free). Set aside.

In a large pot, combine 1½ cups (350ml) water and the milk and slowly bring to a boil over medium-low heat. Add the chicken, frozen vegetables, celery, onion, mushrooms, stock, thyme and black pepper to taste and return to a boil. Partially cover, reduce the heat to low and simmer 15 minutes. Remove the chicken and set it aside. Continue to cook the soup until the vegetables are soft, about 5 more minutes. Add the potatoes and cook until soft, about 5 minutes.

Meanwhile, chop or shred the chicken into small pieces. Add the chicken to the soup and slowly stir in the slurry. Cook until the soup thickens, 2 to 3 minutes. Adjust salt and black pepper to taste and serve.

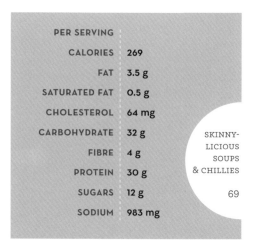

PER SERVING	
CALORIES	269
FAT	3.5 g
SATURATED FAT	0.5 g
CHOLESTEROL	64 mg
CARBOHYDRATE	32 g
FIBRE	4 g
PROTEIN	30 g
SUGARS	12 g
SODIUM	983 mg

SKINNY-
LICIOUS
SOUPS
& CHILLIES

69

Rustic Italian Gnocchi Soup

SERVES 8

Let's test your memory. Think back to school science lessons: how many different tastes are there? If you remember that there were four (bitter, sweet, salty and sour), you'd be wrong today. There's actually a fifth flavour called *umami*, a Japanese word used to describe something savoury. This hearty bowl of soup is bursting with umami. Using a Parmesan rind is a must when I want to add the subtle umami flavour to soups. I always save my rinds when I'm done with my cheese, keeping them in the freezer until I need them.

3 tablespoons plain flour

400g fresh sweet Italian chicken sausages, casings removed†

4½ cups (1 litre) low-salt chicken stock

1 cup (225ml) skimmed milk

1 small onion, chopped

1 celery stalk, chopped

1 carrot, chopped

4 garlic cloves, crushed

Rind from Parmesan (optional)

2 large roasted red peppers, jarred or homemade (see page 233)

½ teaspoon freshly ground black pepper, plus more as needed

450g gnocchi

3 cups (135g) baby spinach, chopped

2 tablespoons chopped fresh basil

Freshly grated Parmesan, for serving (optional)

skinny**scoop**

To save time, I buy fresh gnocchi at a nearby Italian deli in my neighbourhood, but you can find refrigerated, dried or frozen gnocchi in the supermarket. And if you really want to speed this up, you can also use jarred roasted peppers.

PER SERVING	
CALORIES	203
FAT	8 g
SATURATED FAT	3.5 g
CHOLESTEROL	49 mg
CARBOHYDRATE	20 g
FIBRE	2 g
PROTEIN	13 g
SUGARS	5 g
SODIUM	860 mg

In a small bowl, make a slurry by whisking together ½ cup (120ml) cold water and the flour.

Heat a large nonstick pot over medium heat. Add the sausage and cook, using a wooden spoon to break the meat into small pieces, until cooked through and slightly browned, 4 minutes.

Add ½ cup (120ml) water, stock and milk and bring to a boil. Add the onion, celery, carrot, garlic, Parmesan rind (if using), roasted peppers and black pepper and return to a boil. Partially cover the pot, reduce the heat to low and simmer until the vegetables are soft, 15 to 20 minutes. Uncover, slowly stir in the slurry and continue stirring while the soup returns to a boil.

Add the gnocchi, spinach and basil. Cook until the gnocchi start to float to the top and become puffy (or according to the gnocchi packet directions) and the soup thickens. Season with pepper to taste. Discard the Parmesan rind. To serve, ladle the soup into bowls and sprinkle with grated Parmesan, if desired.

† If you can't find Italian chicken sausages, another kind of chicken sausage or reduced-fat pork sausages will work well.

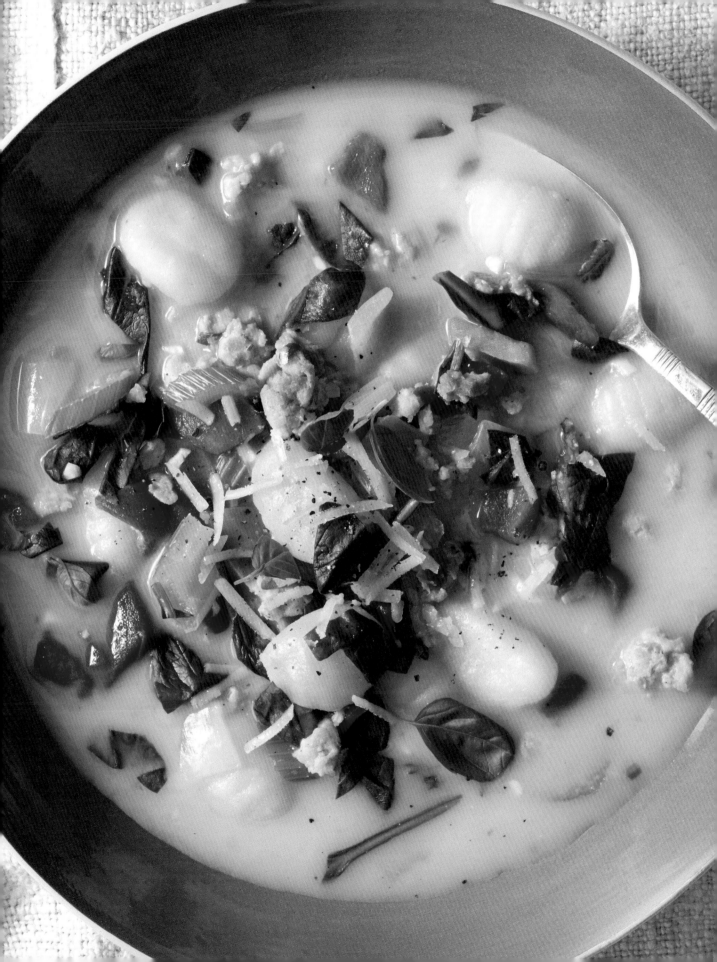

Katia's Caldo Gallego

SERVES 8

A magnificent hearty soup, *caldo gallego* is from the Galician region of Spain. It's the kind of soup that will stick to your bones on chilly winter nights. This recipe comes from my cousin Katia, who is a terrific cook. I asked Katia to share her recipe, and together we brainstormed ways to slim down the already healthy dish, including replacing fatty cuts of meat with leaner ones. We were able to re-create the same great taste without losing the integrity of her original.

3 medium baking potatoes, peeled

100g chorizo sausage, cut crosswise into 5mm-thick slices

400g boneless, skinless chicken thighs, trimmed of all fat, cut into 2 to 3cm chunks

1 beef bone marrow, about 10cm long

½ large head green cabbage, cored and roughly chopped

1 medium onion, finely chopped

2 garlic cloves, crushed

1 (410g) tin haricot beans,* rinsed and drained

1 bunch spring greens, stemmed and cut into 1cm strips

1 teaspoon smoked paprika

2 teaspoons sea salt

Freshly ground black pepper

*Read the label to be sure this product is gluten-free.

Cut one of the potatoes in half, put it into a large pot and add the chorizo, chicken thighs and beef bone. Add 8½ cups (2 litres) water and bring to a boil over medium-high heat. Reduce the heat to medium. Cut the remaining potatoes into cubes (to help thicken the soup) and add to the pot. Add the cabbage, onion and garlic. Cover and cook for 15 minutes. Add the beans, spring greens, paprika, salt and black pepper to taste. Reduce the heat to low, cover and simmer until the greens are tender, about 20 minutes. Discard the bone and serve.

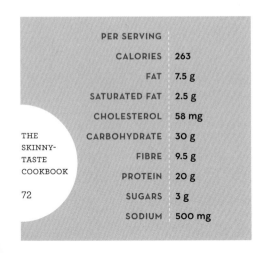

PER SERVING	
CALORIES	263
FAT	7.5 g
SATURATED FAT	2.5 g
CHOLESTEROL	58 mg
CARBOHYDRATE	30 g
FIBRE	9.5 g
PROTEIN	20 g
SUGARS	3 g
SODIUM	500 mg

Slow-Cooker Santa Fe Chicken

SERVES 8

This recipe is one of the most popular recipes on *Skinnytaste*, probably because it has everything you could want in a slow-cooker dish: it requires no prep or precooking; it's inexpensive, healthy, kid-friendly; and it's delicious. I use lots of fresh herbs and spices to boost the flavours without adding extra fat or sodium. Plus, some herbs contain antioxidants, which help fight off a variety of diseases.

STEW

1¾ cups (400ml) low-salt chicken stock*

1 (400g) tin low-salt black beans,* rinsed and drained

2 cups (225g) frozen sweetcorn kernels

1 (400g) tin chopped tomatoes

¼ cup (7g) chopped fresh coriander

3 spring onions, chopped

1 teaspoon garlic powder

1 teaspoon onion powder

1¼ teaspoons ground cumin

1 teaspoon cayenne pepper

¼ teaspoon sea salt

675g boneless, skinless chicken breasts

TOPPINGS

½ cup (60g) chopped spring onions

¼ cup (7g) chopped fresh coriander

Read the label to be sure this product is gluten-free.

For the stew: In a slow cooker, combine the stock, beans, sweetcorn, tomatoes, coriander, spring onions, garlic powder, onion powder, cumin and cayenne. Season the chicken with salt and lay it on top. Cover and cook on low for 10 hours or high for 6 hours.

Thirty minutes before serving, remove the chicken, shred it with two forks and return it to the slow cooker.

For the toppings: To serve, divide the soup among 8 bowls and top with the spring onions and coriander.

PERFECT PAIRINGS
Top this dish with a little soured cream and reduced-fat cheddar; spoon it over coriander-lime rice (combine ¾ cup (150g) cooked brown rice with a squeeze of lime juice and a tablespoon chopped fresh coriander); sprinkle it over baked tortilla chips and top with reduced-fat cheese and jalapeños; or serve it over greens as a salad. (Psst! It's also great as a filling for enchiladas: see page 171 for my awesome enchilada sauce recipe.)

skinny**scoop**

Beat the morning rush by preparing all the ingredients the night before. Then, all you have to do is add them to the slow cooker in the morning and turn it on!

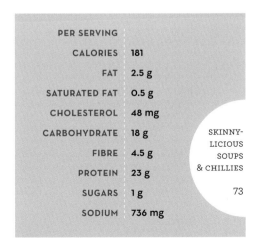

PER SERVING	
CALORIES	181
FAT	2.5 g
SATURATED FAT	0.5 g
CHOLESTEROL	48 mg
CARBOHYDRATE	18 g
FIBRE	4.5 g
PROTEIN	23 g
SUGARS	1 g
SODIUM	736 mg

SKINNY-LICIOUS SOUPS & CHILLIES

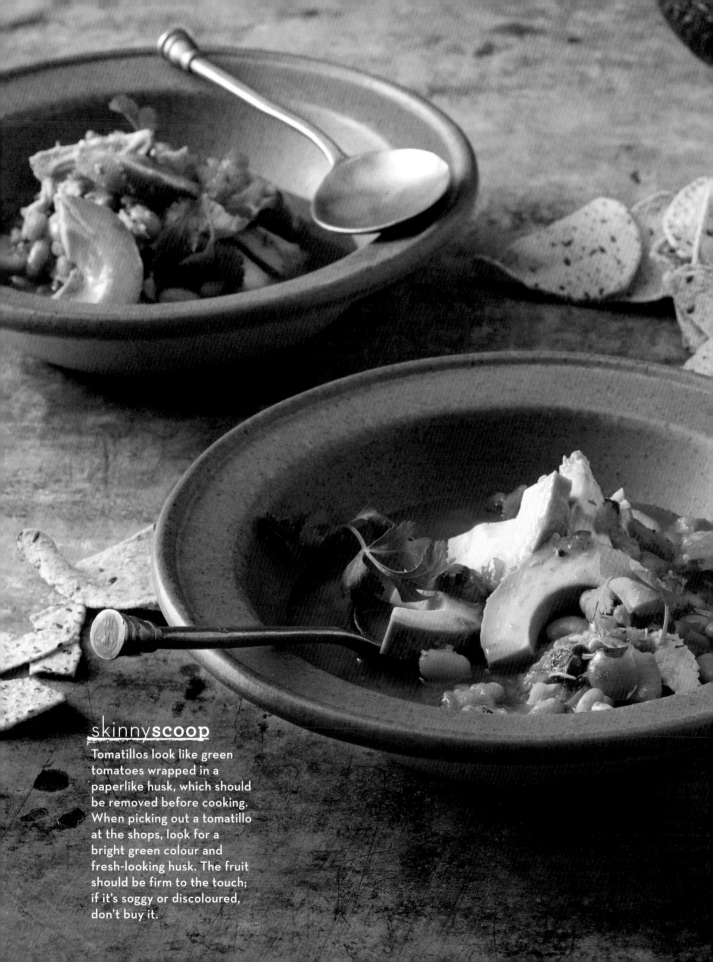

skinnyscoop

Tomatillos look like green tomatoes wrapped in a paperlike husk, which should be removed before cooking. When picking out a tomatillo at the shops, look for a bright green colour and fresh-looking husk. The fruit should be firm to the touch; if it's soggy or discoloured, don't buy it.

Slow-Cooker White Bean Chicken Chilli Verde

SERVES 6

In this lighter twist on the classic Mexican chilli verde, chicken is used in place of pork along with white beans simmered in a rich, spicy sauce. I like using sweet banana-shaped peppers for their milder flavour, which doesn't overpower the other flavours in this dish. Since slow cookers mellow out the flavours of spices, it's always best to taste your dishes at the very end and adjust the spices as needed. Leftovers are even better the next day, so don't worry if you think you've made too much. . You can even freeze whatever you don't plan to eat right away.

1 teaspoon olive oil

1 small onion, chopped

1 cup (180g) chopped sweet peppers

3 medium tomatillos, chopped

3 garlic cloves, crushed

2¾ teaspoons ground cumin

2 (410g) tins cannellini or haricot beans,* rinsed and drained

1 (200g) tin fire-roasted chopped green chillies†

¼ cup (30g) chopped jalapeño or other green chilli, fresh or pickled (remove seeds if you prefer mild heat)

2½ cups (600ml) low-salt chicken stock*

675g boneless, skinless chicken breasts

¼ cup (7g) chopped fresh coriander

1 teaspoon dried oregano

¼ teaspoon chilli powder*

2 bay leaves

¼ teaspoon sea salt

¼ cup (30g) finely chopped spring onions or red onion, for serving

PERFECT PAIRINGS
My favourite combination of toppings for this chilli is chopped spring onions and grated cheese. Sometimes, though, I keep it simple and add just a few slices of avocado. My husband prefers his with light soured cream, grated cheese and tortilla chips on the side.

Read the label to be sure this product is gluten-free.

Heat a medium nonstick frying pan over medium heat. Add the oil, then the onions and peppers. Cook, stirring, until golden and soft, about 5 minutes. Add the tomatillos, garlic and 2½ teaspoons of the cumin and cook for 2 more minutes. Transfer the mixture to the slow cooker and add the beans, green chillies, jalapeño, stock, chicken breasts, coriander, oregano, chilli powder and bay leaves.

Cover and cook on low for 8 hours or high for 4 hours. Remove the chicken from the broth, shred with 2 forks and return it to the slow cooker.

Season with the salt and the remaining ¼ teaspoon cumin, or to taste, and discard the bay leaves. To serve, ladle the chilli into bowls and top with the spring onions.

† If you can't find fire-roasted green chillies, you can use mild fresh green chillies instead.

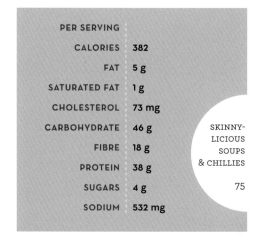

PER SERVING	
CALORIES	382
FAT	5 g
SATURATED FAT	1 g
CHOLESTEROL	73 mg
CARBOHYDRATE	46 g
FIBRE	18 g
PROTEIN	38 g
SUGARS	4 g
SODIUM	532 mg

SKINNY-LICIOUS
SOUPS
& CHILLIES

75

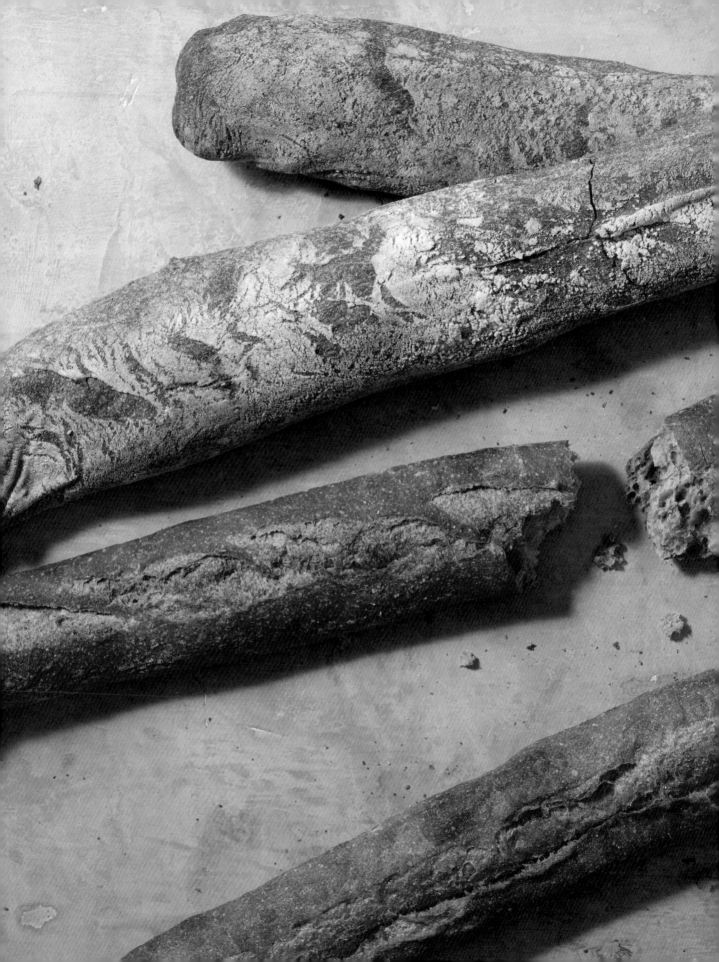

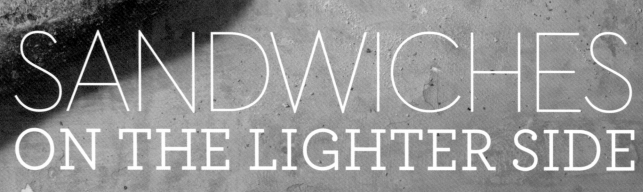

SANDWICHES
ON THE LIGHTER SIDE

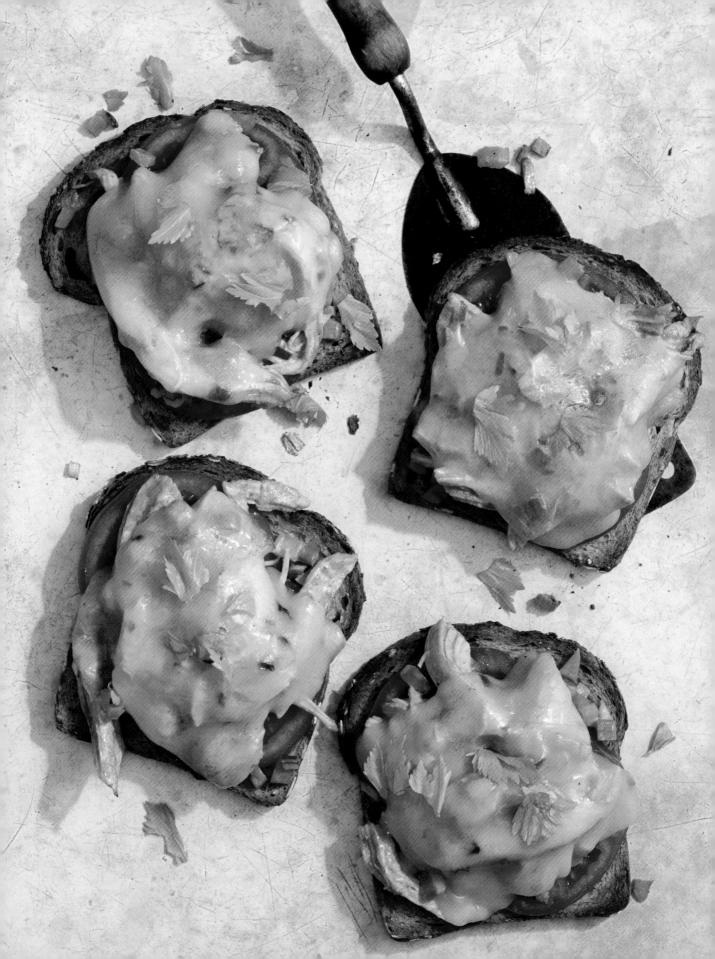

Buffalo Chicken Melts

SERVES 4

I grew up on tuna melts, and now I often make them for my kids. I love this spicier twist on the classic: in place of tuna I use chicken salad made with a hot sauce and chopped carrots, celery and onions. It's served open-face on toasted whole-grain bread and topped with thin slices of tomatoes and melted cheese.

1½ cups (200g) Convenient Slow-Cooker Shredded Chicken (recipe follows) or breast meat from a shop-bought rotisserie chicken

¼ cup (40g) finely chopped carrots

¼ cup (40g) finely chopped celery

1 tablespoon finely chopped red onion

1 tablespoon light mayonnaise such as Hellmann's

2½ tablespoons hot pepper sauce

Pinch of cayenne pepper (optional)

4 slices multigrain bread, lightly toasted

8 thin slices tomato

4 slices (70g total) reduced-fat pepper Jack cheese†

Preheat the grill.

In a medium bowl, combine the chicken, carrots, celery, red onion, mayonnaise, hot sauce and cayenne (if using).

Arrange the toast on a baking sheet and put 2 slices of tomato on each. Divide the chicken salad evenly among the slices and top with 1 slice of cheese. Grill until the cheese is golden and bubbling, about 2 minutes, keeping a close eye on it to avoid burning. Serve hot.

† If you can't get hold of pepper Jack, another lighter cheese of your choice would work well.

(recipe continues)

PER SERVING	
CALORIES	230
FAT	8 g
SATURATED FAT	3 g
CHOLESTEROL	45 mg
CARBOHYDRATE	13 g
FIBRE	2.5 g
PROTEIN	25 g
SUGARS	3 g
SODIUM	414 mg

SAND-
WICHES
ON THE
LIGHTER
SIDE

79

Convenient Slow-Cooker Shredded Chicken

MAKES 500G · SERVES 6

Wanna know my secret to making quick weeknight meals? I use my slow cooker to make shredded chicken. It's my favourite technique because the chicken gets so tender that it just falls apart and it requires almost no attention whatsoever.

I opt for organic chicken and buy chicken breasts in bulk to save money. I throw 3 pieces in my slow cooker and wrap the rest in clingfilm to freeze for another day. A few hours later, the chicken easily shreds into pieces. You can use chicken stock to add more flavour or just use water with salt instead. If I have some herbs, celery or parsley in my refrigerator, I may even throw them in. There are really no rules – use whatever you have to hand.

3 boneless, skinless chicken breasts, trimmed of all fat (675g total)

3 cups (725ml) low-salt chicken stock* (or water)

1 onion, quartered (optional)

1 celery stalk (optional)

1 sprig of fresh parsley (optional)

Read the label to be sure this product is gluten-free.

In a slow cooker, combine the chicken breast, just enough stock (or water) to cover the chicken, and onion, celery and parsley, if using. Cover and cook on high for 4 hours.

Remove the chicken and shred it with two forks. Discard the remaining liquid and vegetables. Use the shredded chicken in any recipe that calls for it, or refrigerate it for up to 3 days.

PER SERVING	
CALORIES	66
FAT	1.5 g
SATURATED FAT	0.5 g
CHOLESTEROL	31 mg
CARBOHYDRATE	2 g
FIBRE	0 g
PROTEIN	11 g
SUGARS	1 g
SODIUM	300 mg

Roast Beef Sandwiches
with Creamy Horseradish Spread

SERVES 4

I distinctly remember the first time I tried a roast beef sandwich with watercress and cucumber. From my very first bite, I thought it was a magical combination. I've been making roast beef sandwiches this way ever since. The horseradish spread really gives this an extra punch of flavour!

HORSERADISH CREAM

3 tablespoons light soured cream

1 tablespoon horseradish sauce

1 tablespoon Dijon mustard

1 tablespoon finely chopped fresh chives

Sea salt and freshly ground black pepper

SANDWICHES

225g wholemeal baguette, cut into 4 pieces

225g thinly sliced lean roast beef

1 cup (30g) watercress or rocket

20 thin slices cucumber (50g)

Sea salt and freshly ground black pepper

For the horseradish cream: In a small bowl, combine the soured cream, horseradish, mustard and chives. Season with a pinch of salt and black pepper.

For the sandwiches: Split each piece of baguette in half lengthwise and spread the horseradish cream onto the bread. Layer each sandwich with a quarter of the roast beef and watercress and 5 slices cucumber. Season each with a pinch of salt and black pepper and serve.

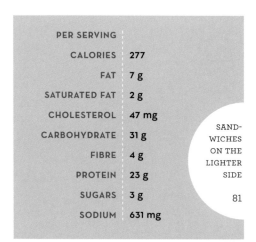

PER SERVING	
CALORIES	277
FAT	7 g
SATURATED FAT	2 g
CHOLESTEROL	47 mg
CARBOHYDRATE	31 g
FIBRE	4 g
PROTEIN	23 g
SUGARS	3 g
SODIUM	631 mg

SAND-
WICHES
ON THE
LIGHTER
SIDE

Greek Salad Pitta Pizzas

SERVES 4

Greek goodness – that's what I call these personal salad pitta pizzas. I came up with the idea after tasting a savoury Greek tart at the farmers' market. The flavours were so fresh and tasty that I wanted to come up with a quick, lighter way anyone could enjoy it. This is so easy to make and takes less than 5 minutes to put together!

2 teaspoons red wine vinegar

1 teaspoon extra-virgin olive oil

3 tablespoons chopped Kalamata olives

1 tablespoon chopped red onion

¾ cup (165g) hummus, homemade (see page 111) or shop-bought

4 (25g) small wholemeal pittas, unsplit and toasted

4 thin slices tomato

⅓ cup (60g) seeded and chopped cucumber

⅓ cup (60g) chopped orange pepper

2 tablespoons crumbled feta cheese

skinnyscoop

Look for small wholemeal pittas that are about 25g each, or cut a larger one in half.

In a small bowl, whisk together the vinegar and olive oil. Stir in the olives and onion.

Spread 2 tablespoons hummus on the top of each toasted pitta. Top each with a slice of tomato, spread with 1 more tablespoon hummus in the centre of the tomato and top with the cucumber, pepper, onion-olive mixture and feta.

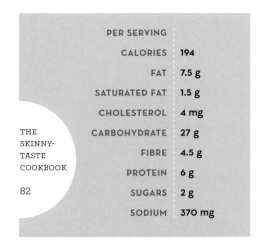

PER SERVING	
CALORIES	194
FAT	7.5 g
SATURATED FAT	1.5 g
CHOLESTEROL	4 mg
CARBOHYDRATE	27 g
FIBRE	4.5 g
PROTEIN	6 g
SUGARS	2 g
SODIUM	370 mg

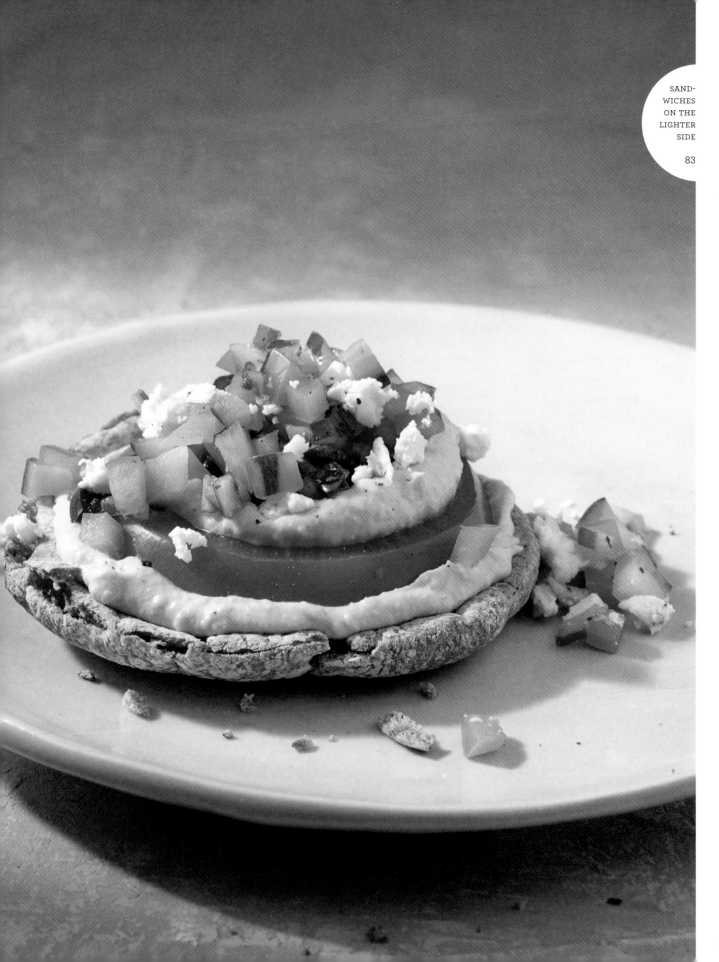

Chicken Philly Cheesesteaks

SERVES 4

I must confess, I have a real weakness for cheesesteaks. I used to work near a sandwich shop that made a pretty decent Philly chicken sub. Whenever I'd walk by during my lunch break, I'd have a hard time passing one up. But at more than 500 calories and 15 grams of fat per sub (yikes!), I always felt guilty if I ordered one. So I made up my own leaner version. It's so good and only about 350 calories!

275g boneless, skinless thin chicken breasts

½ teaspoon garlic powder

Sea salt

Freshly ground black pepper

Cooking spray or oil mister

1 teaspoon olive oil

½ medium green pepper, thinly sliced

½ large onion, halved and thinly sliced

225g mushrooms, sliced

225g wholemeal French or Italian bread, split horizontally and cut crosswise into 4 pieces

4 (25g) slices reduced-fat provolone cheese†

Preheat the oven to 220°C/200°C fan/Gas 7 or the grill to low.

Season the chicken with the garlic powder, ¼ teaspoon salt and black pepper to taste. Heat a large nonstick frying pan over high heat. When hot, spray the frying pan with oil and add half of the chicken, making sure you don't overcrowd the pan. Cook until browned, about 1 minute, turn the chicken over and cook the second side for 1 additional minute. Transfer to a large dish. Repeat with the remaining chicken.

Add ½ teaspoon of the oil to the hot pan. Add the pepper and onion and season with a pinch of salt and black pepper. Cook 1 minute, stir and then cook until the onions are golden and slightly browned, 4 to 5 minutes. Transfer to the plate of chicken.

† If you can't find provolone cheese, another lighter cheese would also work well.

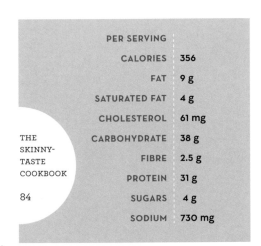

PER SERVING	
CALORIES	356
FAT	9 g
SATURATED FAT	4 g
CHOLESTEROL	61 mg
CARBOHYDRATE	38 g
FIBRE	2.5 g
PROTEIN	31 g
SUGARS	4 g
SODIUM	730 mg

Reduce the heat to medium and add the remaining ½ teaspoon olive oil to the pan. Add the mushrooms, season with ⅛ teaspoon salt and a pinch of black pepper and cook until the mushrooms are slightly browned on one side, 1 to 2 minutes. Turn the mushrooms over and cook until soft, 1 to 2 more minutes. Transfer to the plate of chicken, onions and peppers.

Divide the chicken and vegetables evenly among the bottom halves of the bread and top each with a slice of cheese. Place the sandwiches on a baking sheet.

Heat the sandwiches in the oven or under the grill until the cheese melts, 2 to 3 minutes, being careful not to burn the cheese if using the grill. Remove from the oven, close the sandwiches and serve.

Go Topless

EMBRACING THE OPEN-FACE SANDWICH

A tartine is an open-face sandwich that's often made with a rich spread. Leaving the top piece of bread off cuts calories, making a slimmer sandwich. And topping it with fruit, veggies, healthy fats and more good-for-you ingredients allows you to create a truly healthy bite. Try one of these deliciously skinny, quick tartines, each of which is 300 calories or less.

Top a 50g slice of crusty wholemeal bread with . . .

- 2 sliced vine-ripened tomatoes, finely shredded fresh basil and 1 teaspoon olive oil drizzled on top (211 calories)

- 75g (about ½ cup) mashed avocado and a sprinkle of salt and freshly ground black pepper (276 CALORIES)

- 2 tablespoons light cream cheese, diced spring onions and sliced tomatoes and cucumbers (221 CALORIES)

- 1 chopped hard-boiled egg, thinly sliced red onion, capers and 1 teaspoon olive oil drizzled on top (261 CALORIES)

- 50g tuna (packed in spring water), ¼ medium sliced avocado, chopped tomatoes and a handful of sprouted seeds (300 CALORIES)

Turkey Panini with Avocado, Spinach and Roasted Peppers

SERVES 4

Looking for a fresh way to dress your sandwich? Try mashed avocado seasoned with a touch of salt and black pepper. The spread adds a nice flavour to this crisp, warm panini made with lean turkey breast, sweet roasted peppers and wilted baby spinach pressed between two slices of ciabatta bread.

½ cup (115g) mashed avocado

4 pieces (75g each) ciabatta bread, sliced open

Sea salt and freshly ground black pepper

2 cups (90g) baby spinach

225g thinly sliced turkey breast

8 thin slices roasted red peppers, jarred (not oil-packed) or homemade (see page 233)

Olive oil spray or oil mister

skinny**scoop**

No panini press? No problem. Place the sandwich onto a heated frying pan or griddle, top with a weight, such as another heavy pan, and push down on the weight to press and crisp the sandwich. When the bread is toasted, flip the sandwich and toast the other side.

Preheat a panini press.

Spread 2 tablespoons of the avocado on the top of each piece of ciabatta bread. Season the avocado with a pinch of salt and black pepper. Place a quarter of the spinach on the bottom of each sandwich and top each with a quarter of the turkey and 2 slices roasted pepper. Close the sandwiches and lightly spray the tops with a little olive oil.

Place the sandwiches one at a time on the hot panini press and close. Cook until the bread is toasted and crisp, about 5 minutes. Cut the sandwiches in half diagonally and serve immediately.

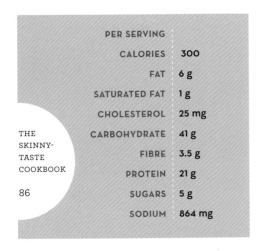

PER SERVING	
CALORIES	300
FAT	6 g
SATURATED FAT	1 g
CHOLESTEROL	25 mg
CARBOHYDRATE	41 g
FIBRE	3.5 g
PROTEIN	21 g
SUGARS	5 g
SODIUM	864 mg

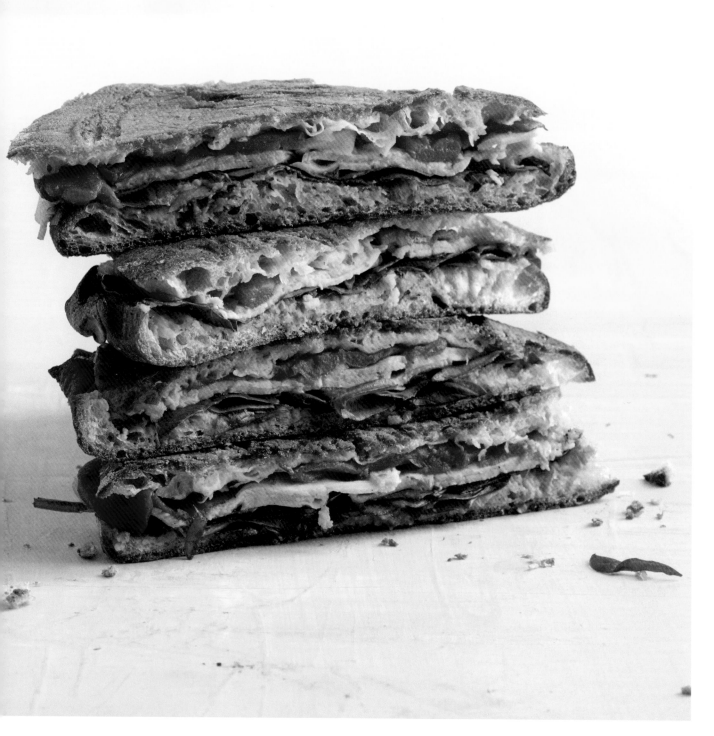

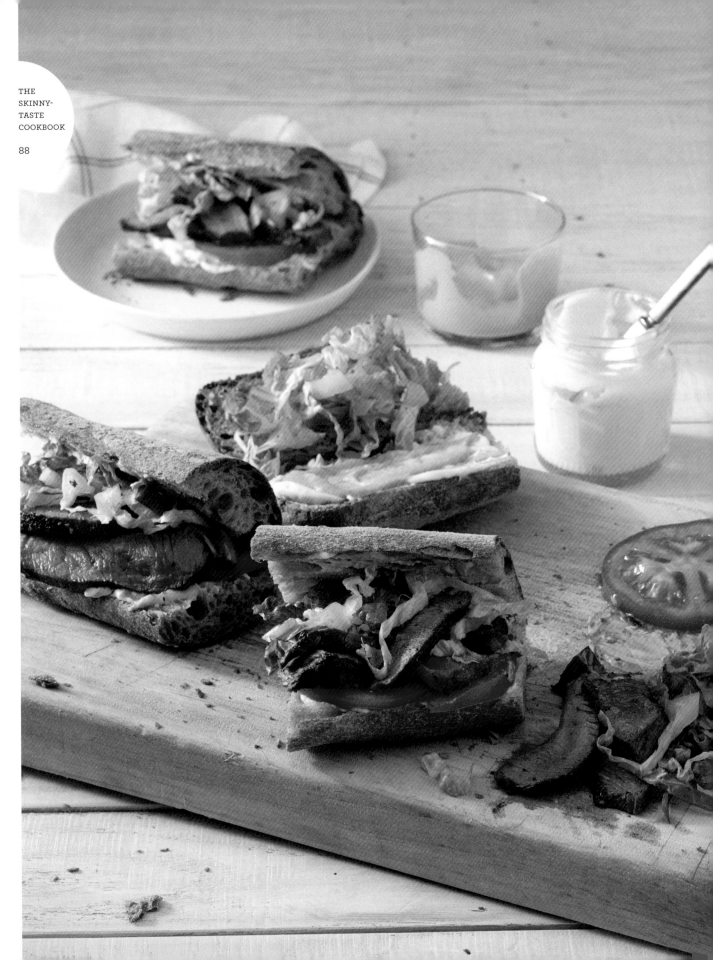

Grilled Steak Sandwiches

SERVES 4

These steak sandwiches are simple – you probably already have most of the ingredients in your cupboards – but put them all together and you have yourself a pretty darn good sandwich. Cook lean sirloin steaks on the grill, top with juicy tomatoes and crisp lettuce, and serve on a wholemeal baguette. Dinner is ready in less than 15 minutes and it's absolutely delicious!

STEAK

400g sirloin steak, trimmed of fat

½ teaspoon garlic powder

¼ teaspoon sea salt

Freshly ground black pepper

Cooking spray or oil mister

SANDWICHES

225g wholemeal baguette, cut into 4 pieces

2 tablespoons American mustard

¼ cup (60g) light mayonnaise

2 cups (100g) shredded romaine lettuce

1 large tomato, sliced

For the steak: Season the sirloin with the garlic powder, salt and black pepper to taste.

Preheat a barbecue (or preheat a grill pan over high heat). Lightly rub the grates with oil or spray a grill pan with oil and add the steaks. Grill for about 3 minutes, turn the steaks over and grill another 3 minutes for medium (cook longer or less according to your preference). Transfer the steak to a chopping board to rest for 5 minutes.

For the sandwiches: Split open each piece of bread, then spread each with ½ tablespoon mustard and 1 tablespoon mayonnaise. Divide the lettuce and tomatoes among the sandwiches.

Thinly slice the steak and divide it among the sandwiches and serve.

skinnyscoop

Always let cooked steak rest for at least 5 minutes before slicing so that you don't lose all those delicious juices. I'd rather keep them in my sandwich than let them collect on the chopping board.

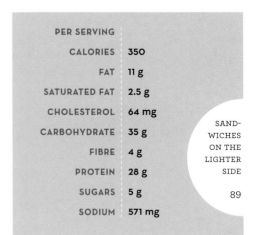

PER SERVING	
CALORIES	350
FAT	11 g
SATURATED FAT	2.5 g
CHOLESTEROL	64 mg
CARBOHYDRATE	35 g
FIBRE	4 g
PROTEIN	28 g
SUGARS	5 g
SODIUM	571 mg

SAND-
WICHES
ON THE
LIGHTER
SIDE

Egg, Tomato and Spring Onion Sandwiches

SERVES 4

Prior to making *Skinnytaste* my full-time career, I worked in Manhattan as a digital photo retoucher. In the lobby of the building where I worked, there was a small café that served a simple egg sandwich. My friend Tricia and I were absolutely hooked. It calls for only a few common ingredients, but the combination is just delicious! I had to remake it at home.

4 large eggs, hard-boiled, peeled and sliced

4 wholemeal rolls

4 thick slices tomato

¼ cup (30g) chopped spring onions

Sea salt and freshly ground black pepper

¼ cup (60g) light mayonnaise

Assemble the sandwiches by placing one sliced egg on the bottom of each roll. Top it with a tomato slice and 1 tablespoon spring onions. Season each with a pinch of salt and black pepper. Spread 1 tablespoon of mayonnaise on the top of each roll, put the tops on the sandwiches and serve.

skinny**scoop**

Here's a foolproof way to make perfect hard-boiled eggs every time: place eggs in a pot, cover with cold water and bring to a rolling boil. Cover the pot, remove it from the heat and let it sit for 20 minutes without opening the lid. Drain the hot water, quickly rinse the eggs under cold water and peel.

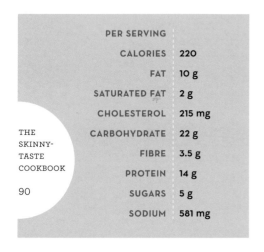

PER SERVING	
CALORIES	220
FAT	10 g
SATURATED FAT	2 g
CHOLESTEROL	215 mg
CARBOHYDRATE	22 g
FIBRE	3.5 g
PROTEIN	14 g
SUGARS	5 g
SODIUM	581 mg

Pear and Brie Grilled Cheese

SERVES 4

Have you ever had baked Brie? If not, you're totally missing out. And if you have, then you'll understand why this grilled cheese sandwich works. I love the salty-sweet combination of ripe pears and Brie. Adding a touch of fig butter – a fruit spread not to be confused with butter – to this grilled cheese sandwich enhances the sweetness of the pears and makes it a real adult treat.

8 slices multigrain bread

4 tablespoons fruit butter such as fig or apple†

1 pear, peeled and thinly sliced

170g light Brie, rind removed and sliced

Olive oil spray or oil mister

Heat a frying pan over medium-low heat.

Spread each slice of bread with ½ tablespoon fig or apple butter. Top 4 of the slices with the pear and Brie, then top with the remaining slices of bread. Spray both sides of the sandwiches with a little oil.

Place the sandwiches, one at a time, in the hot frying pan and cook until the bread is golden and the cheese starts to melt, about 2 minutes on each side. (Alternatively, use a panini press.) Serve hot.

† If you can't find fruit butter, a fruit chutney or quince jelly will work well.

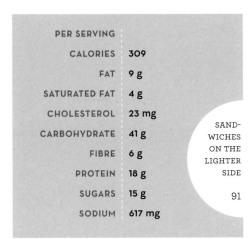

PER SERVING	
CALORIES	309
FAT	9 g
SATURATED FAT	4 g
CHOLESTEROL	23 mg
CARBOHYDRATE	41 g
FIBRE	6 g
PROTEIN	18 g
SUGARS	15 g
SODIUM	617 mg

SAND-
WICHES
ON THE
LIGHTER
SIDE

91

French Bread Pizza Supreme

SERVES 4

French bread pizza reminds me of my high-school days when I would come home from school ravenous and turn French bread into an awesome after-school meal. I still make such pizzas today, although now I sneak in some whole grains and top them with tons of veggies. It's perfect because everyone can customize their toppings to their taste. I've always liked the classic combination of pepperoni, mushrooms, peppers and onions, but you can use any vegetables or leftovers you have, including broccoli, sliced turkey, meatballs, spinach – the possibilities are endless!

1 (275g) loaf wholemeal French bread

1 cup (250g) tomato sauce, homemade (recipe follows) or shop-bought

2 mushrooms, thinly sliced

1 thinly sliced red onion, separated into rings

8 thin slices green pepper

1 cup (110g) light mozzarella cheese, grated

¼ cup (25g) grated Parmesan cheese

8 turkey pepperoni slices, cut in half†

Preheat the oven to 220°C/200°C fan/Gas 7.

Split the bread horizontally lengthwise, then cut each half crosswise into 2 pieces to give you 4 pieces total. Scoop out the centre of the bread, keeping only the crust (each should weigh about 50g).

Place the bread, cut side up, on a baking sheet. Spread each piece with a quarter of the tomato sauce. Divide the mushrooms, onion rings, pepper slices, mozzarella and Parmesan among the pieces, then top with pepperoni.

Bake until the cheese is melted and bubbling, and the bread is crisp, about 10 minutes.

† If you can't find turkey pepperoni, any pepperoni will work well.

PER SERVING	
CALORIES	310
FAT	8 g
SATURATED FAT	4 g
CHOLESTEROL	20 mg
CARBOHYDRATE	42 g
FIBRE	4.5 g
PROTEIN	16 g
SUGARS	4 g
SODIUM	756 mg

(recipe continues)

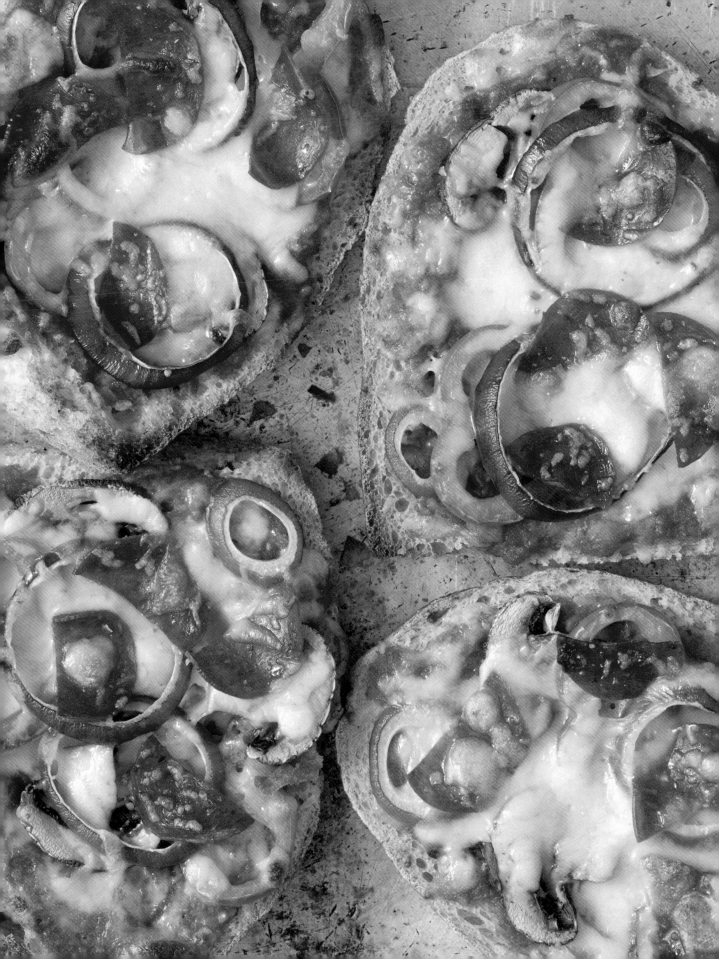

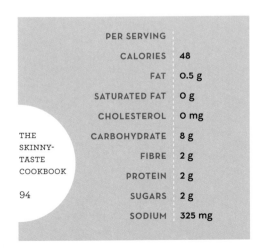

skinny**scoop**

This sauce can be stored in the refrigerator for up to 3 days, or in the freezer for up to 4 months. To freeze, let the sauce cool and transfer it to 1-litre ziplock bags. Label the bags with the name, portion size and date, and lay them flat in the freezer. To thaw, transfer the sauce to the refrigerator 1 to 2 days before you plan to use it, or you can heat the frozen sauce over low heat on the hob.

Quickest Tomato Sauce

MAKES ABOUT 1.5KG

This easy-to-whip-up sauce works well for a variety of quick meals, from pizza to pasta to chicken parmigiana, which you can throw together on a busy weeknight. The secret to the perfect sauce is buying the right tomatoes. Not all tinned tomatoes are created equal; you should look for a brand you like.

2 teaspoons olive oil

5 garlic cloves, smashed

4 (400g) tins chopped tomatoes

¾ teaspoon sea salt, plus more as needed

Freshly ground black pepper

¼ cup (15g) roughly chopped fresh basil

Heat a medium-large saucepan over medium heat. Add the oil and garlic and cook, stirring, until golden, about 2 minutes. (Tip: Because I don't use a lot of oil, I tilt my pan to one side so the garlic is submerged in the oil and cooks evenly.) Add ¼ cup (50ml) water, the tomatoes and salt and season with black pepper to taste. Cover the pot, bring to a boil, reduce the heat to medium-low and simmer until the sauce is heated through, about 10 minutes. Remove the pan from the heat, stir in the basil and adjust salt and pepper to taste if needed.

PER SERVING	
CALORIES	48
FAT	0.5 g
SATURATED FAT	0 g
CHOLESTEROL	0 mg
CARBOHYDRATE	8 g
FIBRE	2 g
PROTEIN	2 g
SUGARS	2 g
SODIUM	325 mg

Grilled Vegetable Sandwiches with Pesto Mayonnaise

SERVES 4

Summer is my favourite season – I love the warm weather, the beach, the long hours of daylight and the abundance of fresh produce available at farmers' markets. This is the ideal quickie weeknight summer dinner. What really makes a sandwich is the bread it's made on – good bread is worth seeking out. For this sandwich, I like to use a crusty, wholemeal or multigrain rustic-style loaf, which you can find in any good bakery or supermarket.

PESTO MAYONNAISE

1 cup (50g) fresh basil leaves

1 garlic clove

2 tablespoons grated Parmesan cheese

Freshly ground black pepper

¼ cup (60g) light mayonnaise (I prefer Hellmann's Light)

SANDWICHES

1 medium aubergine, cut lengthwise into 5mm-thick slabs

2 medium courgettes, sliced lengthwise 5mm thin

Olive oil spray or mister

2 tablespoons balsamic vinegar

¼ teaspoon dried oregano

¼ teaspoon sea salt

Freshly ground black pepper

8 (25g) slices bread from a multigrain round country loaf

1 large tomato, thinly sliced

For the pesto mayonnaise: In a food processor, combine the basil, garlic, Parmesan and black pepper to taste and pulse until smooth. Add the mayonnaise and pulse a few times.

For the sandwiches: Preheat a grill to medium (or preheat a grill pan over medium heat).

Spray the sliced vegetables generously with olive oil and drizzle on the balsamic vinegar. Season with the oregano, salt and black pepper to taste. Grill the vegetables until lightly browned and tender, 5 to 6 minutes on each side.

Toast the bread under the grill for about 1 minute per side. Spread the pesto mayonnaise on the bread. Divide the grilled vegetables among 4 of the bread slices, layer the sliced tomatoes on the vegetables and then top with the remaining 4 slices of bread.

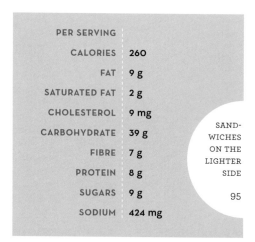

PER SERVING	
CALORIES	260
FAT	9 g
SATURATED FAT	2 g
CHOLESTEROL	9 mg
CARBOHYDRATE	39 g
FIBRE	7 g
PROTEIN	8 g
SUGARS	9 g
SODIUM	424 mg

SAND-
WICHES
ON THE
LIGHTER
SIDE

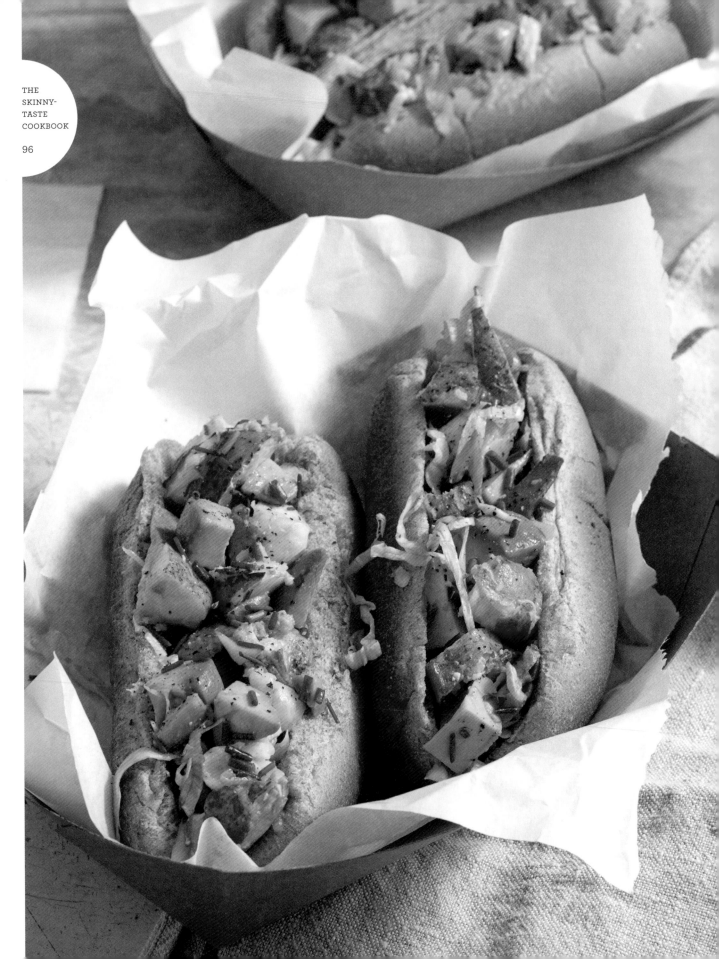

Summer Lobster Rolls

SERVES 4

Lobster rolls always remind me of Fire Island, New York. In the summer I love taking day trips by ferry out to this barrier island off the south shore of Long Island and often treat myself to a lobster roll for lunch. But it's usually swimming in fatty mayonnaise, or worse, melted butter. Here, I remake this favourite summer sandwich so that it's a bit healthier. The fresh avocado gives it a creamy texture, plus a dose of heart-healthy fat.

If you want to eliminate the carbs, bypass the bread and serve this in a fancy martini glass instead. If fresh lobster isn't available to you, you can use crabmeat instead.

250g fresh cooked lobster meat (from two 675g live lobsters), chopped

1 medium (110g) avocado, chopped

Juice of 1 large lemon

1 teaspoon olive oil

2 teaspoons finely chopped fresh chives

Sea salt and freshly ground black pepper

4 wholemeal hot dog rolls

1 cup (50g) shredded lettuce

In a medium bowl, combine the lobster meat, avocado, lemon juice, olive oil and chives, and season with a pinch of salt and black pepper.

Open the hot dog rolls and put the shredded lettuce inside. Top with the lobster salad and serve.

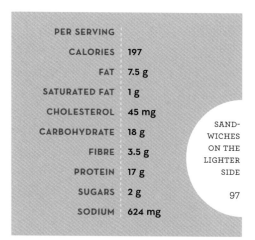

PER SERVING	
CALORIES	197
FAT	7.5 g
SATURATED FAT	1 g
CHOLESTEROL	45 mg
CARBOHYDRATE	18 g
FIBRE	3.5 g
PROTEIN	17 g
SUGARS	2 g
SODIUM	624 mg

SAND-
WICHES
ON THE
LIGHTER
SIDE

97

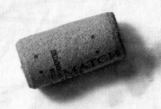

SKINNY BITES

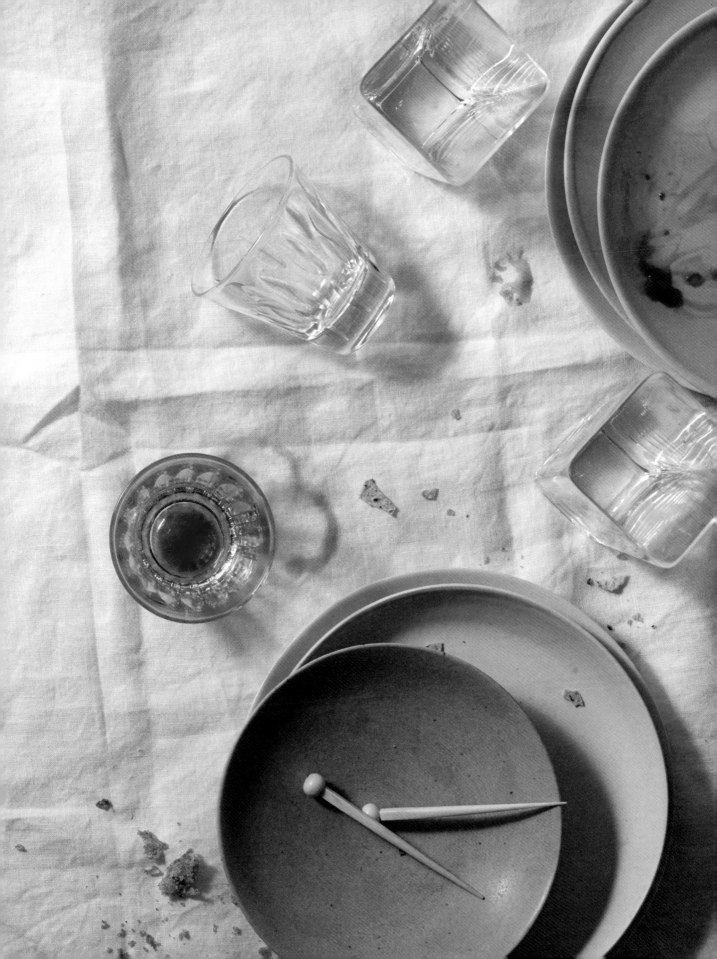

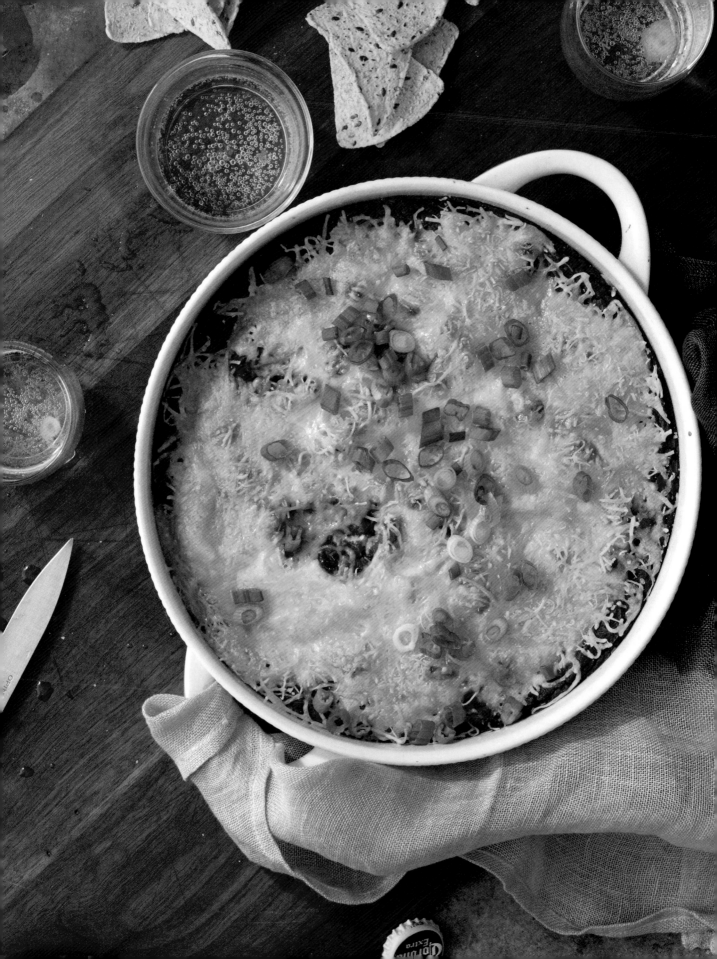

Caliente Bean and Queso Dip

SERVES 14

Melted cheese is my weakness, but I believe in everything in moderation. Plus, there *are* some health perks associated with cheese: it's a complete protein with the right amount of amino acids to give our bodies a protein fix, and it's rich in calcium, vitamin A and folate. Cheesy days are always happier than cheeseless days for me, so to make it work calorie-wise, I look for reduced-fat or light cheese options.

Cooking spray or oil mister

1 (425g) tin refried beans*

1 tablespoon taco seasoning mix*

1¼ cups (310g) jarred mild tomato salsa

1 (110g) tin diced green chillies†

1½ cups (170g) grated reduced-fat Mexican cheese blend‡

1 teaspoon chopped fresh coriander

Read the labels to be sure these products are gluten-free.

Preheat the oven to 180°C/160°C fan/Gas 4. Spray a 23 x 23cm baking dish with oil.

In a small bowl, combine the refried beans and taco seasoning and spread the mixture evenly over the bottom of the baking dish. Pour the salsa and green chillies on top of the beans.

Bake until the edges begin to bubble, about 30 minutes. Remove from the oven, top with the cheese and return to the oven. Bake just long enough to melt the cheese, 5 to 6 minutes. Remove from the oven and sprinkle with coriander.

† If you can't get hold of tinned green chillies, you can use pickled jalapeños instead – although the results will be much hotter!

‡ If you can't find Mexican cheese, lighter cheddar will work well.

PERFECT PAIRING
I like to serve this dip with baked tortilla chips.

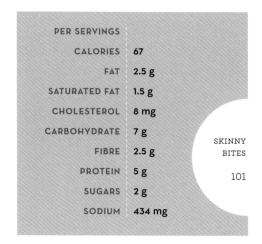

PER SERVINGS	
CALORIES	67
FAT	2.5 g
SATURATED FAT	1.5 g
CHOLESTEROL	8 mg
CARBOHYDRATE	7 g
FIBRE	2.5 g
PROTEIN	5 g
SUGARS	2 g
SODIUM	434 mg

SKINNY BITES

101

Guiltless Sausage-Stuffed Mushrooms

MAKES 12 TO 14 MUSHROOMS · SERVES 6 OR 7

It's pretty hard to resist popping these bite-size sausage-stuffed mushrooms into your mouth – believe me, I know. When I was testing these out, I probably ate half of them in one sitting for lunch. Good thing these glorious snacks are made with ingredients I feel good about. But don't be fooled by their lack of fat and calories. If you serve these to company, no one would ever notice they were 'light'!

400g button mushrooms

75g fresh sweet Italian chicken sausages, casings removed†

1 teaspoon olive oil

⅓ cup (50g) finely chopped onion

1 celery stalk, finely chopped

¼ teaspoon sea salt, plus more as needed

Freshly ground black pepper

2 tablespoons seasoned wholemeal bread crumbs, homemade (see page 110) or shop-bought

2 tablespoons grated Parmesan cheese

Cooking spray or oil mister

skinny**scoop**

For this recipe, I prefer the smaller mushrooms as opposed to the larger ones that are actually meant for stuffing because they taste better, they hold together better, and there's nothing better than popping those little suckers right into your mouth. If you're making these for a large party, you can prep them ahead of time and bake them in the oven when your guests arrive.

Preheat the oven to 200°C/180°C fan/Gas 6.

Stem the mushrooms, finely chop the stems and set aside.

Heat a medium nonstick frying pan over medium heat. Add the sausage and cook, using a wooden spoon to break the meat into small pieces, until cooked through and browned, 3 to 4 minutes. Transfer to a plate and set aside.

Add the olive oil to the pan, then add the onion. Cook, stirring, for 1 minute, then add the celery. Reduce the heat to medium and cook, stirring, until the celery is soft, about 12 minutes. Add the chopped mushroom stems to the pan, season with the salt and a pinch of black pepper and cook, stirring, until soft, 4 to 5 minutes. Add the cooked sausage, stir in the bread crumbs and Parmesan, then set aside.

Lightly season the inside of the mushroom caps with a pinch of salt. Fill each mushroom with about 1 heaped tablespoon sausage stuffing, rounding off the tops. It's easy to do this right over the pan one at a time. Place them in a baking dish and lightly spray the tops with oil.

Bake until golden brown, about 20 minutes. Serve hot.

† If you can't find Italian chicken sausages, another kind of chicken sausage or reduced-fat pork sausages will work well.

PER SERVING	
CALORIES	63
FAT	3 g
SATURATED FAT	1 g
CHOLESTEROL	13 mg
CARBOHYDRATE	5 g
FIBRE	1 g
PROTEIN	5 g
SUGARS	2 g
SODIUM	162 mg

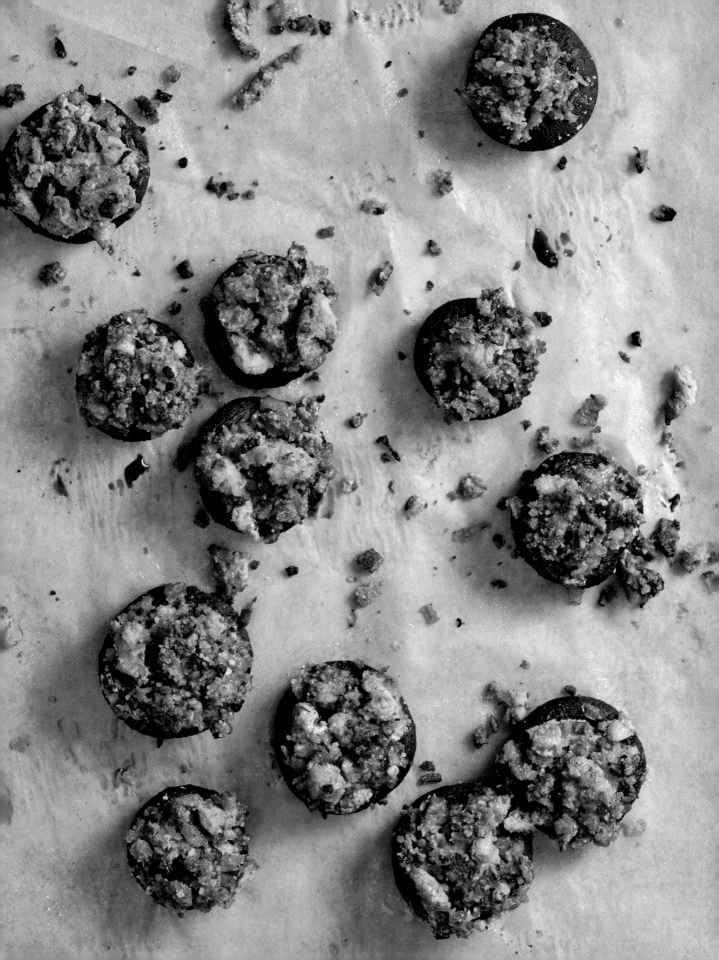

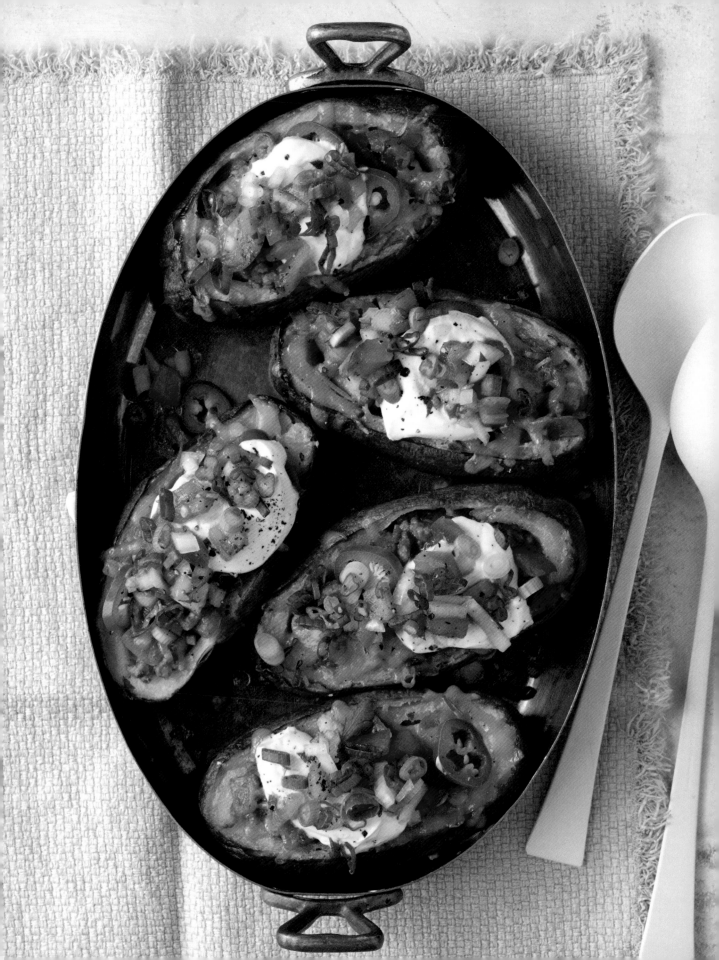

Loaded 'Nacho' Potato Skins

SERVES 16

I took two of my favourite party foods – loaded nachos and potato skins – and combined them into one ultimate starter! Thanks to the surge of low- or no-carb diets, the potato has got a bad rap. But the humble spud is far from 'bad'. In fact, it's a whole food that's packed with nutrients, as well as fibre if the skins are left intact. Here, I even splurged and used full-fat cheddar to top them off. After all, these are potato skins, so they need to be cheesy.

8 small baking potatoes
(about 1kg total)

QUICK CHILLI FILLING

170g turkey breast mince

¼ teaspoon sea salt

¼ cup (40g) chopped onion

¼ cup (45g) chopped red pepper

1 garlic clove, crushed

⅓ cup (90g) tinned chopped tomatoes with chillies

½ cup (115g) tinned refried beans*

¾ teaspoon ground cumin

¼ teaspoon chilli powder

¼ teaspoon smoked paprika

POTATO SKIN TOPPINGS

Cooking spray or oil mister

⅛ teaspoon sea salt

Freshly ground black pepper

1 cup (110g) grated mature cheddar cheese

¼ cup (35g) pickled jalapeño slices

½ cup (125g) light soured cream

½ cup (125g) pico de gallo, homemade (see page 120) or shop-bought fresh salsa

¼ cup (30g) chopped spring onions

Read the label to be sure this product is gluten-free.

Pierce each potato several times with a fork. Microwave on high for about 12 minutes, or until the potatoes are cooked through. (Alternatively, bake them in a 200°C/180°C fan/Gas 6 oven directly on the rack until the skins are crisp and a knife easily pierces the potatoes, about 50 minutes.) Transfer to a wire rack and leave until cool enough to handle, about 10 minutes.

(recipe continues)

PER SERVING	
CALORIES	75
FAT	3 g
SATURATED FAT	1.5 g
CHOLESTEROL	15 mg
CARBOHYDRATE	7 g
FIBRE	1 g
PROTEIN	5 g
SUGARS	1 g
SODIUM	172 mg

SKINNY
BITES

Preheat the grill.

For the quick chilli filling: Heat a medium frying pan over medium-high heat. Add the turkey and cook, using a wooden spoon to break the meat into small pieces, until no longer pink, 4 to 5 minutes. Season with the salt. Add the onion, pepper and garlic and cook for 2 to 3 minutes. Add the tomatoes, refried beans, cumin, chilli powder and paprika. Reduce the heat to low, cover and simmer for 7 to 8 minutes to blend the flavours.

For the potato skin toppings: Slice each potato in half lengthwise. Using a spoon, scoop out the flesh, leaving about 5mm intact. Lightly coat the insides and skin sides of the potatoes with oil, and season both sides with the salt and black pepper to taste. Arrange the potato shells on a baking sheet and grill until the skins start to crisp and brown, 2 to 3 minutes on each side. Preheat the oven to 200°C/180°C fan/Gas 6.

Divide the chilli evenly among the potato skins and top with the cheese and jalapeño slices. Return to the oven and heat until the cheese is melted, 2 to 3 minutes. Remove from the oven and top with the soured cream, salsa and spring onions. Serve immediately.

Roasted Edamame with Sea Salt

SERVES 4

When my daughter Madison was about one and started growing her first few teeth, one of her favourite solid foods was edamame. She would ask for it all the time, which always made me laugh – I created a foodie at the young age of one! As she got older, I would buy packets of dehydrated edamame as a snack. But a small packet was so expensive that I decided to try roasting edamame myself. They turned out nutty and crunchy and, I find, a bit addictive if seasoned with a little sea salt.

350g fresh or frozen shelled edamame

Cooking spray or oil mister

¼ teaspoon sea salt

If the edamame are frozen, thaw and dry them well with kitchen paper.

Preheat the oven to 220°C/200°C fan/Gas 7. Spray a large baking sheet with oil.

Spread the edamame out on the baking sheet, spray with a little more oil, and season with the sea salt. Bake until golden and crisp through the centre, shaking the pan every 10 minutes or so to brown evenly, 28 to 38 minutes. Allow to cool completely.

PER SERVING	
CALORIES	120
FAT	5.5 g
SATURATED FAT	0.5 g
CHOLESTEROL	0 mg
CARBOHYDRATE	9 g
FIBRE	3.5 g
PROTEIN	11 g
SUGARS	0 g
SODIUM	353 mg

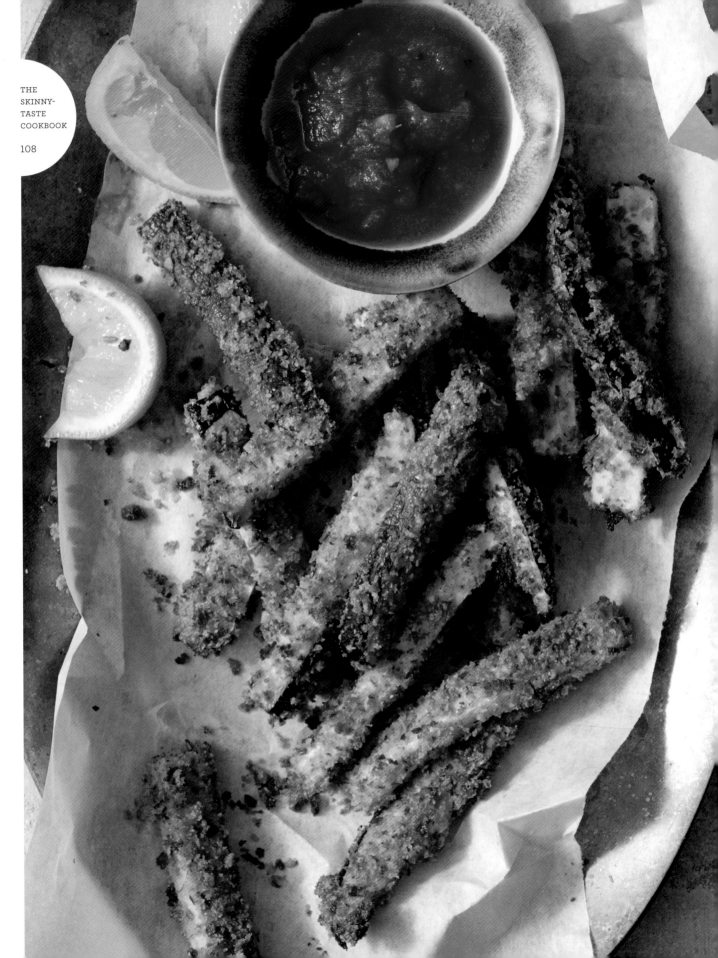

Baked Courgette Sticks

SERVES 4

I guarantee that even the pickiest of eaters will love these! In fact, when my daughter Karina (a very picky eater) was younger, this was her favourite way to eat courgettes. The only complaint I used to get when I made these was that I never made enough, so if you think this is a lot for four people, keep in mind they shrink a bit when they cook.

Cooking spray or oil mister

4 medium courgettes, ends trimmed

3 large egg whites

¼ teaspoon sea salt

Freshly ground black pepper

1 cup (80g) seasoned wholemeal bread crumbs, homemade (recipe follows) or shop-bought

2 tablespoons grated Pecorino Romano cheese

¼ teaspoon garlic powder

Preheat the oven to 220°C/200°C fan/Gas 7. Spray 2 large baking sheets with oil.

Cut each courgette into 16 sticks about 10cm long and about 1cm thick for a total of 64 sticks and put them on kitchen paper to blot excess moisture.

In a small bowl, season the egg whites with the salt and black pepper to taste and beat well. In a medium shallow bowl, combine the bread crumbs, Romano and garlic powder. Dip the courgette sticks into the egg whites and then into the bread crumbs, turning to coat well. Place the breaded courgette sticks in a single layer on the prepared baking sheets and spray the tops with more oil.

Bake until golden brown and tender in the centre, 23 to 25 minutes.

PERFECT PAIRINGS
Serve this with warm **Quickest Tomato Sauce (page 94)** on the side for dipping.

skinnyscoop

For best results, bread the courgettes in two batches so the crumbs don't clump up. Divide the bread crumbs in half. Bread the first two courgettes, then use the remaining crumbs to finish breading the last two.

(recipe continues)

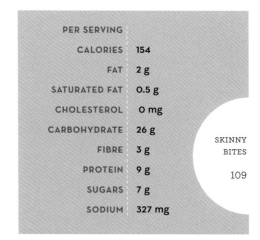

PER SERVING	
CALORIES	154
FAT	2 g
SATURATED FAT	0.5 g
CHOLESTEROL	0 mg
CARBOHYDRATE	26 g
FIBRE	3 g
PROTEIN	9 g
SUGARS	7 g
SODIUM	327 mg

SKINNY BITES

Seasoned Wholemeal Bread Crumbs

MAKES ABOUT 100G

My parents are pretty old-school. I grew up in a home where nothing went to waste. For instance, stale bread in the hands of my mother usually turned into bread crumbs. Any time I have unused wholemeal French bread sitting around (especially when I make sandwiches), I turn it into these delicious seasoned bread crumbs. Mom totally rubbed off on me!

skinny**scoop**

This works best with very stale bread that's a few days old. If your bread is only a day old and you want to make it right away, cut the bread into cubes and toast it in the oven at 150°C/130°C fan/Gas 2 for a few minutes to dry it out.

110g stale wholemeal French bread, cut into bite-size pieces

3 tablespoons grated Pecorino Romano cheese

1 teaspoon dried parsley

½ teaspoon Italian seasoning

½ teaspoon garlic powder

½ teaspoon onion powder

½ teaspoon sea salt

Put the bread pieces in a blender or food processor and pulse until they turn into crumbs.

Put the crumbs in a medium bowl and add the Romano, parsley, Italian seasoning, garlic powder, onion powder and salt. Store in an airtight container for up to 3 weeks and use in any recipe calling for seasoned bread crumbs.

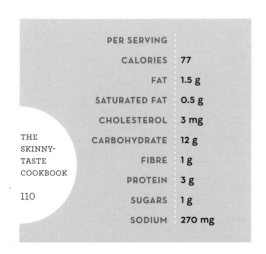

PER SERVING	
CALORIES	77
FAT	1.5 g
SATURATED FAT	0.5 g
CHOLESTEROL	3 mg
CARBOHYDRATE	12 g
FIBRE	1 g
PROTEIN	3 g
SUGARS	1 g
SODIUM	270 mg

Lemony Herb Hummus

SERVES 10

Hummus is a Middle Eastern dip made from chickpeas, tahini (sesame seed paste) and a lot of oil to make it smooth. I created a lighter version by using a lot less oil and adding white beans to help make it extra creamy. Another trick for making extra-smooth hummus: when using tinned chickpeas (or beans), bring them to a boil and blend them while they're warm. It helps soften the skin and produces a silkier texture, rather than the grainy texture you get with cold tinned chickpeas. Serve this with freshly cut vegetables or baked pitta chips.

1 (400g) tin chickpeas,* rinsed and drained

1 (400g) tin cannellini beans,* rinsed and drained

1 garlic clove, crushed

1 tablespoon tahini

Pinch of grated lemon zest

5 tablespoons fresh lemon juice

2 tablespoons chopped fresh parsley

1½ teaspoons sea salt

¼ teaspoon freshly ground black pepper, plus more for garnish

1 tablespoon extra-virgin olive oil

Pinch of paprika or ground cumin, for garnish

Sprig of fresh parsley, for garnish

Read the label to be sure this product is gluten-free.

Put the chickpeas and beans in a medium pot and add just enough water to cover. Set the pot over high heat and bring the mixture to a boil. Simmer about 1 minute, then drain the beans, reserving some of the water.

Transfer the chickpeas and beans and 2 to 3 tablespoons of the reserved water to a food processor. Pulse a few times.

In a medium bowl, combine the garlic, tahini, lemon zest, lemon juice, parsley, salt and black pepper. Add the mixture to the food processor and blitz until smooth and creamy, 5 to 7 minutes. If it's too thick, add more of the reserved water.

Transfer to a serving dish and smooth the top with the back of a spoon. Drizzle the olive oil over the top, sprinkle with black pepper and paprika and put the sprig of parsley on top.

skinnyscoop

This dish will stay refrigerated for up to 4 days. To serve, bring it back to room temperature.

PER SERVING	
CALORIES	131
FAT	3.5 g
SATURATED FAT	0.5 g
CHOLESTEROL	0 mg
CARBOHYDRATE	20 g
FIBRE	2 g
PROTEIN	6 g
SUGARS	0 g
SODIUM	277 mg

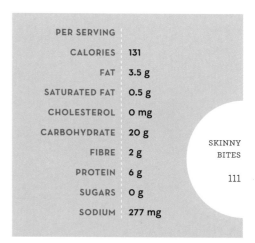

SKINNY BITES

111

Cheesy 'Fried' Mozzarella Bites

SERVES 12

These fun, tasty treats are great for kids and adults alike. I mean, who doesn't love 'fried' mozzarella? These bites are better for you than standard mozzarella sticks because they're made with low-fat cheese and are baked instead of fried. These actually need to be baked when they're completely frozen so they don't melt in the oven before they turn golden on the outside. For this reason, I like to prep them ahead of time and keep them ready in my freezer.

12 sticks reduced-salt light mozzarella cheese (250g)

1 large egg

2 tablespoons plain flour

5 tablespoons seasoned wholemeal bread crumbs, homemade (see page 110) or shop-bought

5 tablespoons panko bread crumbs

1 tablespoon grated Parmesan cheese

1 tablespoon dried parsley

Olive oil spray or oil mister

PERFECT PAIRINGS
Serve this with warm **Quickest Tomato Sauce** (page 94) for dipping.

Cut each piece of mozzarella into quarters, place the pieces on a baking sheet and freeze for at least 8 hours, or overnight.

In a small bowl, beat the egg. Put the flour in a second small bowl. In a third medium bowl, combine the seasoned bread crumbs, panko, Parmesan and parsley.

Line a baking sheet with greaseproof paper. Dip the frozen cheese into the flour, shaking off any excess, then into the egg, and lastly coat with the bread-crumb mixture. Put the breaded cheese on the baking sheet. Freeze the breaded cheese for at least 1 hour (this is a must or they will melt in the oven before browning).

Preheat the oven to 220°C/200°C fan/Gas 7. Lightly spray a baking sheet with olive oil.

Place the frozen cheese bites on the prepared baking sheet and lightly spray the tops with a little oil. Bake for 3 minutes, turn them over and bake until melted inside and golden on the outside, watching them closely so the cheese doesn't come out of the bread crumbs, about 2 minutes. Serve immediately as baked mozzarella hardens quicker than fried.

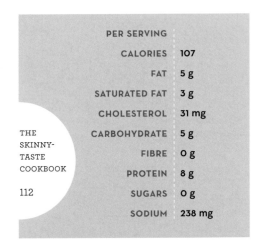

PER SERVING	
CALORIES	107
FAT	5 g
SATURATED FAT	3 g
CHOLESTEROL	31 mg
CARBOHYDRATE	5 g
FIBRE	0 g
PROTEIN	8 g
SUGARS	0 g
SODIUM	238 mg

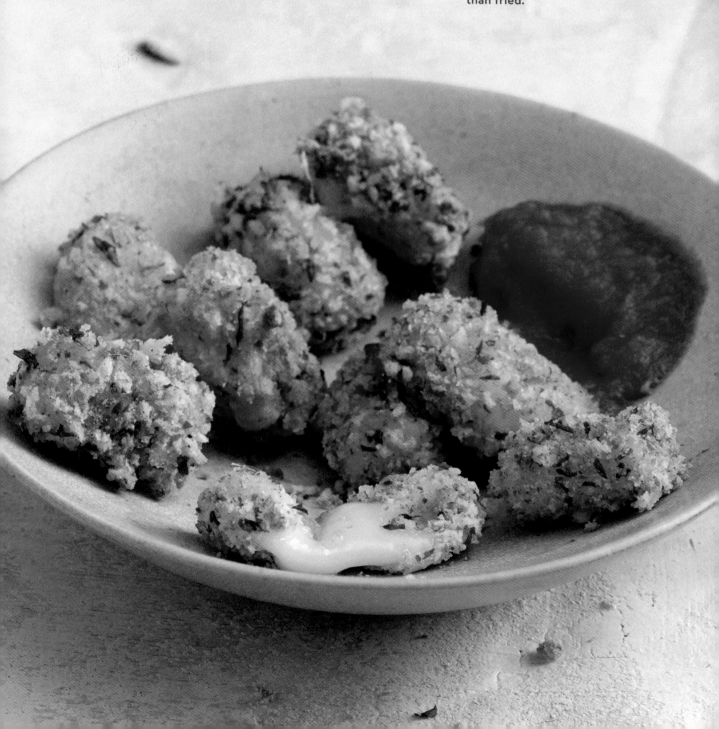

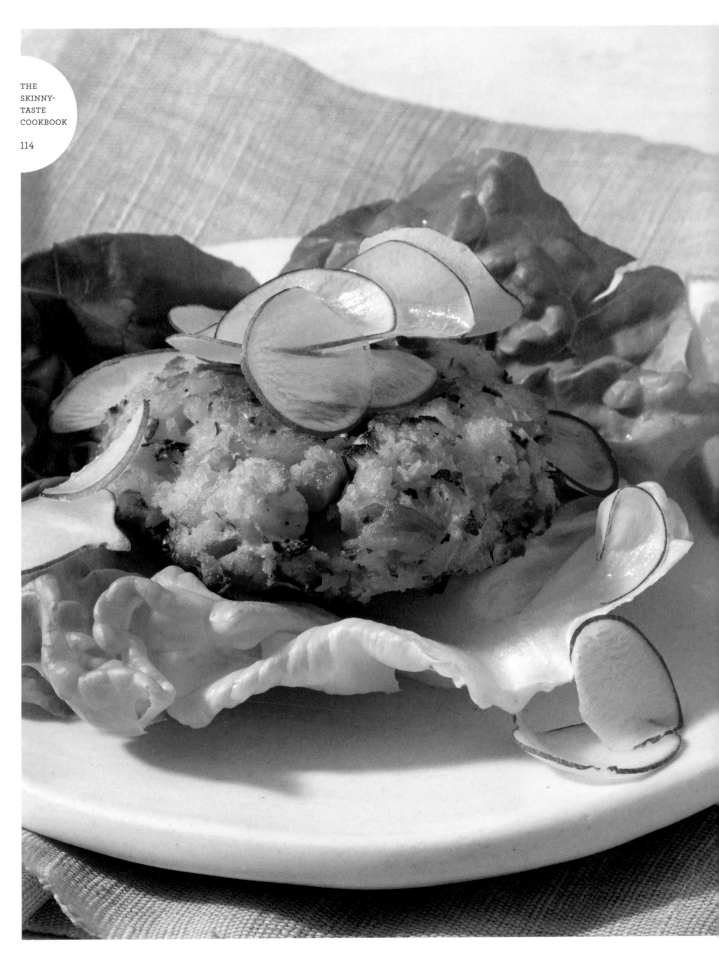

Petite Baked Crab Cakes

SERVES 8

Fresh crab is quite plentiful here on Long Island – you can get it just about everywhere. In the warmer months, you can even see people crabbing off the side of the road. I have access to some really great fresh seafood vendors, so I usually buy crabmeat from a trusted source. I've had great success with everything from snow crab to king crab legs, so use whatever is freshest for you. I don't, however, recommend using crab from a tin, as the taste and smell is a bit fishy and metallic, and the price is much the same as fresh. For a pretty presentation, serve the crab cakes on large leaves of lettuce, topped with thinly sliced radishes.

½ cup (30g) panko bread crumbs

1 large egg

1 large egg white

2 tablespoons finely chopped shallots

2 tablespoons finely chopped red pepper

1 tablespoon light mayonnaise

2 tablespoons finely chopped fresh parsley

1 tablespoon fresh lemon juice

A few dashes of Tabasco sauce

Sea salt

⅛ teaspoon freshly ground black pepper

250g crabmeat

Cooking spray or oil mister

8 small lemon wedges, for serving

In a large bowl, combine the panko, whole egg, egg white, shallots, pepper, mayonnaise, parsley, lemon juice, Tabasco, ¼ teaspoon plus ⅛ teaspoon salt and black pepper. Pick over the crabmeat to remove any bits of shell, then fold the meat into the panko mixture, being careful not to overmix. Gently shape into 8 round patties with your hands, about ¼ cup each. Refrigerate for at least 30 minutes before baking.

Preheat the oven to 220°C/200°C fan/Gas 7. Spray a nonstick baking sheet with oil and arrange the crab cakes on it. Bake until golden, turning once, 8 to 10 minutes on each side. Serve with lemon wedges for squeezing.

skinnyscoop

You can form the patties ahead of time and keep them refrigerated until you're ready to bake. These are perfect as a starter or as a main course for four if served with a large salad.

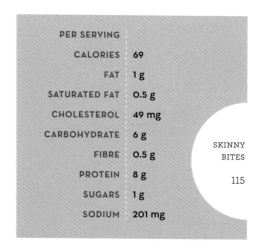

PER SERVING	
CALORIES	69
FAT	1 g
SATURATED FAT	0.5 g
CHOLESTEROL	49 mg
CARBOHYDRATE	6 g
FIBRE	0.5 g
PROTEIN	8 g
SUGARS	1 g
SODIUM	201 mg

SKINNY
BITES

115

Bangin' Good Shrimp

SERVES 4

I've never been to the Bonefish Grill, but fans begged me for a recipe makeover from the popular seafood chain restaurant. They would say things like, 'We order Bang Bang Shrimp *every time* we go, but it's really bad for you,' or 'Holy Cow! We love that shrimp. Please make it lighter,' and so on. Receiving *that* many e-mails, I took notice. The biggest problems with the original dish are that it's deep-fried and smothered in a fatty mayonnaise sauce. Once I made my skinny fixes, it became one of the most popular starters on my website. Whether you eat them as a starter or serve them over rice to make them a main dish, these shrimp are bangin' good!

5 tablespoons light mayonnaise (I prefer Hellmann's Light)

3 tablespoons Thai sweet chilli sauce

1 to 2 teaspoons Sriracha hot chilli sauce, or to taste

450g shelled and deveined large prawns

2 teaspoons cornflour

1 teaspoon rapeseed oil

3 cups (150g) shredded iceberg lettuce

1 cup (75g) shredded red cabbage

6 or 7 coriander leaves

¼ cup (15g) diagonally sliced spring onions

In a medium bowl, combine the mayonnaise, sweet chilli sauce and Sriracha.

Toss the prawns with the cornflour, mixing well with your hands. Heat a large nonstick frying pan or wok over high heat. Add the oil and prawns and cook through, stirring, about 3 minutes. Transfer the prawns to the bowl of sauce and toss well.

In a large bowl, combine the lettuce, cabbage and coriander and divide among 4 plates. Divide the prawns among the plates; garnish with the spring onions and serve immediately.

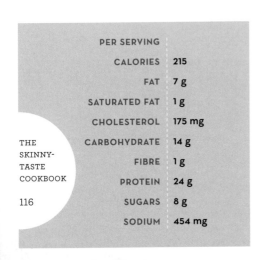

PER SERVING	
CALORIES	215
FAT	7 g
SATURATED FAT	1 g
CHOLESTEROL	175 mg
CARBOHYDRATE	14 g
FIBRE	1 g
PROTEIN	24 g
SUGARS	8 g
SODIUM	454 mg

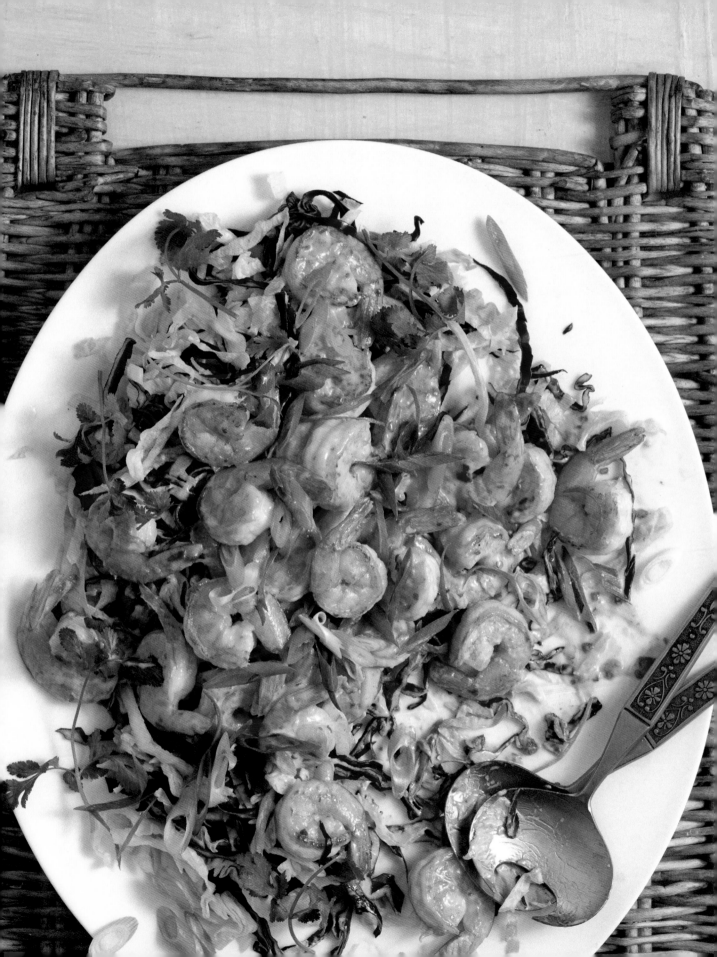

Less-Guilt Zesty Mango Guacamole

SERVES 8

My avocado obsession is so strong that I created an entire Pinterest board devoted to it. I love their taste and texture, but I also love how nutrient-rich avocados are: they're loaded with healthy fats, fibre, vitamins and potassium. Adding mango to guacamole is brilliant; it adds a touch of sweetness which complements the savoury flavours of the dip, and it gives more volume to the dish without adding any fat or a lot of calories.

2 medium (225g) avocados, chopped

2 large mangoes, chopped

1 small jalapeño or other green chilli, finely chopped (include the seeds if you want it spicy)

¼ cup (40g) chopped red onion

2 tablespoons chopped fresh coriander

2½ tablespoons fresh lime juice

¼ teaspoon sea salt

⅛ teaspoon freshly ground black pepper

Place the avocados in a medium bowl and mash with a fork, leaving some large chunks. Add the mango, jalapeño, onion, coriander, lime juice, salt and black pepper.

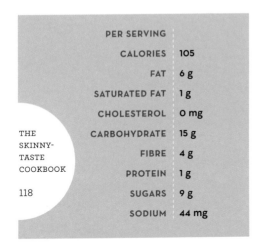

PER SERVING	
CALORIES	105
FAT	6 g
SATURATED FAT	1 g
CHOLESTEROL	0 mg
CARBOHYDRATE	15 g
FIBRE	4 g
PROTEIN	1 g
SUGARS	9 g
SODIUM	44 mg

Skinny Green Goddess Dip

SERVES 5

This recipe is the perfect excuse to round up fresh herbs from the garden and make the most of them. I lightened it up by using Greek yoghurt (in place of mayo) and some creamy mashed avocado, which adds healthy fat, makes it greener and gives it a great texture. I've tried this with many different herbs, but as a basil lover I like to use a big bunch of the summery ingredient. It tastes even better the next day, so it's great to make a day in advance.

½ cup (125g) fat-free Greek yoghurt

¼ cup (60g) light mayonnaise (I prefer Hellmann's Light)

¼ cup (60g) mashed avocado

½ cup packed (30g) chopped fresh basil

¼ cup (15g) chopped fresh chives

¼ cup (15g) chopped fresh parsley

2 anchovy fillets, rinsed and patted dry

1 garlic clove, chopped

1 tablespoon fresh lemon juice

⅛ teaspoon sea salt

Freshly ground black pepper

In a blender, combine the yoghurt, mayonnaise, avocado, basil, chives, parsley, anchovy, garlic, lemon juice, salt and pepper to taste. Process until smooth, then transfer the dip to a bowl. Keep refrigerated, covered, until ready to serve. This can be made up to a day in advance.

PERFECT PAIRING
Serve this dip with crisp, colourful vegetables cut into strips. I love using peppers (yellow, orange and red), cucumbers, baby carrots, sugar snap peas and courgettes. You can even include some jumbo cooked prawns.

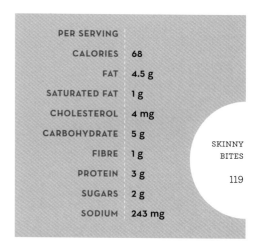

PER SERVING	
CALORIES	68
FAT	4.5 g
SATURATED FAT	1 g
CHOLESTEROL	4 mg
CARBOHYDRATE	5 g
FIBRE	1 g
PROTEIN	3 g
SUGARS	2 g
SODIUM	243 mg

Garden Pico de Gallo

SERVES 8

Pico de gallo is a bright, fresh salsa made from diced tomatoes, onions, cucumbers, jalapeños, coriander and lime juice. It's perfect served as a starter with baked chips, but I also love it as a condiment over tacos, tostadas, grilled meats and salads. In the spring, I plant tomatoes, peppers, jalapeños and fresh herbs, so that I can use them throughout the summer. This quick, fresh salsa is one way to make use of those tasty vegetables.

4 medium tomatoes, chopped

⅓ cup (40g) chopped jalapeño or other green chillies (about 2)

⅓ cup (60g) chopped cucumber

¼ cup (40g) chopped white onion

¼ cup (7g) finely chopped fresh coriander leaves

1 garlic clove, crushed

2 tablespoons fresh lime juice

¾ teaspoon sea salt

⅛ teaspoon freshly ground black pepper

In a large bowl, combine the tomatoes, jalapeños, cucumber, onion, coriander, garlic, lime juice, salt and black pepper. Let the salsa marinate in the refrigerator for at least 1 hour before eating.

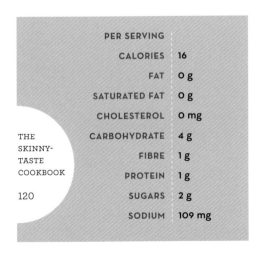

PER SERVING	
CALORIES	16
FAT	0 g
SATURATED FAT	0 g
CHOLESTEROL	0 mg
CARBOHYDRATE	4 g
FIBRE	1 g
PROTEIN	1 g
SUGARS	2 g
SODIUM	109 mg

Crave-Worthy Snacks

Slimming snacks don't have to taste like cardboard, and they shouldn't be loaded with processed junk! My real food snacks clock in at 150 calories or less and are easy to assemble at home or at the office – no cooking (or cardboard crackers) required.

- **PARMESAN POPCORN**
  2 cups (15g) air-popped popcorn topped with 2 tablespoons grated Parmesan (110 calories)

- **HARD-BOILED EGG & CHIVES**
  1 large hard-boiled egg with snipped chives and a pinch of salt (80 calories)

- **HUMMUS & VEGGIES**
  ¼ cup (25g) sugar snap peas and ¼ cup (65g) baby carrots dipped in ¼ cup Lemony Herb Hummus (page 111) (150 calories)

- **APPLES & CHEDDAR**
  ½ sliced apple with 25g cheddar (150 calories)

- **PEARS & BLUE**
  ½ sliced pear with 25g blue cheese (150 calories)

- **GRAPES & GRUYERE**
  ½ cup (90g) grapes with 25g Gruyère cheese (150 calories)

- **CHIPS & GUAC**
  10 baked tortilla chips and ½ cup (90g) red pepper strips dipped in ¼ cup Less-Guilt Zesty Mango Guacamole (page 118) (130 calories)

- **NUTTY BANANA**
  Spread 1 medium banana with ½ tablespoon almond butter (150 calories)

- **CHERRIES & PISTACHIOS**
  1 cup (140g) cherries mixed with 1 tablespoon shelled pistachios (130 calories)

- **ALMOND BUTTER & APPLE**
  ½ tablespoon almond butter spread on 1 apple, sliced (120 calories)

- **BANANA ICE CREAM**
  Freeze 1 large ripe banana and purée in a food processor until smooth (120 calories)

- **CREAMY BERRIES**
  170g fat-free Greek yoghurt topped with 1 cup (220g) berries (150 calories)

- **SKINNY DIP**
  ¼ cup Skinny Green Goddess Dip (page 119) with 1 cup (60g) broccoli florets and 1 cup (250g) baby carrots (140 calories)

- **FRESH FRUIT & NUTS**
  1 medium-size fruit (apple, pear, peach, orange, banana, etc.) with 1 tablespoon unsalted nuts (130 calories)

- **FETA & WATERMELON**
  2 cups (300g) cubed watermelon with 1 tablespoon crumbled feta cheese and 1 tablespoon chopped mint (120 calories)

- **GREEK TREAT**
  170g fat-free Greek yoghurt mixed with 1 tablespoon shaved dark chocolate and ½ tablespoon raspberry jam (140 calories)

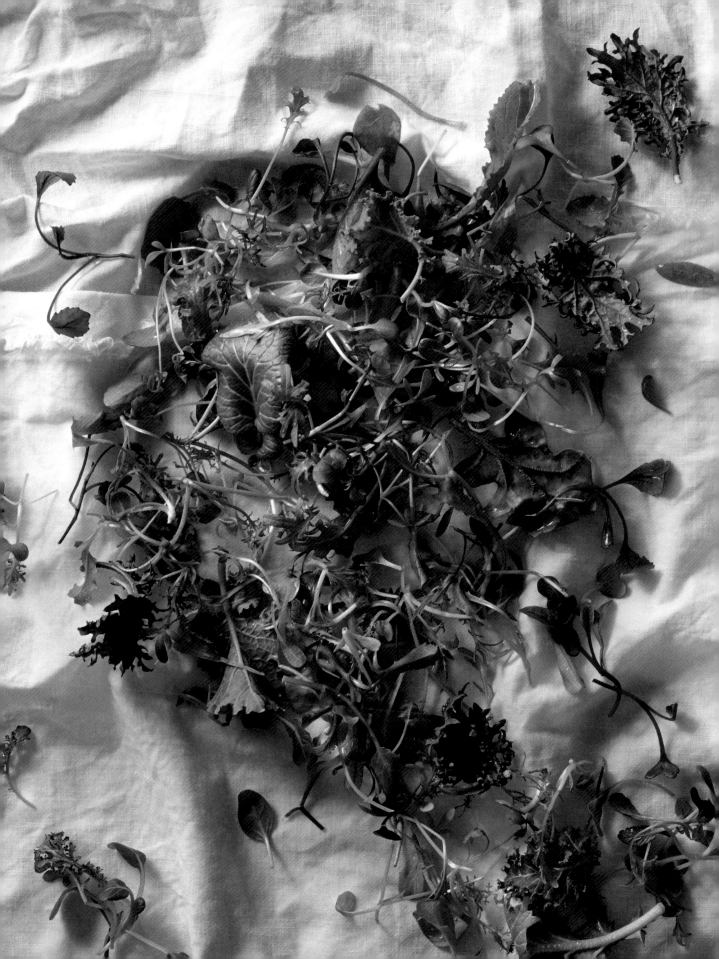

FABULOUS MAIN-DISH SALADS

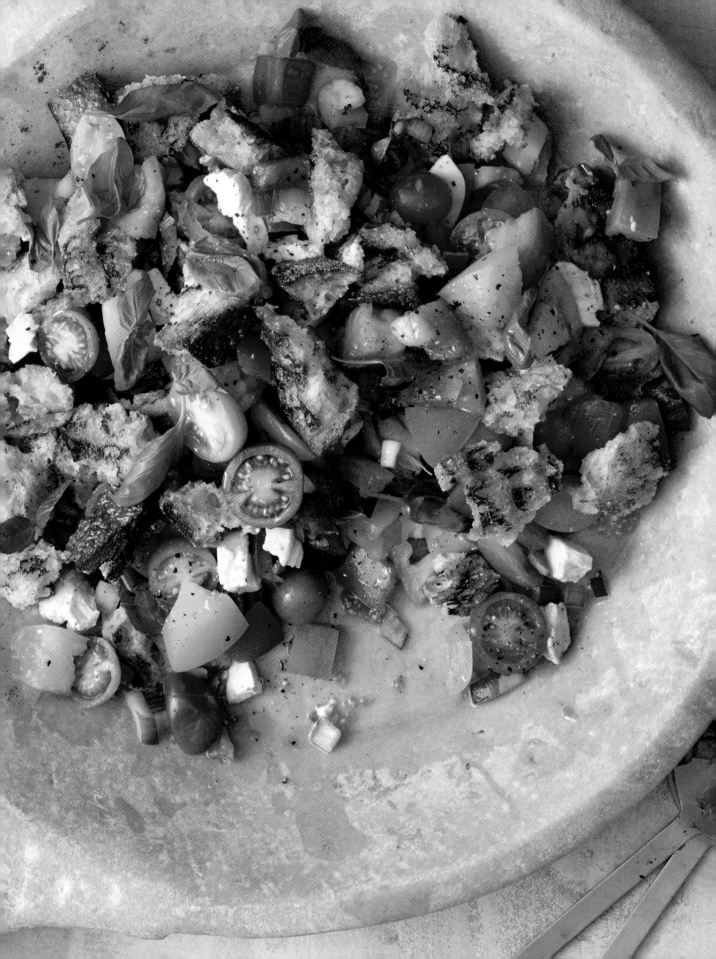

Tuscan Panzanella Salad with Grilled Garlic Bread

SERVES 4

My husband, who's half-Italian, makes this simple salad by combining just a few quality ingredients. But here's the secret: before adding the bread, he lets the other flavours marinate for 30 minutes at room temperature. It makes quite a difference! The bread is important, too. You'll want to look for a rustic loaf with a crunchy crust. Wholemeal bread would also be great for a whole-grain option.

8 cups (1.6kg) vine-ripened tomatoes, cut into 2 to 3cm cubes

½ cup (80g) chopped red onion

8 to 10 basil leaves, cut into thin strips (chiffonade)

1 tablespoon extra-virgin olive oil

1½ teaspoons sea salt, plus more as needed

Freshly ground black pepper

Olive oil spray or oil mister

170g artisanal bread, cut into 1cm slices

1 garlic clove, halved

110g fresh mozzarella, cut into 5mm cubes

In a large bowl, combine the tomatoes, onion, basil, olive oil and salt, and season with a few turns of freshly ground black pepper. Allow to sit at room temperature until the flavours have blended (the juices from the tomatoes will release and create a kind of dressing), 20 to 25 minutes.

Meanwhile, preheat a grill to medium.

Lightly spray each bread slice with olive oil and season with a pinch of salt. Grill the slices until slightly toasted and golden brown on each side, about 1 minute per side. Remove from the heat and rub the toasted bread all over with the garlic. Cut the bread into 1cm cubes and set aside.

When ready to serve, toss the tomato mixture with the mozzarella and grilled bread and divide among 4 bowls. Eat immediately so the bread doesn't get soggy.

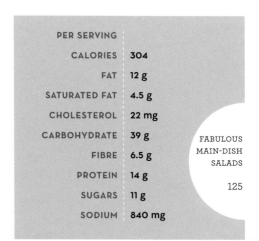

PER SERVING	
CALORIES	304
FAT	12 g
SATURATED FAT	4.5 g
CHOLESTEROL	22 mg
CARBOHYDRATE	39 g
FIBRE	6.5 g
PROTEIN	14 g
SUGARS	11 g
SODIUM	840 mg

FABULOUS MAIN-DISH SALADS

Coconut Chicken Salad with Warm Honey-Mustard Vinaigrette

SERVES 4

I created this recipe a few years back after someone requested a makeover for a fatty deep-fried version they had on vacation. Call me loco for coco, because I love all things coconut. I happily got busy in my kitchen and played around with a faux-fried crispy coating for my chicken that is oven-baked at a high temperature to make you feel like you're eating fried.

VINAIGRETTE

1 tablespoon Dijon mustard

4 teaspoons extra-virgin olive oil

4 teaspoons honey

4 teaspoons white vinegar

CHICKEN

Olive oil spray or oil mister

½ cup (30g) sweetened desiccated coconut

⅓ cup (20g) panko bread crumbs

3 tablespoons crushed cornflake crumbs

¼ teaspoon sea salt, plus more as needed

3 large egg whites

8 chicken mini fillets (about 450g total)

SALAD

8 cups (600g) mixed salad leaves

1 cup (155g) grated carrots

1 large vine-ripened tomato, thinly sliced

1 medium cucumber, sliced

For the vinaigrette: In a medium bowl, whisk together the mustard, oil, honey, vinegar and 2 teaspoons water. Set aside.

For the chicken: Preheat the oven to 190°C/170°C fan/Gas 5. Spray a large nonstick baking sheet with olive oil.

In a medium bowl, combine the coconut, panko, cornflake crumbs and a pinch of salt. In a second medium bowl, beat the egg whites.

Season the chicken with the remaining salt. Dip the chicken in the egg whites, then in the coconut-crumb mixture. Place the chicken on the prepared baking sheet. Lightly spray the top of the chicken with olive oil.

(recipe continues)

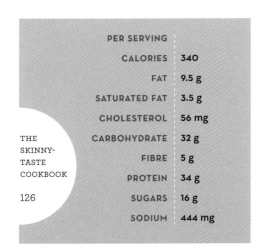

PER SERVING	
CALORIES	340
FAT	9.5 g
SATURATED FAT	3.5 g
CHOLESTEROL	56 mg
CARBOHYDRATE	32 g
FIBRE	5 g
PROTEIN	34 g
SUGARS	16 g
SODIUM	444 mg

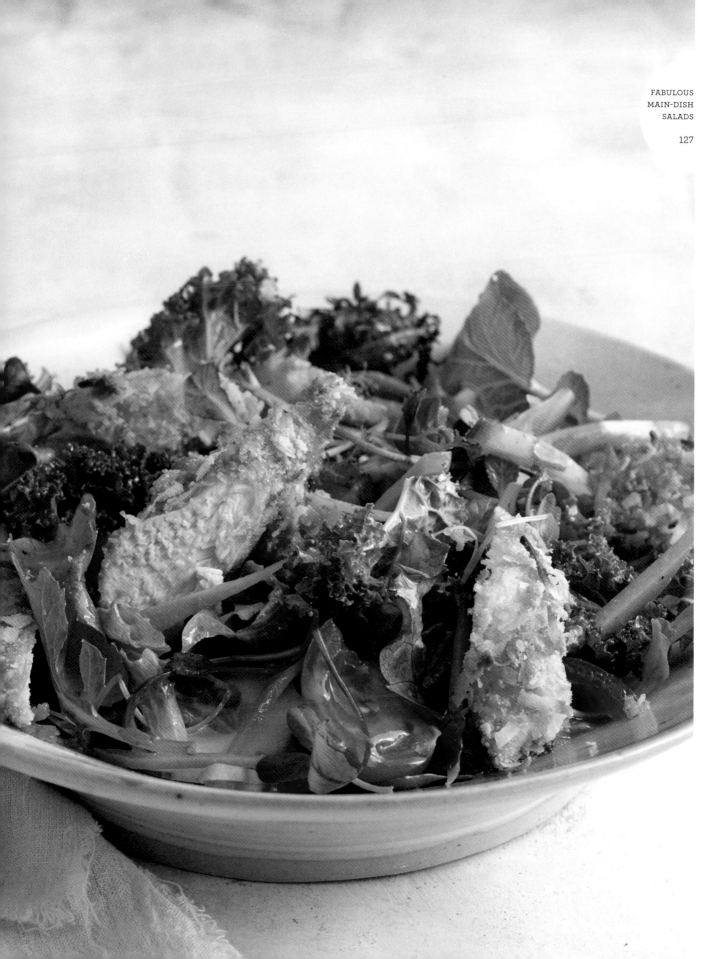

Bake for 15 minutes, flip and cook until the chicken is cooked through, 15 more minutes.

For the salad: Place a quarter of the salad leaves on each of 4 plates. Divide the carrots, tomato slices and cucumber slices among the plates. Slice the chicken at an angle and place on top of the greens. Heat the dressing in the microwave for a few seconds and divide it among the salads.

8 Heart-Healthy Oils

Ready to give your salads and dishes a health and flavour boost? This handy primer will tell you everything you need to know about the eight healthiest oils on the shelf.

AVOCADO OIL Just like the fruit it's made from, avocado oil is rich in monounsaturated fat and antioxidants, which research suggests helps counter some of the effects of damaging free radicals that can cause diabetes and other diseases.

RAPESEED OIL Rapeseed oil is the lowest in saturated fat of all common cooking oils, and it's rich in heart-healthy omega-3s and vitamin E, an antioxidant that protects your cells from damage and plays a role in immune function.

FLAXSEED (LINSEED) OIL A delicate oil with a low smoke point, flaxseed oil is a great source of omega-3 alpha-linolenic acid (ALA). ALA appears to have anti-inflammatory properties and may also help lower blood pressure. Since flaxseed oil doesn't hold up in heat, use it in cold dishes like pesto and salads.

GRAPESEED OIL A by-product of wine-making, this oil is high in polyunsaturated fats – which can help improve cholesterol levels and reduce your risk of heart disease – as well as vitamin E.

OLIVE OIL Olive oil has earned superfood status, as it's one of the foods credited for the many health benefits associated with the Mediterranean diet. Its makeup consists mostly of monounsaturated fats, which may help lower the risk of heart disease, normalize blood clotting and aid in blood sugar control. Extra-virgin and virgin olive oils have more antioxidants than refined olive oils.

SESAME OIL (LIGHT AND DARK) Herbalists often use sesame oil for its anti-cancer, antibacterial and anti-inflammatory properties. Dark sesame oil has a uniquely strong, nutty flavour and should be used sparingly because a little goes a long way.

SUNFLOWER OIL Sunflower oil has more of the antioxidant vitamin E in one tablespoon than any of the other common cooking oils.

WALNUT OIL Walnut oil may reduce the risk of cardiovascular disease by improving blood vessel function, which is especially helpful for people with cardiovascular disease. Walnut oil has a strong flavour, so it's meant to be used on finished dishes.

Buffalo Chicken Salad

SERVES 4

When I was in my late teens and early twenties, I loved going out to dinner with the girls to order strictly off the starters menu. We'd share all kinds of typical American starters, like Buffalo wings, complete with celery and blue cheese dressing. I don't think I realized – or cared – just how fattening those deep-fried wings smothered in butter actually were. Now, after having children and my metabolism has slowed a bit, I skip the fattening wings in favour of this salad, which has everything I love about Buffalo wings, but in a healthy form.

SKINNY BLUE CHEESE DRESSING

½ cup (60g) crumbled blue cheese

140g fat-free Greek yoghurt

2 tablespoons buttermilk

1 tablespoon light mayonnaise (I prefer Hellmann's Light)

1 tablespoon white balsamic vinegar

½ tablespoon fresh lemon juice

½ teaspoon dried parsley

⅛ teaspoon garlic powder

⅛ teaspoon sea salt

Freshly ground black pepper

CHICKEN

450g chicken mini fillets

½ teaspoon chilli powder*

½ teaspoon garlic powder

⅛ teaspoon freshly ground black pepper

Cooking spray or oil mister

⅓ cup (85ml) cayenne hot sauce

SALAD

1 medium red leaf lettuce

1 cucumber, sliced 5mm thick and halved

1 cup (155g) grated carrots

2 medium celery stalks, sliced 5mm thick (½ cup)

1 medium tomato, chopped

¼ cup (30g) crumbled blue cheese

Read the label to be sure this product is gluten-free.

For the skinny blue cheese dressing: In a small bowl, mash the blue cheese and yoghurt together with a fork. Stir in the buttermilk, mayonnaise, vinegar, lemon juice, dried parsley and garlic powder. Season with the salt and a pinch of black pepper.

For the chicken: Season the chicken with the chilli powder, garlic powder and black pepper.

(recipe continues)

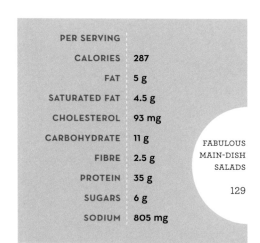

PER SERVING	
CALORIES	287
FAT	5 g
SATURATED FAT	4.5 g
CHOLESTEROL	93 mg
CARBOHYDRATE	11 g
FIBRE	2.5 g
PROTEIN	35 g
SUGARS	6 g
SODIUM	805 mg

FABULOUS MAIN-DISH SALADS

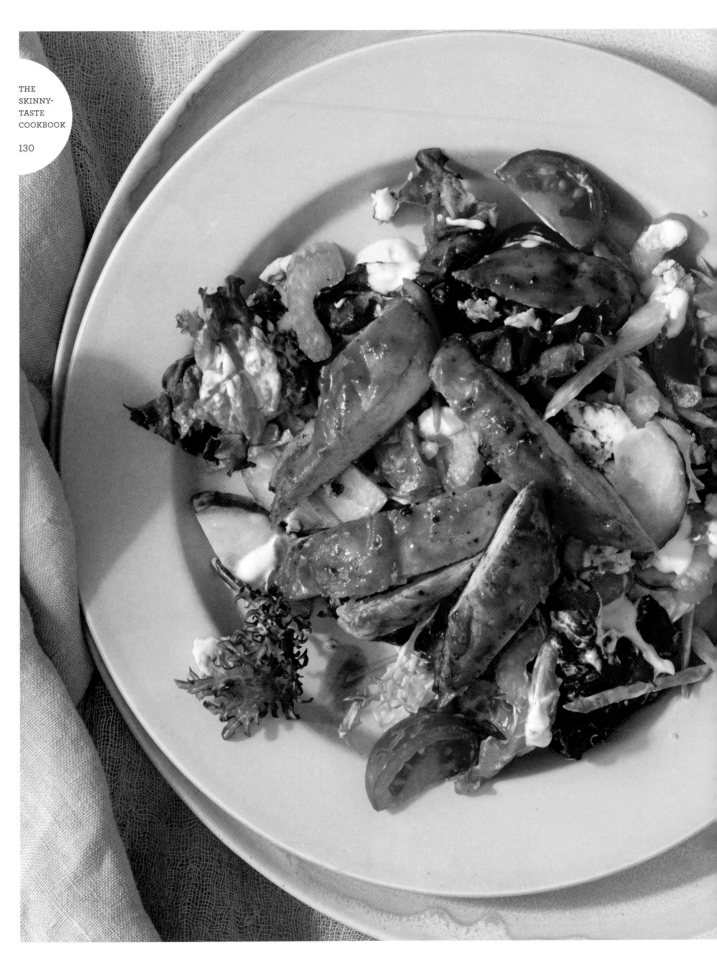

Heat a large nonstick frying pan over high heat. Spray the pan with oil. Add the chicken and cook until browned on each side and no longer pink, 6 to 8 minutes. Remove the pan from the heat and pour the hot sauce over the chicken, turning to coat well. Slice on an angle and set aside.

For the salad: Tear the lettuce into bite-size pieces. Put it into a large bowl with half the dressing and toss. Divide the lettuce among 4 plates. Top with the cucumbers, carrots, celery and tomatoes, and drizzle the remaining dressing on top. Top the salad with the sliced chicken and sprinkle with the blue cheese crumbs.

FOOD FACTS **heating things up**

Adding a little spice to your foods may help you eat less. Capsaicin, the component that gives chillies their kick, has been shown to rev metabolism and increase body temperature, both of which can help burn more calories. Research also suggests that it helps quell appetite, cut cravings and reduce the number of calories consumed at a meal. However, many of these benefits were seen in people who don't normally consume capsaicin – so if you normally like it hot, you may not reap all these chilli perks.

skinny**scoop**

Leftover buttermilk? Freeze it! Then thaw it overnight in the refrigerator or defrost it in the microwave. Freezing may cause the milk to separate. Before using in your recipe, be sure to mix it well to reincorporate.

Curried Chicken Salad

SERVES 5

The first time I made this chicken salad, I dreamed about it for the next few days. It's spicy, savoury and sweet, and has lots of great texture. The best part is that it's made with fat-free Greek yoghurt instead of mayonnaise, so there's no guilt! And it's even better the next day, so it's perfect to make ahead for lunch during the week.

2 teaspoons olive oil

¼ cup (40g) chopped onion

½ tablespoon curry powder*

450g boneless, skinless chicken breasts, cut into 1cm cubes

¼ teaspoon sea salt

Freshly ground black pepper

2 tablespoons fat-free Greek yoghurt

¼ teaspoon ground cinnamon

¾ cup (90g) dried cranberries*

1 large sweet apple, peeled and finely chopped

¼ cup (30g) slivered or flaked almonds

2 tablespoons chopped fresh coriander

¼ cup (15g) sliced spring onions

PERFECT PAIRINGS
I like to serve this chicken salad cold on a large romaine lettuce leaf, which adds a nice amount of crunch and stands in for bread. You can also serve it over a bed of salad leaves or in a wholemeal wrap.

Read the label to be sure this product is gluten-free.

In a large, heavy nonstick frying pan, heat the olive oil over medium heat. Add the onion and curry powder and cook, stirring, until golden, 3 to 4 minutes. Increase the heat to medium-high, add the chicken, salt and a pinch of black pepper and cook, stirring frequently, until just cooked through, about 5 minutes. Transfer the chicken to a large bowl and let cool.

When cool, add the yoghurt, cinnamon, cranberries, apple, almonds, coriander and spring onions. Toss together to coat.

PER SERVING	
CALORIES	233
FAT	7 g
SATURATED FAT	1 g
CHOLESTEROL	58 mg
CARBOHYDRATE	22 g
FIBRE	2.5 g
PROTEIN	21 g
SUGARS	16 g
SODIUM	168 mg

Wild Salmon Salad with Balsamic-Caper Vinaigrette

SERVES 4

Wild salmon, green beans, capers and salad leaves topped with shaved Parmesan and balsamic vinegar – it's a heart-healthy salad loaded with mega omegas! I try to eat salmon at least once a week, and if there are any leftovers from the night before, this is usually what's for lunch the next day! When I worked full-time in the city, this was one of my favourite go-to lunches. I would pack the shaved Parmesan cheese and dressing on the side and anxiously await lunchtime.

BALSAMIC-CAPER VINAIGRETTE

8 teaspoons balsamic vinegar

4 teaspoons extra-virgin olive oil

⅛ teaspoon sea salt

Freshly ground black pepper

4 teaspoons capers, drained

SALAD

¾ teaspoon sea salt

225g green beans, trimmed and halved

450g skin-on wild salmon fillet, cut into 4 pieces

Freshly ground black pepper

Cooking spray or oil mister

6 cups (180g) mixed watercress, rocket and spinach

¼ cup (25g) shaved Parmesan cheese

For the balsamic-caper vinaigrette: In a small bowl, whisk together the vinegar and oil. Season with the salt and a pinch of black pepper. Toss in the capers and set aside.

For the salad: Bring a medium pot of water with ½ teaspoon of the salt to a boil. Add the green beans and cook until crisp-tender, 8 to 10 minutes. Drain and run under cold water to stop the cooking. Drain again and set aside.

Heat a frying pan or griddle over high heat. Season the salmon with the remaining ¼ teaspoon salt and a pinch of black pepper, lightly spray the pan with oil and put the salmon in the pan. Sauté until cooked through, about 5 minutes on each side. Transfer to a plate and remove the skin.

Place a quarter of the salad leaves on each of 4 plates. Divide the green beans among the plates, sprinkle with the Parmesan and put a piece of salmon on top. Drizzle the dressing over the top of each salad.

skinny**scoop**

If you're pressed for time, you can use tinned salmon or even tuna in place of the wild salmon.

PER SERVING	
CALORIES	262
FAT	13.5 g
SATURATED FAT	2.5 g
CHOLESTEROL	62 mg
CARBOHYDRATE	9 g
FIBRE	3.5 g
PROTEIN	27 g
SUGARS	3 g
SODIUM	305 mg

FABULOUS MAIN-DISH SALADS

133

BLT Salad with Avocado

SERVES 4

I have a confession: I LOVE bacon. (Really, who doesn't?) I find a way to work bacon into my life whenever a craving strikes. This salad is the answer to my BLT-loving prayers, with all the best flavours of the sandwich and none of the added calories of the bread. When I bring home the bacon (pun intended!), I always look for centre-cut or back bacon – it's leaner than streaky bacon.

12 slices lean centre-cut or back bacon, at room temperature

4 vine-ripened tomatoes, chopped

¼ cup (60g) light mayonnaise (I prefer Hellmann's Light)

⅛ teaspoon sea salt

Freshly ground black pepper

6 cups (300g) chopped romaine lettuce

1 medium (110g) avocado, chopped

PERFECT PAIRINGS
This salad is perfect as is for lunch, but if you want to make this a light dinner, toss in 170g of chopped grilled chicken (250 calories).

Put the bacon in a large frying pan and set the pan over low heat. Cook the bacon, turning often, until crisp. Transfer to kitchen paper to drain and cool. Crumble the bacon.

In a medium bowl, combine the tomatoes and mayonnaise and season with the salt and a pinch of black pepper. Set aside for about 10 minutes to let the tomatoes release their juices as this will be the 'dressing' to your salad.

To serve, place a quarter of the lettuce on each plate, then top each with about a quarter of the tomato mixture. Top with the avocado and bacon.

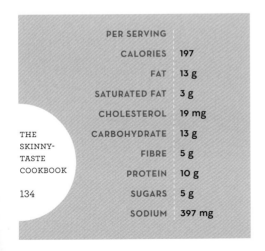

PER SERVING	
CALORIES	197
FAT	13 g
SATURATED FAT	3 g
CHOLESTEROL	19 mg
CARBOHYDRATE	13 g
FIBRE	5 g
PROTEIN	10 g
SUGARS	5 g
SODIUM	397 mg

THE
SKINNY-
TASTE
COOKBOOK

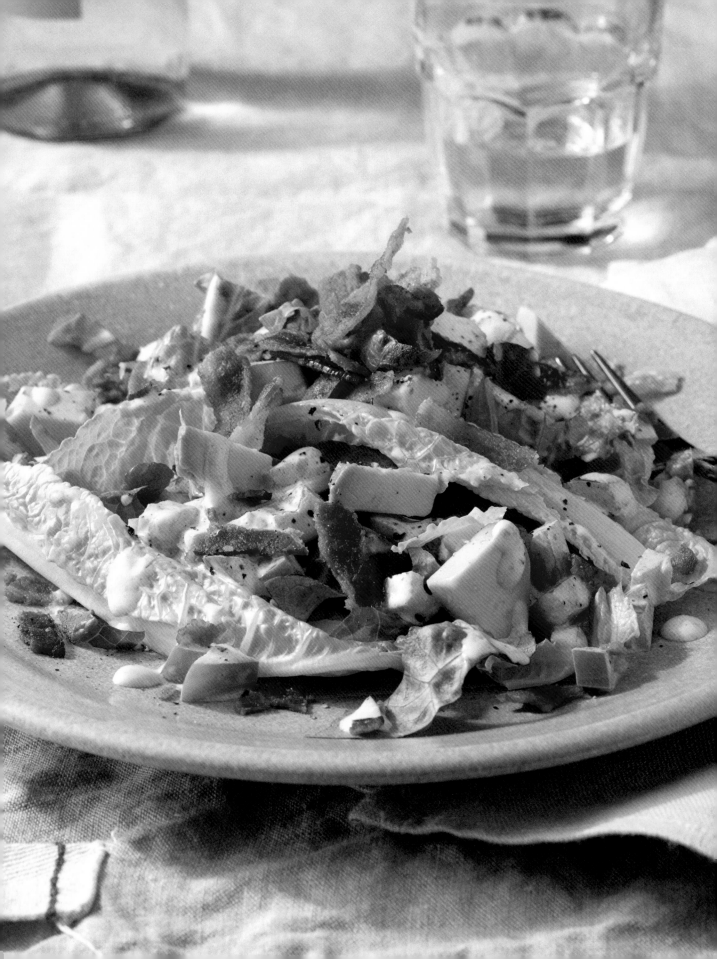

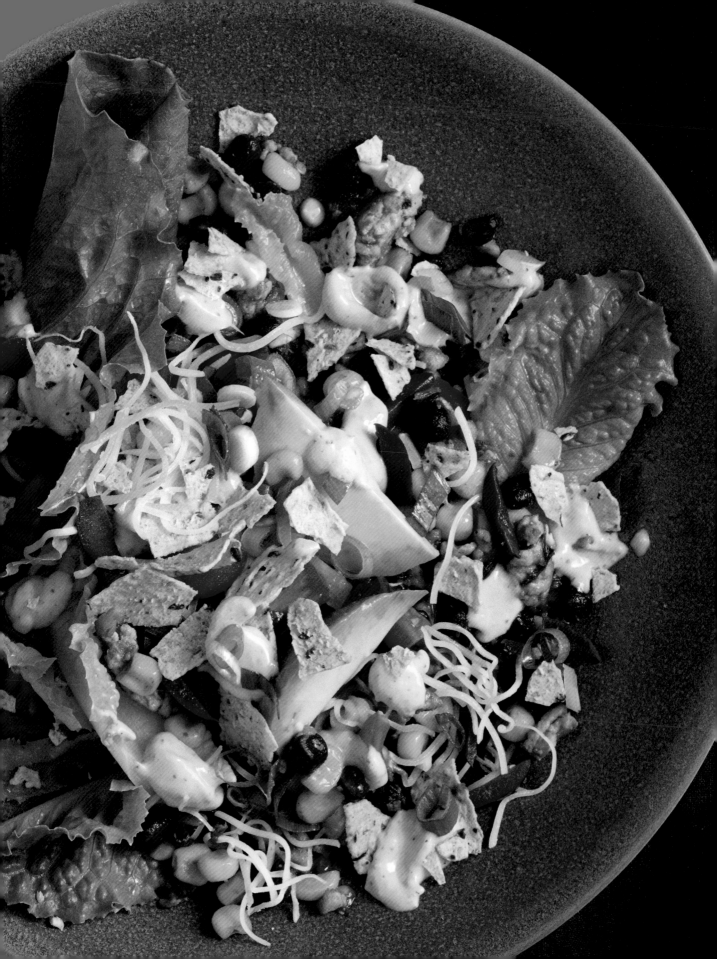

Turkey Santa Fe Taco Salad with Avocado Crema

SERVES 4

Each bite of this salad is a fiesta in your mouth! Colour, crunch, flavour and spice – this is the whole package. But in my opinion, what really makes it fresh and new is the zesty avocado crema. Not to mention, this satisfying dish is loaded with fibre and protein. The turkey-bean topping is so good that I usually double it and use the extras as a filling the next day for stuffed peppers, enchiladas or even mixed in with some scrambled egg whites – delish!

TURKEY-BEAN TOPPING

225g turkey breast mince

½ teaspoon sea salt

½ cup (115g) tinned black beans,* rinsed and drained

2 tablespoons chopped pickled jalapeño pepper (or more to taste)

1 large tomato, chopped

1 garlic clove, crushed

3 tablespoons chopped onion

2 tablespoons chopped fresh coriander, plus more for garnish

1¼ teaspoons ground cumin

¾ cup (110g) frozen sweetcorn kernels

AVOCADO CREMA

1 medium (110g) avocado, chopped

¼ cup (60g) light soured cream

1 tablespoon fresh lime juice

1 medium jalapeño or other green chilli, chopped

1½ tablespoons chopped fresh coriander

¼ teaspoon plus ⅛ teaspoon sea salt

Freshly ground black pepper

SALAD

5 cups (250g) shredded green leaf lettuce

½ cup (60g) grated reduced-fat Mexican cheese blend†

1 cup (200g) chopped tomatoes

2 tablespoons sliced black olives

2 tablespoons chopped spring onions

25g baked tortilla chips, crushed

Read the label to be sure this product is gluten-free.

For the turkey-bean topping: Heat a large frying pan over medium-high heat. Add the turkey, season with ¼ teaspoon salt and cook, using a wooden spoon to break the meat into small pieces, until no longer pink, 4 to 5 minutes. Add the beans, pickled jalapeño, tomato, garlic, onion, coriander and cumin. Stir well, reduce the heat to low, cover and cook for 20 minutes to blend the flavours. Uncover and add the sweetcorn

(recipe continues)

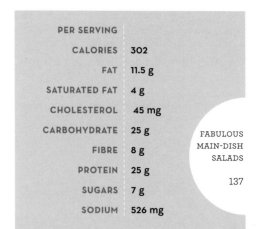

PER SERVING	
CALORIES	302
FAT	11.5 g
SATURATED FAT	4 g
CHOLESTEROL	45 mg
CARBOHYDRATE	25 g
FIBRE	8 g
PROTEIN	25 g
SUGARS	7 g
SODIUM	526 mg

FABULOUS MAIN-DISH SALADS

and ¼ teaspoon salt. Simmer until the liquid reduces and the sweetcorn is cooked through, 5 more minutes.

For the avocado crema: In a blender, combine half the avocado (reserve the other half for the salad), the soured cream, lime juice, ¼ cup (50ml) water, the jalapeño, coriander, salt and black pepper to taste. Blend until smooth.

For the salad: Divide the lettuce among 4 plates. Add the turkey-bean topping, cheese, tomatoes, olives, spring onions and remaining avocado. Top with the avocado crema and crushed tortilla chips.

† If you can't find Mexican cheese, lighter cheddar will work well.

The Salad Solution

Want to add more vegetables and vitamins into your day? There's a simple solution: eat more salads! Here are a few tips to keep in mind:

GO GREEN The darker the leaf, the more phytonutrients it contains. That means spinach greens are more antioxidant-packed than romaine lettuce, which is more nutritious than iceberg lettuce. Don't be afraid to try new greens or go for a mix of different leaves.

BE COLOURFUL Phytochemicals, the beneficial nutrients in plants that offer a variety of health benefits, are what give plants their colour, and each colour represents a different health benefit. To make sure you're covering your bases, opt for a colourful spread in your salad bowl.

EAT SEASONALLY Eating what's in season offers a number of perks. In-season fruits and veggies are usually tastier because they're fresher. They can also be cheaper because they don't have to travel great distances to get to your plate.

PICK YOUR PROTEIN Make your salad more satisfying by topping it with some lean protein, which is shown to be more satiating than fat or carbs. Some healthy picks to consider: tofu, edamame, chicken, fish, egg whites and beans.

ADD SOME CRUNCH Satisfy your senses by sprinkling on nuts or seeds; slicing up some sweet apples or pears; or going with radishes, peppers or water chestnuts.

GET YOUR HEALTHY FAT FIX Fat not only makes a salad more satisfying, it can also help boost your absorption of certain nutrients. Good sources of healthy fat include avocados, olive oil, nuts and seeds, and fatty fish like salmon.

GO FOR WHOLE GRAINS Get an extra hit of fibre and B vitamins by topping your salad with grains like quinoa, farro, barley or couscous.

Baja Grilled Flank Steak Salad

SERVES 4

Flank steak is a great choice for steak salads because it's lean and full-flavoured. But because it's so lean, to get melt-in-your-mouth results, cook it medium-rare and thinly slice it across the grain. Although I really love veggies, I could probably never become a vegetarian because I love steak, too! But that's okay – I believe in everything in moderation, and by choosing lean beef I know I'm getting a good dose of iron and nutrients without all the saturated fat I'd get from fattier cuts.

SPICE RUB

1 teaspoon garlic powder

¾ teaspoon sea salt

½ teaspoon ground cumin

½ teaspoon sweet paprika

¼ teaspoon dried oregano

¼ teaspoon chipotle chilli powder or cayenne pepper

450g flank steak, trimmed of all external fat

LEMON-LIME DRESSING

2 tablespoons fresh lime juice

1 tablespoon fresh lemon juice

1 tablespoon extra-virgin olive oil

1 tablespoon finely chopped spring onions

1 tablespoon finely chopped fresh coriander

⅛ teaspoon sea salt

Freshly ground black pepper

SALAD

2 medium ears fresh sweetcorn or 1 cup (150g) thawed frozen sweetcorn kernels

1 large head romaine lettuce, cut lengthwise into 4 wedges

1 medium (110g) avocado, thinly sliced

1 cup (200g) vine-ripened cherry tomatoes, halved

¼ cup (35g) crumbled queso fresco or cotija cheese†

For the spice rub: In a small bowl, combine the garlic powder, salt, cumin, paprika, oregano and chipotle powder.

Generously season each side of the steak with the dry rub and, using your hands, rub it into the meat. Allow to sit for about 10 minutes.

For the lemon-lime dressing: In a medium bowl, whisk together the lime juice, lemon juice, olive oil, spring onions, coriander, salt and a pinch of black pepper. Set aside.

Preheat a grill to medium-high (or preheat a grill pan over medium-high heat).

(recipe continues)

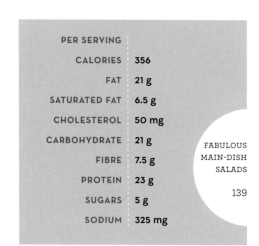

PER SERVING	
CALORIES	356
FAT	21 g
SATURATED FAT	6.5 g
CHOLESTEROL	50 mg
CARBOHYDRATE	21 g
FIBRE	7.5 g
PROTEIN	23 g
SUGARS	5 g
SODIUM	325 mg

skinny scoop

Summer sweetcorn is so sweet and delicious, you barely have to cook it – you can basically eat it raw, or just toss it on the grill for a minute or two. But if it's out of season, you can use thawed frozen sweetcorn in its place.

For the salad: If using fresh sweetcorn, grill, turning often, until charred on all sides, 20 to 25 minutes. Set aside to cool.

Increase the heat of the grill or grill pan to high. Grill the steak for 5 to 7 minutes on each side for medium-rare, or longer to your taste. Remove the steak from the grill, cover and allow to rest for 5 minutes. Cut the sweetcorn kernels off the cob and set aside.

Thinly slice the steak 5mm thick, across the grain and at an angle to the chopping board, then cut it crosswise into 1cm pieces.

Put a romaine wedge on each plate and top each with a quarter of the grilled steak. Dividing evenly, top with the avocado, sweetcorn, tomatoes and cheese. Drizzle the dressing over the salads.

✝ If you are unable to find either of these cheeses, light feta also works well.

FOOD FACTS like it lean?
Flank is nutrient-rich because it packs a powerhouse of essential nutrients (iron, niacin and potassium) in a reasonable number of calories: a 100g serving of cooked flank steak has 155 calories, 7 grams of total fat and about 3 grams of saturated fat.

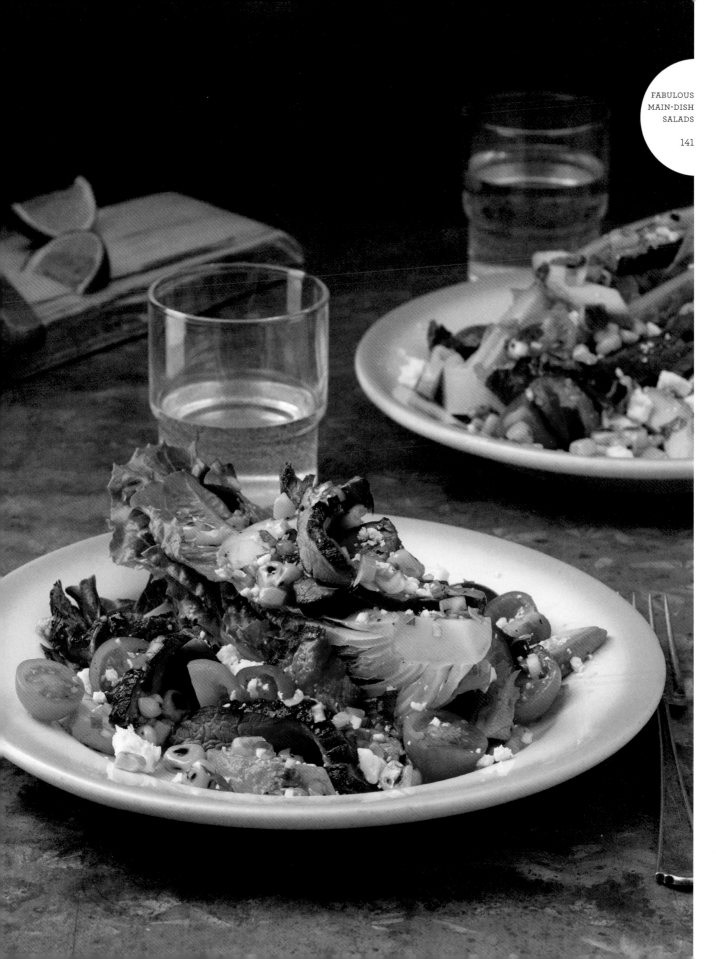

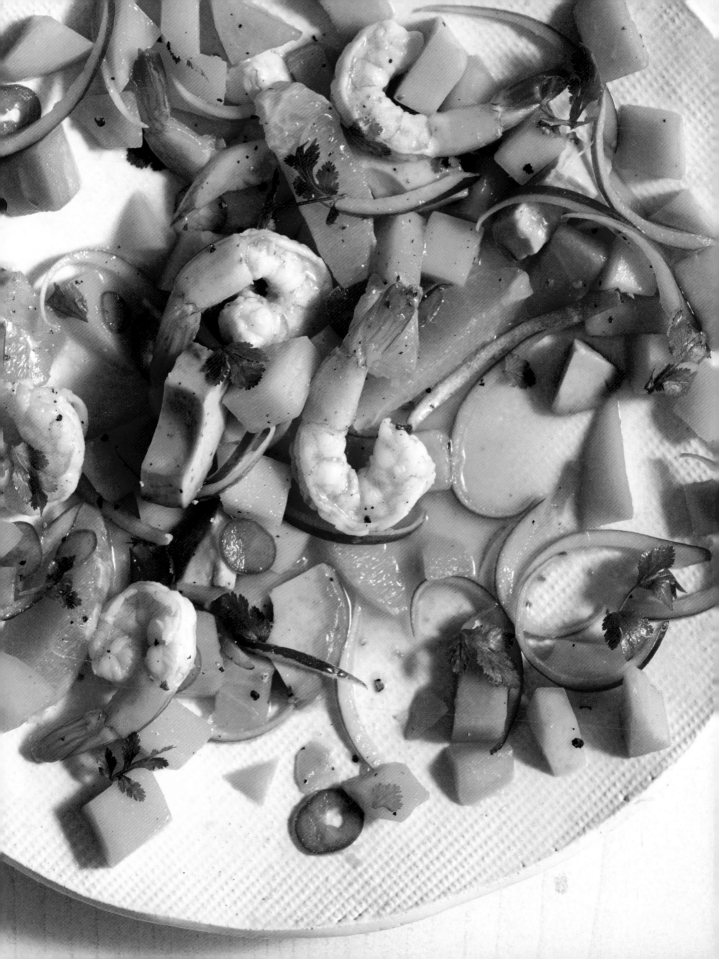

Chilled Caribbean Prawn Salad

SERVES 5

Easy, delicious and no cooking involved – this is the perfect dish for those warm summer nights when you don't want to heat up the kitchen. I'm a big fan of tropical fruit, probably because I spent many of my summers as a teen in Puerto Rico, where I fell in love with the island, culture and, especially, the tropical fruit. Mangoes used to litter my cousin's backyard, and I would eat them every chance I could.

¼ medium red onion, thinly sliced

Sea salt

1 tablespoon extra-virgin olive oil

2½ tablespoons fresh lime juice

2 oranges, peeled and divided into segments

450g cooked and peeled large prawns

1 mango, cut into 2 to 3cm chunks

1½ cups (270g) chopped fresh papaya

1 medium jalapeño or other green chilli, thinly sliced

2 tablespoons chopped fresh coriander

1 medium (110g) avocado, cut into 2 to 3cm chunks

Freshly ground black pepper

Put the onions in a large bowl and season with ¼ teaspoon salt. Add the olive oil and lime juice. Set aside for 5 minutes.

Set aside 3 segments of the orange, then put the remaining orange pieces in the bowl with onions. Add the prawns, mango, papaya, jalapeño and coriander and season with another ¼ teaspoon of salt and black pepper to taste.

Squeeze the juice from the remaining orange segments over the salad and refrigerate until chilled, at least 30 minutes. When ready to serve, sprinkle a pinch of salt and pepper over the avocado and gently toss into the salad.

FOOD FACTS **a plus for papayas**
Papayas, which can range in size from 500g to 9kg, are loaded with nutrients, including potassium, vitamins A and C and fibre. One cup (180g) of papaya contains enough vitamin E to satisfy both a man's and a woman's daily requirements.

skinny**scoop**

To make this ahead, simply leave out the avocado, then add it just before you're ready to serve. If you can't find papaya, try substituting cantaloupe or honeydew melon.

PER SERVING	
CALORIES	236
FAT	7.5 g
SATURATED FAT	1 g
CHOLESTEROL	177 mg
CARBOHYDRATE	24 g
FIBRE	5 g
PROTEIN	21 g
SUGARS	17 g
SODIUM	347 mg

FABULOUS
MAIN-DISH
SALADS

143

Roast Beef and Watercress Pasta Salad

SERVES 4

Yesterday's roast is transformed into a fabulous (and mayo-less) pasta salad! Karina, my older daughter, loves when I make Sunday Night Roast Beef (page 211) for dinner, so I usually try to make it for her when she's home from college. But unless we're having company to join us for dinner, a whole roast is usually too large for our family of four to eat in one night, so I came up with this recipe as a quick way to turn leftovers into a new meal. If I don't have leftovers, I still make this recipe, using sliced roast beef from the deli instead.

110g uncooked fusilli pasta (use brown rice pasta for gluten-free*)

¼ teaspoon sea salt, plus more for the pot

1 tablespoon extra-virgin olive oil

4 cups (60g) watercress or rocket

170g thinly sliced roast beef, cut into strips

1 cup (200g) halved cherry tomatoes

3 tablespoons capers, drained

2½ tablespoons balsamic vinegar

⅛ teaspoon freshly ground black pepper

¼ cup (25g) freshly shaved Parmesan cheese

Read the label to be sure this product is gluten-free.

Cook the pasta to al dente in a pot of salted boiling water according to packet directions. Drain and rinse under cold water.

Transfer the pasta to a large bowl and toss with the olive oil. Add the watercress, roast beef, tomatoes, capers, vinegar, salt and black pepper. Just before serving, top with shaved Parmesan.

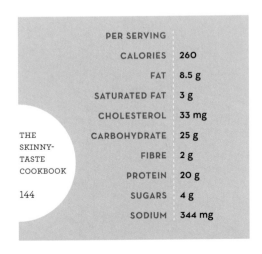

PER SERVING	
CALORIES	260
FAT	8.5 g
SATURATED FAT	3 g
CHOLESTEROL	33 mg
CARBOHYDRATE	25 g
FIBRE	2 g
PROTEIN	20 g
SUGARS	4 g
SODIUM	344 mg

Grilled Portobello Spinach Salad

SERVES 4

There's a fabulous family-style Italian restaurant in my neighbourhood called Nick's that makes the best salads and brick-oven pizzas. One of the salads I love is made with grilled portobello mushrooms topped with freshly shaved Parmesan. That's where I got the inspiration for this salad. Portobello mushrooms are large and substantial, so they make a great meat substitution.

MUSHROOMS

¼ cup (50ml) balsamic vinegar

1 tablespoon olive oil, plus more for the grill

1 teaspoon dried basil

1 teaspoon dried oregano

1 tablespoon crushed garlic

⅛ teaspoon sea salt

Freshly ground black pepper

4 portobello mushroom caps (350g total)

BALSAMIC VINAIGRETTE

1 tablespoons balsamic vinegar

3 tablespoons olive oil

⅛ teaspoon sea salt

Freshly ground black pepper

SALAD

6 cups (350g) baby spinach

⅛ teaspoon sea salt

Freshly ground black pepper

¼ cup (35g) sun-dried tomatoes (not oil-packed), thinly sliced

½ cup (50g) shaved Parmesan cheese

For the mushrooms: In a large bowl, whisk together the vinegar, olive oil, basil, oregano, garlic, salt and black pepper to taste. Add the mushroom caps and toss well. Allow to sit at room temperature for about 30 minutes, turning a few times.

For the balsamic vinaigrette: In a medium bowl, whisk together the vinegar, olive oil, salt and black pepper to taste.

Preheat a grill to medium (or preheat a grill pan over medium heat). Brush the grill grate or spray the pan with oil. Put the mushrooms on the grill, reserving the marinade for basting. Grill until tender, basting frequently, 5 to 7 minutes on each side. Transfer to a chopping board.

For the salad: In a large bowl, toss the spinach with the balsamic vinaigrette and season with the salt and black pepper to taste. Divide the spinach among 4 plates and top with the sun-dried tomatoes. Slice the mushroom caps at an angle, put one on each salad and then top with the Parmesan.

PERFECT PAIRINGS

I like to serve this over baby spinach, but it would also be great over rocket or mixed salad leaves. If you like, you can grill some chicken breasts along with the mushrooms to add to the salad.

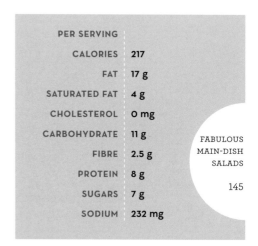

PER SERVING	
CALORIES	217
FAT	17 g
SATURATED FAT	4 g
CHOLESTEROL	0 mg
CARBOHYDRATE	11 g
FIBRE	2.5 g
PROTEIN	8 g
SUGARS	7 g
SODIUM	232 mg

FABULOUS
MAIN-DISH
SALADS

Greek Chickpea Salad

SERVES 4

Believe it or not, I started including chickpeas in my salads only a few years ago, but now it's a regular thing! They add great texture to this Mediterranean-inspired salad and make it a great meatless option. I chop all the vegetables the same size as the chickpeas and let them marinate for a few hours or overnight so they absorb all the flavours from the lemon, herbs and olives. Just before serving, I add the cucumbers and top it with feta so the cucumbers stay crunchy and the feta doesn't get lost.

2 garlic cloves, crushed

1 tablespoon olive oil

3 tablespoons fresh lemon juice

½ teaspoon sea salt

2 cups (400g) tinned chickpeas,* rinsed and drained

¼ cup (40g) chopped red onion

1 cup (200g) quartered cherry tomatoes

½ cup (90g) chopped orange pepper

2 tablespoons chopped fresh parsley

½ teaspoon fresh oregano leaves or ¼ teaspoon dried

¼ cup (40g) Kalamata olives, stoned and chopped

1½ cups (265g) seeded, chopped cucumber

⅓ cup (50g) crumbled feta cheese

Read the label to be sure this product is gluten-free.

In a large bowl, combine the garlic, olive oil, lemon juice and salt. Add the chickpeas, red onion, tomatoes, pepper, parsley, oregano and olives and toss well. For best results, marinate for a few hours or overnight in the refrigerator to allow the flavours to meld. Just before serving, toss in the cucumbers and feta cheese.

FOOD FACTS **chickpeas boost satiety**

Chickpeas are loaded with fibre and protein – the right combo to help tame your appetite. In a study done by Australian researchers, people who ate a diet rich in chickpeas – 100 grams (about ½ cup) per day – for 3 months reported feeling more satiated and consumed fewer calories during that time. Once the study participants resumed their normal diet again, they consumed more processed snack food.

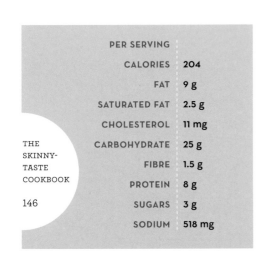

PER SERVING	
CALORIES	204
FAT	9 g
SATURATED FAT	2.5 g
CHOLESTEROL	11 mg
CARBOHYDRATE	25 g
FIBRE	1.5 g
PROTEIN	8 g
SUGARS	3 g
SODIUM	518 mg

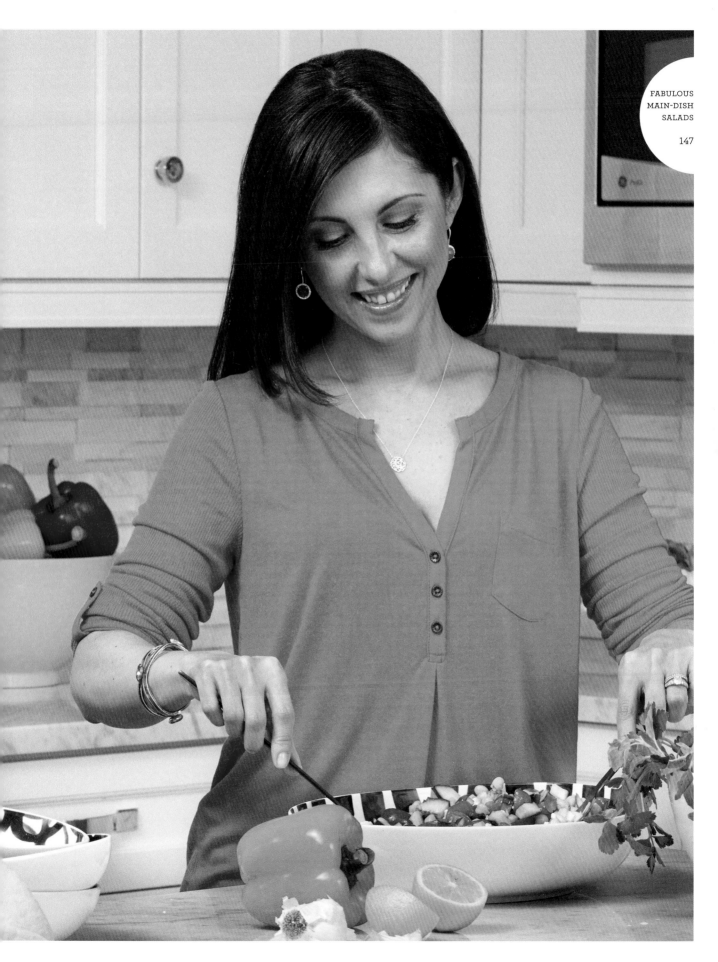

PERFECT POULTRY

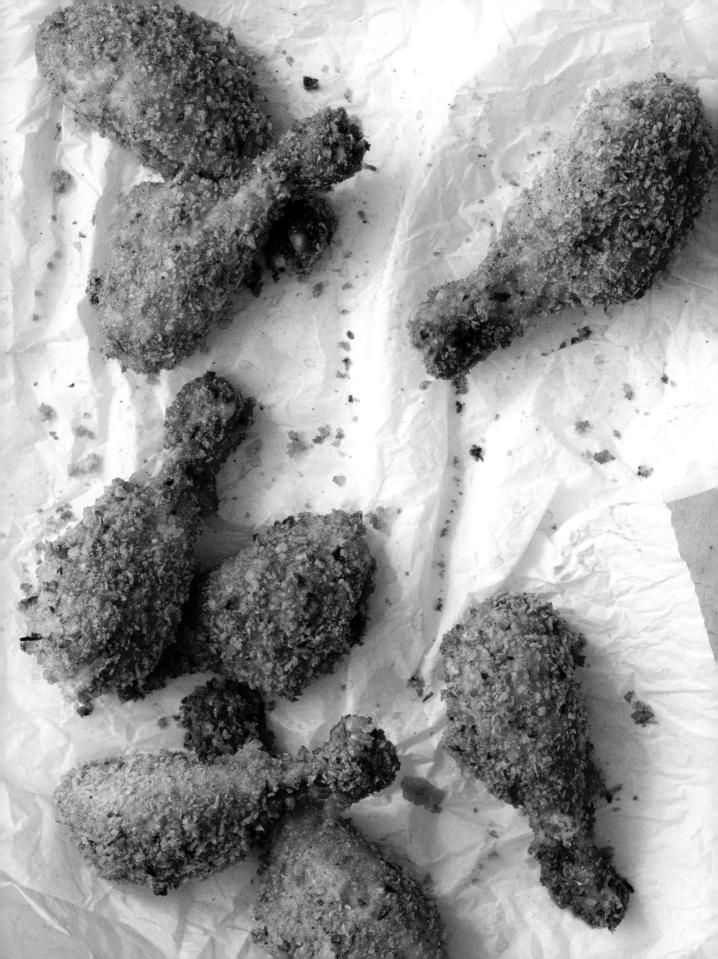

Buttermilk Oven 'Fried' Chicken

SERVES 4

Fried chicken is one of my biggest weaknesses, so naturally I've been perfecting this lighter version for years. I've managed to achieve the same crispy golden texture you get from frying from my oven. Yep, it's skinnier, easier, quicker and (bonus) there's no greasy mess to clean up. Soaking the chicken overnight (sometimes two nights) in a buttermilk bath is a must for meat that's moist and juicy. To easily remove the skin from the drumsticks, use one paper towel to grasp the joint end and a second one to pull off the skin.

CHICKEN

8 chicken drumsticks (about 100g each), skinned

½ teaspoon sea salt

½ teaspoon sweet paprika

½ teaspoon chicken seasoning

¼ teaspoon garlic powder

⅛ teaspoon freshly ground black pepper

1 cup (225ml) buttermilk

Juice of ½ lemon

Cooking spray or oil mister

COATING

⅔ cup (40g) panko bread crumbs

½ cup (25g) crushed cornflake crumbs

2 tablespoons grated Parmesan cheese

1½ teaspoons sea salt

1 teaspoon dried parsley

1½ teaspoons sweet paprika

½ teaspoon onion powder

½ teaspoon garlic powder

¼ teaspoon chilli powder

For the chicken: In a medium bowl, season the chicken with the salt, paprika, chicken seasoning, garlic powder and black pepper. Pour the buttermilk and lemon juice over the chicken and refrigerate for 6 to 8 hours, preferably overnight.

Preheat the oven to 200°C/180°C fan/Gas 6. Place a rack on a baking sheet and lightly spray with oil.

For the coating: In a shallow bowl, combine the panko, cornflake crumbs, Parmesan, salt, parsley, paprika, onion powder, garlic powder and chilli powder.

Remove the chicken from the buttermilk, dredge each piece in the crumb mixture and put the pieces onto the prepared baking sheet. Spray the tops of the chicken with oil.

Bake until golden brown and cooked through, 40 to 45 minutes.

PERFECT PAIRINGS
Serve this with corn on the cob, **Cheesy Cauliflower 'Mash' (page 269),** or **Seasoned Sweet Potato Wedges (page 277)** and a side of **Confetti Slaw (page 285).**

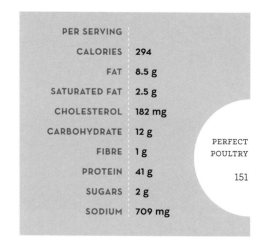

PER SERVING	
CALORIES	294
FAT	8.5 g
SATURATED FAT	2.5 g
CHOLESTEROL	182 mg
CARBOHYDRATE	12 g
FIBRE	1 g
PROTEIN	41 g
SUGARS	2 g
SODIUM	709 mg

Chicken Rollatini Stuffed with Courgette and Mozzarella

SERVES 4

I came up with this recipe a few summers back when my garden produced an overabundance of courgettes. I make stuffed chicken breasts so many different ways, and this is one of my favourites. It's easier than you think – there are no strings or toothpicks required.

Cooking spray or oil mister

1 tablespoon plus 1 teaspoon olive oil

4 garlic cloves, chopped

1½ cups packed (200g) grated courgettes

¼ cup (25g) plus 2 tablespoons grated Parmesan cheese

½ teaspoon plus ⅛ teaspoon sea salt

Freshly ground black pepper

¾ cup (75g) grated light mozzarella

8 thin chicken breasts (110g each)

½ cup (40g) seasoned wholemeal bread crumbs, homemade (see page 110) or shop-bought

Juice of 1 lemon

Preheat the oven to 230°C/210°C fan/Gas 8. Lightly spray a baking dish with oil.

Heat a large frying pan over medium-high heat. Add 1 teaspoon of the oil and the garlic. Cook, stirring, until golden, about 1 minute. Add the courgette, ¼ cup of the Parmesan, ⅛ teaspoon of the salt and black pepper to taste. Cook, stirring, until the courgette is tender, 3 to 4 minutes. Remove the pan from the heat and allow to cool to room temperature. Add the mozzarella and mix well.

Wash and dry the chicken and arrange on a chopping board. Spread each chicken breast with 3 tablespoons courgette-cheese mixture. Loosely roll up and set aside, seam side down.

In a small bowl, combine the bread crumbs and remaining 2 tablespoons Parmesan. In a separate bowl, combine the remaining 1 tablespoon of olive oil, the lemon juice, the remaining ½ teaspoon salt and a pinch of black pepper.

Dip the rolled chicken in the lemon mixture, then into the bread crumbs, rolling to coat evenly. Place the chicken seam side down in the prepared baking dish. Spray the tops of the chicken with oil. Bake until cooked through, 25 to 30 minutes. Serve hot.

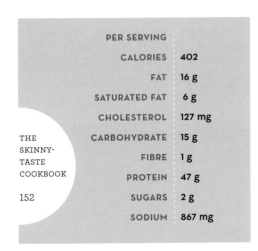

PER SERVING	
CALORIES	402
FAT	16 g
SATURATED FAT	6 g
CHOLESTEROL	127 mg
CARBOHYDRATE	15 g
FIBRE	1 g
PROTEIN	47 g
SUGARS	2 g
SODIUM	867 mg

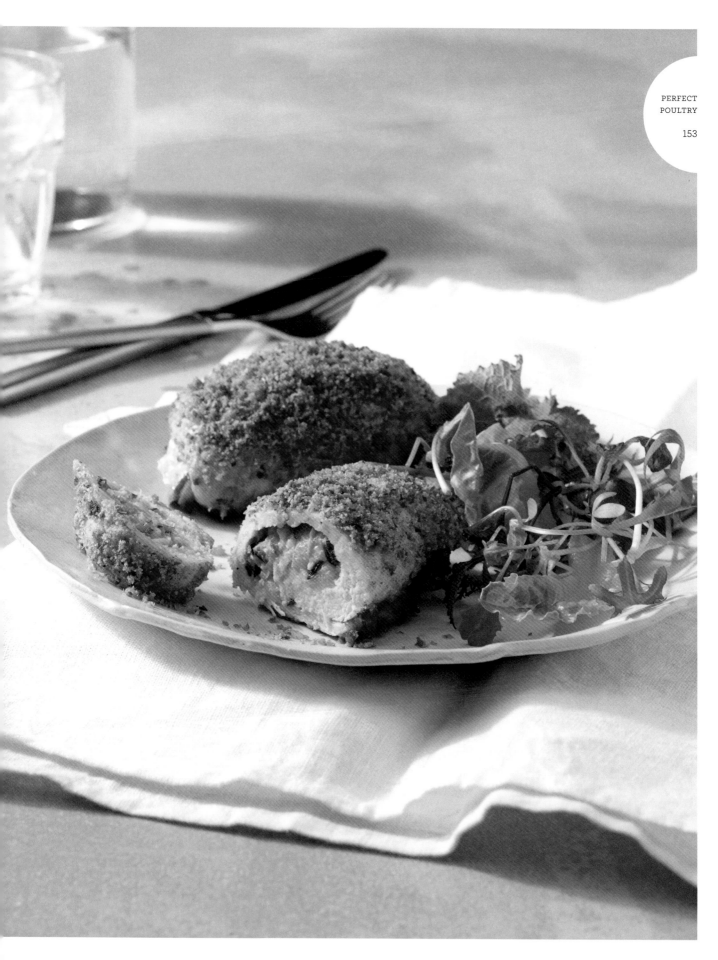

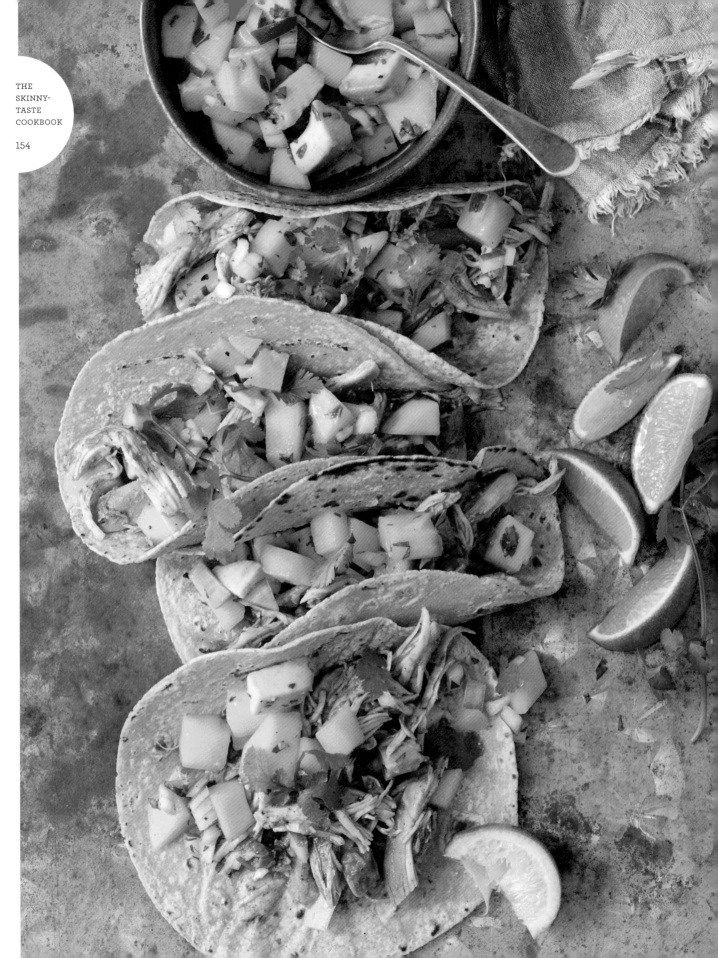

Slow-Cooker Jerk Chicken Tacos with Caribbean Salsa

SERVES 6

GF **SC**

Who says tacos have to be Mexican? These chicken tacos get their heat from the wonderful flavours of Jamaican jerk spices, and then they're topped with a fresh mango-avocado salsa.

CHICKEN

3 garlic cloves, crushed

2 tablespoons jerk seasoning*

Sea salt

675g boneless chicken breasts

1 tablespoon lime juice (from ½ lime)

¼ cup (50ml) fresh orange juice

1 tablespoon chopped fresh coriander

CARIBBEAN SALSA

1 large mango, diced into 1cm pieces

½ medium (50g) avocado, diced into 1cm pieces

1 tablespoon chopped red onion

1 tablespoon chopped fresh coriander

1½ tablespoons fresh lime juice

⅛ teaspoon sea salt

Freshly ground black pepper

12 extra-thin yellow corn tortillas

Read the label to be sure this product is gluten-free.

For the chicken: Combine the garlic, jerk seasoning and ¼ teaspoon salt and spread it over the chicken. Put the chicken, the lime and orange juices and coriander in the slow cooker. Cover and cook on high for 2 hours.

For the Caribbean salsa: Meanwhile, in a medium bowl, combine the mango, avocado, red onion, coriander, lime juice, salt and black pepper to taste. Refrigerate until ready to serve.

Remove the chicken from the slow cooker and shred it with two forks. Pour any liquid in the slow cooker into a bowl, then return the chicken to the slow cooker. Add ½ cup (120ml) of the reserved liquid, just enough to moisten the chicken, and season with ⅛ teaspoon salt and black pepper to taste.

Heat the tortillas in a frying pan set over medium-high heat for about 30 seconds. Fill each with some chicken and 2 tablespoons of salsa.

skinnyscoop

Although any brand of jerk seasoning will do, I really like Walkerswood Jerk Seasoning, which I purchase online. It's very spicy – a little goes a long way! If you don't enjoy too much spice, get the mild variety, which is what I use.

PER SERVING	
CALORIES	272
FAT	6 g
SATURATED FAT	1 g
CHOLESTEROL	73 mg
CARBOHYDRATE	28 g
FIBRE	4.5 g
PROTEIN	27 g
SUGARS	11 g
SODIUM	490 mg

PERFECT POULTRY

155

Naked Persian Turkey Burgers

SERVES 5

This bunless burger isn't just *any* burger. It's a moist, delicious spin on kofta, a Middle Eastern meatball that's full of fresh herbs, spices and even some veggies. My secret to making turkey burgers perfectly moist every time is adding shredded courgette – it works like a charm! To serve them, I place each burger on a bed of lettuce and top it with a chopped salad that's sort of like a Persian salsa.

PERSIAN SALAD

2½ cups (450g) chopped cucumbers

1½ cups (300g) quartered small cherry tomatoes

⅓ cup (50g) chopped red onion

2 teaspoons finely chopped fresh mint

2½ tablespoons fresh lemon juice

1 tablespoon extra-virgin olive oil

¼ teaspoon sea salt

Freshly ground black pepper

BURGERS

¾ cup (100g) grated courgette

575g turkey breast mince

⅓ cup (50g) finely chopped red onion

2 garlic cloves, crushed

¼ cup (20g) unseasoned wholemeal bread crumbs

¼ cup (15g) chopped fresh parsley

1 tablespoon finely chopped fresh mint

1 teaspoon ground cumin

½ teaspoon ground coriander

¼ teaspoon ground allspice

¼ teaspoon chilli powder

¼ teaspoon sea salt

Freshly ground black pepper

Cooking spray or oil mister

5 cups (250g) chopped romaine lettuce

5 tablespoons grated feta cheese

For the Persian salad: In a large bowl, combine the cucumbers, tomatoes, red onion, mint, lemon juice, olive oil, salt and black pepper to taste. Mix well, cover and refrigerate for at least 1 hour.

For the burgers: Squeeze any liquid out of the courgette with kitchen paper. Put the courgette in a large bowl and add the turkey, red onion, garlic, bread crumbs, parsley, mint, cumin, coriander, allspice, chilli powder, salt and black pepper to taste. Form into 5 equal, flattened patties about 2 to 3cm thick. Refrigerate until ready to cook.

(recipe continues)

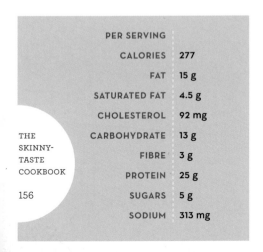

PER SERVING	
CALORIES	277
FAT	15 g
SATURATED FAT	4.5 g
CHOLESTEROL	92 mg
CARBOHYDRATE	13 g
FIBRE	3 g
PROTEIN	25 g
SUGARS	5 g
SODIUM	313 mg

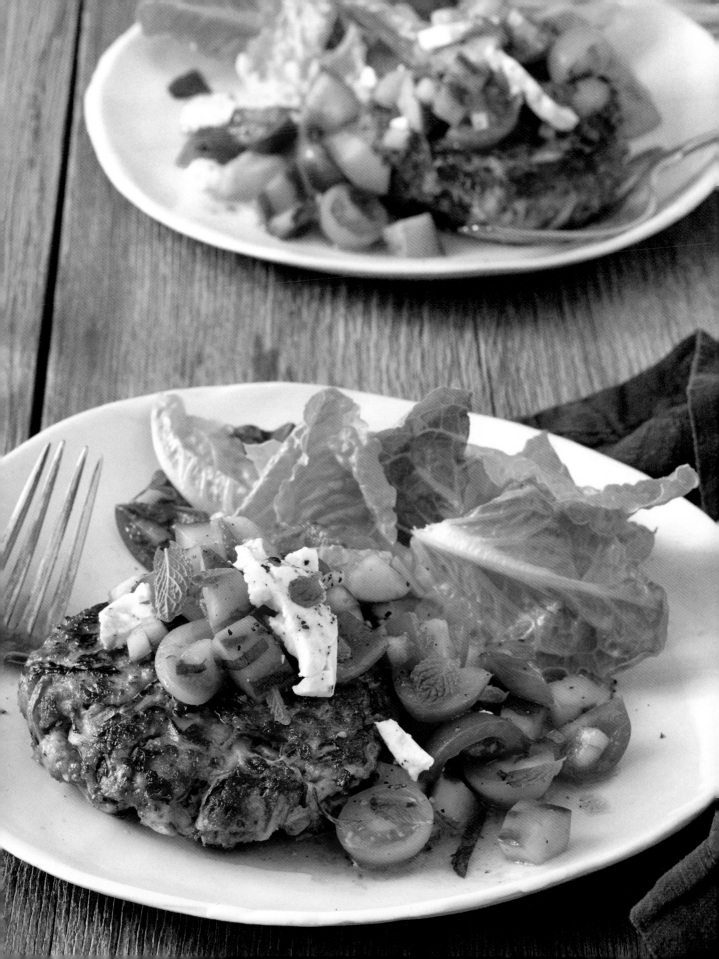

skinnyscoop

I use cherry tomatoes for my Persian salad, which is also known as a salad Shirazi, but you can use any type of tomatoes you like. Just be sure to chop all the vegetables about the same size. Because the burgers are made with courgettes, they work best when they're cooked in a frying pan over medium-low heat so that they don't burn. Leftover patties can be kept in the freezer for future meals.

Heat a large nonstick frying pan over medium-high heat. Lightly spray the pan with oil. Put the burgers in the pan and reduce the heat to medium-low. Cook until browned, about 4 minutes on each side.

To serve, put a fifth of the lettuce on each plate. Put a turkey burger on each plate along with the salad, then sprinkle 1 tablespoon feta on each.

Sausage with Peppers and Onions

SERVES 4

On those busy nights when I've been out all day and have no idea what to make for dinner, I usually wind up making this dish. Whether I make it outside on the barbecue in the summer or indoors in the winter, it's a year-round favourite in my home. I make this lean by swapping fatty pork sausages for leaner chicken sausages, which taste just as good (if not better).

1 teaspoon olive oil

1 large red pepper, cut into 5mm-wide strips

1 large yellow or orange pepper, cut into 5mm-wide strips

1 medium onion, thinly sliced

¼ teaspoon dried oregano

1 sprig of fresh rosemary

Sea salt and freshly ground black pepper

400g fresh sweet or hot Italian sausages*

*Read the label to be sure this product is gluten-free.

Preheat the grill, barbecue or a grill pan to medium heat.

Heat a large frying pan over medium-low heat. Add the olive oil, peppers and onion, tossing to coat well. Add the oregano, rosemary and a pinch of salt and black pepper to taste. Cover the pan and cook, stirring occasionally, until the vegetables are soft, 18 to 20 minutes.

Grill the sausages, turning, until golden and cooked through, 12 to 15 minutes. Transfer to a chopping board and slice into 1cm pieces. Add to the cooked peppers and onions and cover until ready to serve.

† If you can't find Italian chicken sausages, another kind of chicken sausage or reduced-fat pork sausages will work well.

skinny**scoop**

If you want to make the whole thing outside on the barbecue, use a cast-iron pan to cook the onions and peppers (covered and over medium heat), turning every 3 to 5 minutes until they are soft, then grill the sausage until cooked through.

PERFECT PAIRINGS
This can be served with a crusty piece of wholemeal bread and **My House Salad, Made with Love (page 267)**, or turn it into a sandwich by tucking it all into a wholemeal baguette.

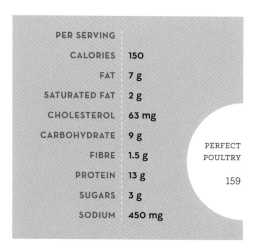

PER SERVING	
CALORIES	150
FAT	7 g
SATURATED FAT	2 g
CHOLESTEROL	63 mg
CARBOHYDRATE	9 g
FIBRE	1.5 g
PROTEIN	13 g
SUGARS	3 g
SODIUM	450 mg

PERFECT POULTRY

159

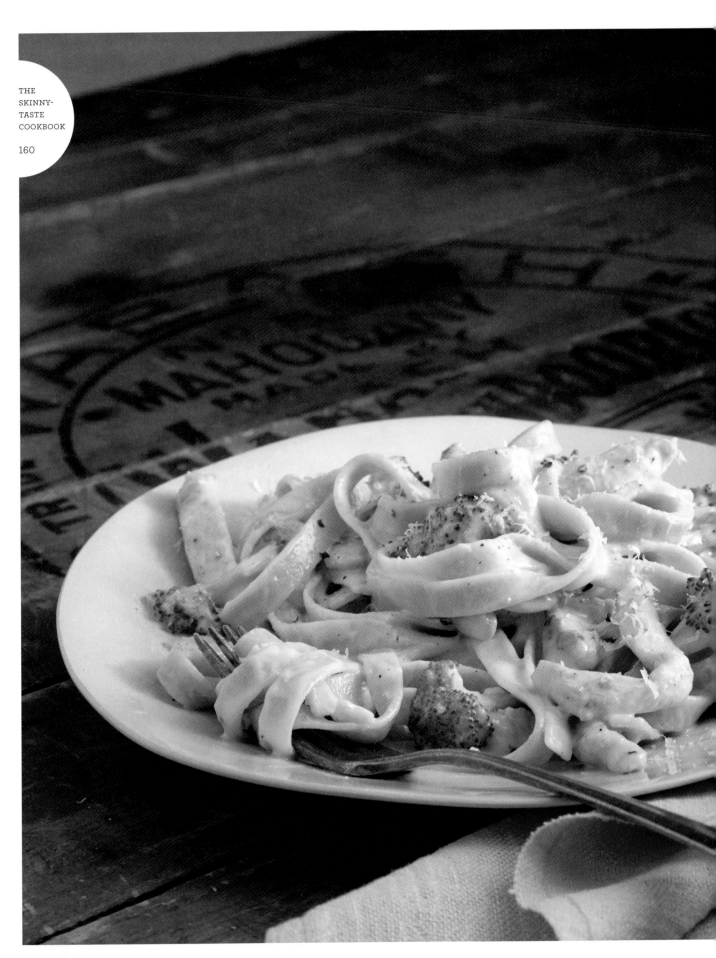

Fettuccine Alfredo with Chicken and Broccoli

SERVES 5

You may not be all that surprised to learn that Fettuccine Alfredo is the most requested recipe makeover on *Skinnytaste*. It's such a decadent, flavourful dish, although certainly not a simple one to skinny-fy, as it traditionally consists of nothing more than butter, cream, pasta and cheese. My skinny solution: use wholewheat pasta, add lean protein and vegetables, and use the best-quality cheese to make up for the lack of butter. That way, you'll feel totally satisfied and you can enjoy a dish that's full of flavour without all the extra fat and calories. I'm *so* confident that you'll love it, because I've put a lot of time, effort and heart into it!

Cooking spray or oil mister

450g thin chicken breasts, cut into thin strips

1 teaspoon garlic salt

Freshly ground black pepper

250g wholewheat fettuccine

2 teaspoons sea salt

3 cups (225g) small broccoli florets

1 cup (225ml) skimmed milk

2 tablespoons light cream cheese

1 tablespoon unsalted butter

1 tablespoon finely chopped shallot

1 garlic clove, crushed

1 tablespoon plain flour

⅔ cup (150ml) low-salt chicken stock

⅓ cup (35g) freshly grated Parmesan cheese

¼ cup (25g) freshly grated Pecorino Romano cheese (plus more for serving, optional)

1 tablespoon finely chopped fresh parsley

Heat a large, deep nonstick frying pan over high heat. Spray the frying pan with oil. Season the chicken with the garlic salt and black pepper to taste, and add half of the chicken to the pan. Cook until the chicken is golden on the outside and cooked through, about 2 to 3 minutes on each side. Transfer to a large plate. Spray the pan and repeat with the remaining chicken and set aside. Remove the frying pan from the heat and allow to cool.

Cook the pasta to al dente in a pot of salted boiling water according to packet directions, adding the broccoli in the last 1½ to 2 minutes of cooking. Reserving ¼ cup (50ml) of the cooking water, drain the pasta and broccoli in a large colander and return it to the cooking pot.

(recipe continues)

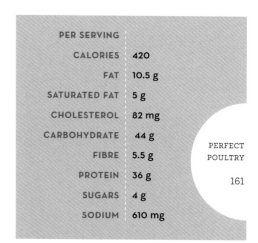

PER SERVING	
CALORIES	420
FAT	10.5 g
SATURATED FAT	5 g
CHOLESTEROL	82 mg
CARBOHYDRATE	44 g
FIBRE	5.5 g
PROTEIN	36 g
SUGARS	4 g
SODIUM	610 mg

While the pasta cooks, in a blender, combine the milk and cream cheese and blend until smooth; set aside.

Set the frying pan over medium-low heat and add the butter. Once melted, add the shallot and garlic and cook, stirring, until golden, about 1 minute. Sprinkle in the flour and cook, stirring, for 1 minute. Whisk in the chicken stock, then whisk in the milk–cream cheese mixture. Increase the heat to medium-high and bring to a boil, whisking occasionally. Reduce the heat to low and simmer the cream sauce until thickened, 2 to 3 minutes.

Once the pasta is cooked and drained, set the pot over medium-high heat and add 2 tablespoons of the reserved pasta water. Add the chicken, cream sauce and Parmesan and toss well. Season with a pinch of black pepper to taste. If needed, add the remaining 2 tablespoons reserved pasta water to loosen the sauce.

Divide the pasta among 5 plates. Sprinkle with the Romano and garnish with the parsley. Serve hot with extra black pepper and grated Romano on the side, if desired.

Chicken Cordon Bleu Meatballs

SERVES 6

Who says meatballs have to be Italian? Not me! I thought it would be fun to use the flavours of Chicken Cordon Bleu in a meatball, and I was right! Each meatball is stuffed with ham and light Swiss cheese and baked in the oven, then finished in a creamy white wine sauce. I'm not sure what I like best – the oozing cheese that comes out from the centre of each meatball or the decadent sauce they're simmered in.

MEATBALLS

Cooking spray or oil mister

675g minced chicken

¼ cup (20g) seasoned wholemeal bread crumbs, homemade (see page 110) or shop-bought

¼ cup (25g) grated Parmesan cheese

¼ cup (15g) finely chopped fresh parsley

1 large egg

1 large garlic clove, crushed

½ teaspoon sea salt

2 (25g) slices lean ham, cut into 6 pieces each

3 slices lighter Swiss cheese, cut into 4 pieces each (55g total)

SAUCE

1 tablespoon unsalted butter

1 tablespoon plain flour

¼ cup (50ml) white wine

1 cup (225ml) low-salt chicken stock

½ cup (120ml) skimmed milk

1 tablespoon Dijon mustard

1 teaspoon fresh lemon juice

⅛ teaspoon sea salt

Freshly ground black pepper

1 teaspoon finely chopped fresh parsley

Preheat the oven to 220°C/200°C fan/Gas 7. Spray a large nonstick baking sheet with oil.

For the meatballs: In a large bowl, combine the chicken, bread crumbs, Parmesan, parsley, egg, garlic and salt. Form 12 meatballs using slightly wet hands to prevent them from sticking. Stuff each meatball by making a hole in the middle and placing one piece each of ham and Swiss cheese in the centre. Seal the meatballs well by pinching them closed. Place on the prepared baking sheet and bake 20 minutes, or until almost cooked through.

(recipe continues)

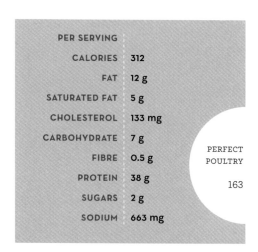

PER SERVING	
CALORIES	312
FAT	12 g
SATURATED FAT	5 g
CHOLESTEROL	133 mg
CARBOHYDRATE	7 g
FIBRE	0.5 g
PROTEIN	38 g
SUGARS	2 g
SODIUM	663 mg

PERFECT
POULTRY

To balance out the richness of this dish, serve it with **Lemon-Roasted Asparagus (page 278)**.

For the sauce: Meanwhile, in a large, deep nonstick pan with a fitted lid, melt the butter over medium heat. Sprinkle in the flour and cook, whisking constantly, for about 1 minute. Whisk in the wine and cook for 1 minute, then whisk in the chicken stock and milk. Bring to a boil, then simmer until it thickens slightly, about 5 minutes. Whisk in the mustard and lemon juice, and season with the salt and a pinch of black pepper; remove from the heat and keep covered.

When the meatballs come out of the oven, add them to the pan with the sauce. Cover and simmer the meatballs over medium-low heat until the meatballs are cooked through and the chicken is no longer pink, about 5 minutes.

To serve, place 2 meatballs on each plate and top with the sauce and parsley.

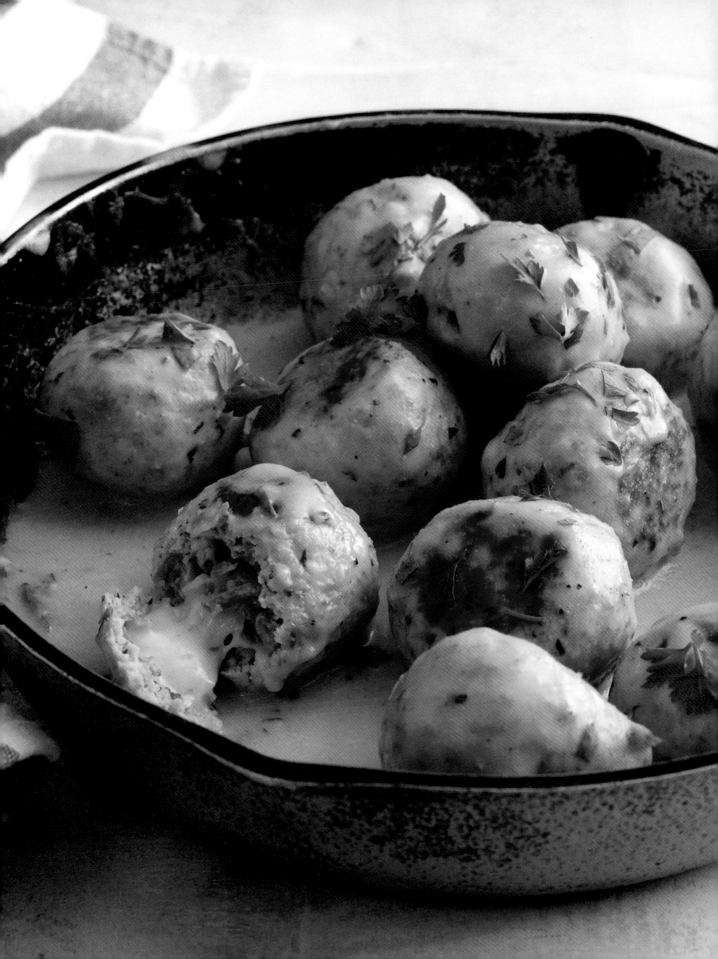

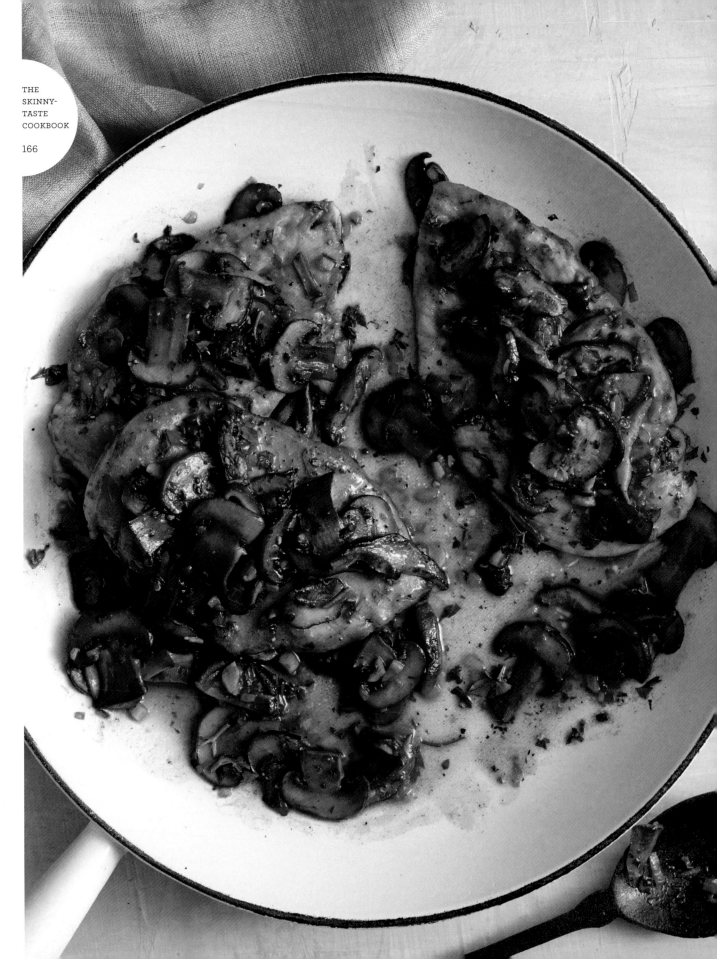

Chicken Marsala on the Lighter Side

SERVES 4

Chicken Marsala is one of those dishes that's found on just about every Italian restaurant menu in the States, but the dish is usually swimming in butter. So I've lightened it up, resulting in a tender chicken dish with a rich pan sauce made with a touch of Marsala wine and fresh parsley. Trust me, you'll be happy you decided not to eat out!

2 large boneless, skinless chicken breasts (225g each)

Sea salt

Freshly ground black pepper

¼ cup plus 1 teaspoon (35g) plain flour

1 tablespoon unsalted butter

2 teaspoons olive oil

3 garlic cloves, crushed

¼ cup (30g) finely chopped shallots

225g sliced mushrooms

75g sliced shiitake mushrooms

⅓ cup (75ml) Marsala wine

½ cup (120ml) low-salt chicken stock

2 tablespoons chopped fresh parsley

Preheat the oven to its lowest setting.

Slice the chicken breasts in half horizontally to make 4 pieces. Put each piece between two sheets of clingfilm and lightly pound them until they are about 5mm thick. Season with ½ teaspoon salt and a pinch of black pepper.

Place a 45cm-long sheet of greaseproof paper on the worktop. Put all but 1 teaspoon of the flour in a shallow bowl and lightly dredge the chicken pieces in the flour, shaking off any excess. Put the chicken on the greaseproof paper; reserve the 1 teaspoon remaining flour to use later.

Heat a large nonstick frying pan over medium-high heat. Add ½ tablespoon of the butter and 1 teaspoon of the olive oil to the pan and swirl the pan until the butter has melted. Add the chicken and cook until slightly golden on both sides, about 3 minutes per side. Transfer to a baking dish and place in the oven to keep warm.

(recipe continues)

PERFECT PAIRINGS
You can serve this with noodles, roasted potatoes or a simple vegetable, such as **Sautéed Rapini with Garlic and Oil (page 284)**.

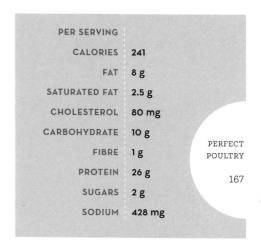

PER SERVING	
CALORIES	241
FAT	8 g
SATURATED FAT	2.5 g
CHOLESTEROL	80 mg
CARBOHYDRATE	10 g
FIBRE	1 g
PROTEIN	26 g
SUGARS	2 g
SODIUM	428 mg

PERFECT POULTRY

Add the remaining ½ tablespoon butter and 1 teaspoon olive oil to the pan. Add the garlic and shallots and cook until soft and golden, about 2 minutes. Add the mushrooms, season with ⅛ teaspoon salt and a pinch of black pepper and cook, stirring occasionally, until golden, about 5 minutes. Sprinkle in the reserved 1 teaspoon of flour and cook, stirring, for about 30 seconds. Add the Marsala wine, chicken stock and parsley. Cook, stirring and scraping up any browned bits from the bottom of the pan with a wooden spoon, until thickened, about 2 minutes.

Return the chicken to the pan with the mushrooms, reduce heat to low, cover and simmer in the sauce to let the flavours blend, about 4 to 5 minutes.

Put a piece of chicken on each plate. Spoon the mushrooms and sauce evenly over the top, and serve hot.

Spaghetti 'Squashta' with Turkey Bolognese

SERVES 6

This quick slimmed-down Bolognese sauce is the perfect topping for spaghetti squash – my favourite low-calorie solution to pasta. A great big bowl of 'squashta', as my husband calls it, is under 250 calories! My kids prefer to have real pasta, so I just boil some pasta for them instead.

50g pancetta, chopped

½ tablespoon unsalted butter

1 small onion, finely chopped

1 celery stalk, finely chopped

1 medium carrot, finely chopped

600g turkey breast mince

Sea salt

Freshly ground black pepper

¼ cup (50ml) white wine

½ tablespoon tomato paste

¾ cup (175ml) skimmed milk

2 (400g) tins chopped tomatoes

1 bay leaf

2 medium spaghetti squash

¼ cup (15g) chopped fresh basil

In a large Dutch oven, sauté the pancetta over medium heat until the fat melts, about 3 minutes. Reduce heat to medium-low, add the butter, onion, celery and carrot and cook until soft, 5 to 6 minutes. Increase the heat to medium-high, add the turkey and season with ¾ teaspoon salt and pepper to taste. Cook until no longer pink, 7 to 8 minutes, breaking up the meat with a wooden spoon. Add the wine and cook until reduced, 2 to 3 minutes. Add the tomato paste, milk, tomatoes and bay leaf. Bring to a boil, reduce heat to low and simmer, covered, 20 to 25 minutes, stirring occasionally.

Meanwhile, using a sharp knife, pierce the squash 8 or 9 times. Microwave on high for 6 minutes. Turn the squash and cook until the shell is tender, 5 to 8 minutes depending on the size. Allow to cool for 5 minutes. Halve the squash lengthwise. (There should be no resistance, but if there is, microwave it for a few more minutes.) Remove the seeds and use a fork to scrape out the spaghetti-like strands of squash.

Remove and discard the bay leaf; stir in the basil. To serve, put the spaghetti squash into bowls and top each with a generous spoonful of sauce.

skinnyscoop

You can also bake the squash in the oven. See page 268 for instructions.

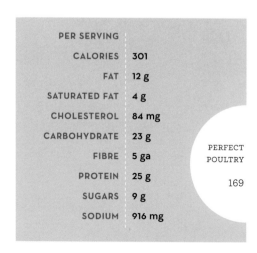

PER SERVING	
CALORIES	301
FAT	12 g
SATURATED FAT	4 g
CHOLESTEROL	84 mg
CARBOHYDRATE	23 g
FIBRE	5 ga
PROTEIN	25 g
SUGARS	9 g
SODIUM	916 mg

PERFECT POULTRY

169

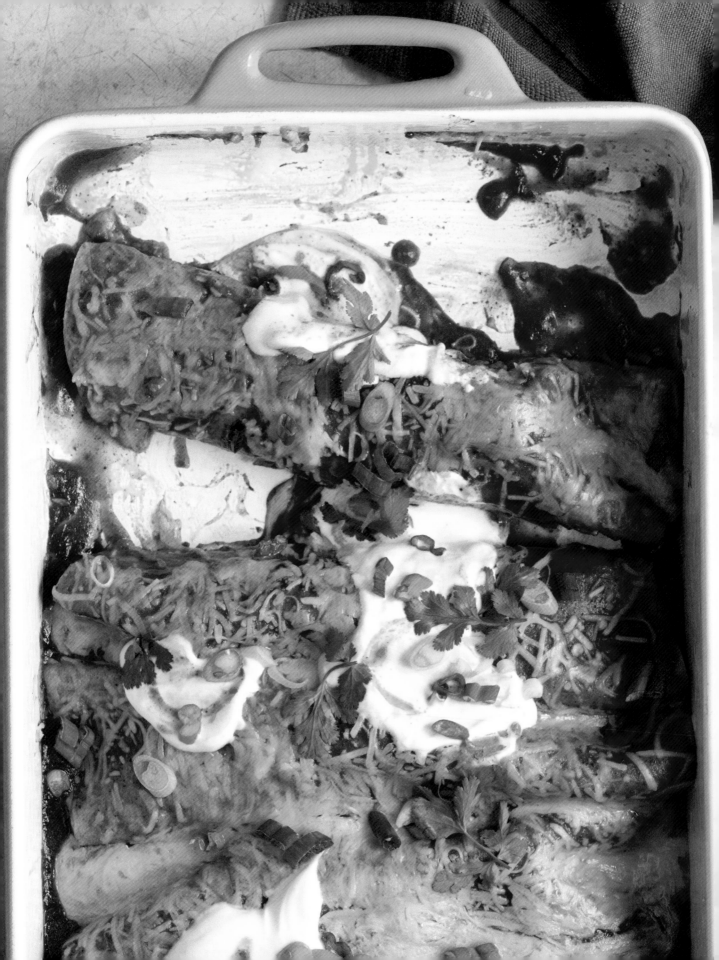

So-Addicted Chicken Enchiladas

SERVES 8

Enchiladas are on my top-three list of Mexican favourites, right along with chiles rellenos and carnitas tacos. Stuffed tortillas smothered in a spicy sauce topped with melted cheese – that's a recipe for delicious! I'm not exactly sure just how authentic my enchiladas are, but I really don't care because they are so darn good. But are they skinny? Of course!

1 teaspoon rapeseed or olive oil

1 cup (155g) chopped onion

2 large garlic cloves, crushed

½ cup (125g) passata

⅓ cup (75ml) low-salt chicken stock

250g cooked, shredded chicken breast (see page 80)

¼ cup plus 1 tablespoon (20g) chopped fresh coriander

1 teaspoon chilli powder

1 teaspoon ground cumin

½ teaspoon dried oregano

¾ teaspoon sea salt

Cooking spray or oil mister

8 low-carb, wholewheat flour tortillas

½ batch of Best Enchilada Sauce from Scratch (recipe follows) or shop-bought sauce

1 cup (125g) grated reduced-fat Mexican cheese†

2 tablespoons chopped spring onions, for garnish

4 tablespoons light soured cream, for serving (optional)

Preheat the oven to 200°C/180°C fan/Gas 6.

In a medium nonstick frying pan, heat the oil over low heat. Add the onion and garlic and cook, stirring, until soft, about 2 minutes. Add the passata, chicken stock, cooked chicken, all but 1 tablespoon of the coriander, the chilli powder, cumin, oregano and salt. Simmer until the flavours blend and the sauce reduces, 4 to 5 minutes. Remove the pan from the heat.

Spray a 23 × 32cm glass baking dish with oil. Put an eighth of the chicken mixture into each tortilla, roll them up and place seam side down in the baking dish. Top with the enchilada sauce, then sprinkle the top with the cheese. Cover the dish with foil, being careful it does not touch the cheese. Bake until hot and the cheese is melted, 20 to 25 minutes.

To serve, put an enchilada on each plate, sprinkle with the spring onions and the remaining 1 tablespoon coriander, and serve with light soured cream on the side, if desired.

† If you can't find Mexican cheese, lighter cheddar will work well.

PERFECT PAIRINGS
I serve these with coriander lime rice – combine ¾ cup (140g) cooked brown rice with a squeeze of lime juice and a tablespoon of chopped fresh coriander – and a simple side salad.

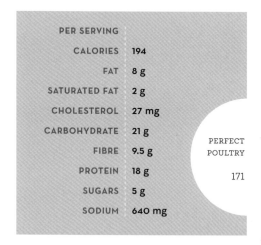

PER SERVING	
CALORIES	194
FAT	8 g
SATURATED FAT	2 g
CHOLESTEROL	27 mg
CARBOHYDRATE	21 g
FIBRE	9.5 g
PROTEIN	18 g
SUGARS	5 g
SODIUM	640 mg

Best Enchilada Sauce from Scratch

MAKES ENOUGH FOR 16 TO 18 ENCHILADAS

I have a serious weakness for enchiladas. As long as I have some tortillas, cheese and my homemade enchilada sauce, I can turn any leftover into a delicious enchilada. Shop-bought sauce is just not an option for me, and you'll see why after you try this simple homemade recipe. It makes enough for 16 to 18 enchiladas, so use what you need and freeze whatever you don't.

skinny**scoop**

I like to freeze this in freezer bags so I can quickly thaw what I need to whip up a Mexican fiesta any time I want!

½ teaspoon olive oil

4 garlic cloves, crushed

1½ cups (350ml) low-salt chicken stock*

3 cups (750g) passata

2 tablespoons chopped chipotle chilli in adobo sauce (or more to taste)†

1 teaspoon chilli powder (or to taste)

1 teaspoon ground cumin

½ teaspoon sea salt

⅛ teaspoon freshly ground black pepper

Read the label to be sure this product is gluten-free.

Heat a medium nonstick saucepan over medium heat. Add the oil and garlic and cook, stirring, until golden, about 1 to 1½ minutes. Add the chicken stock, passata, chipotle chilli, chilli powder, cumin, salt and black pepper. Bring to a boil, reduce the heat to low and simmer until the flavours blend, 7 to 10 minutes. Serve immediately, or allow to cool and refrigerate in an airtight container for up to 3 days, or keep frozen for up to 3 months.

† If you can't find chipotle chilli in adobo sauce, chipotle paste would work well as an alternative.

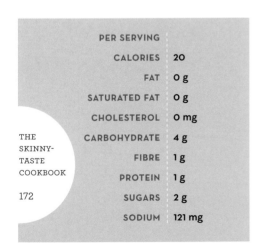

PER SERVING	
CALORIES	20
FAT	0 g
SATURATED FAT	0 g
CHOLESTEROL	0 mg
CARBOHYDRATE	4 g
FIBRE	1 g
PROTEIN	1 g
SUGARS	2 g
SODIUM	121 mg

Roasted Poblanos Rellenos with Chicken

SERVES 5

Meet my new favourite chile relleno! Okay, so this isn't exactly like a traditional chile relleno: stuffed with cheese, battered in egg and deep-fried. I gave these babies a much-needed healthy makeover, and they turned out awesome! This recipe is a little more labour-intensive than others, so I recommend making this on the weekend or when you have more time. You can even prepare it a day ahead and bake when ready to eat – and it freezes well once baked, so it's perfect for make-ahead meals for the week.

5 poblano or large sweet peppers

1 medium jalapeño or other green chilli

SAUCE

4 medium vine-ripened tomatoes, quartered

½ onion, chopped

3 garlic cloves

2 tablespoons chopped fresh coriander

1 teaspoon olive oil

1 teaspoon ground cumin

¾ teaspoon sea salt

FILLING

1 teaspoon olive oil

½ cup (80g) diced onion

4 garlic cloves, crushed

¼ cup (15g) finely chopped fresh coriander

225g cooked, shredded chicken breast (see page 80)

1 cup (180g) tinned haricot beans,* drained and lightly mashed

¾ cup (175ml) low-salt chicken stock*

½ teaspoon ground cumin

½ teaspoon garlic powder

¼ teaspoon sea salt

Freshly ground black pepper

1¼ cups (155g) grated reduced-fat Colby-Jack cheese blend†

2 tablespoons fresh coriander leaves, for garnish

Read the label to be sure this product is gluten-free.

Using a small, sharp knife, cut a slit lengthwise along one side of each pepper, then make a small crosswise slit along the top to create a T-shape, being careful not to cut off the stem. Carefully cut out and remove the core and scoop out the seeds. Holding the peppers with tongs, roast them and the jalapeño over an open flame, such as a barbecue or gas hob, turning often, until the skin is completely blistered and blackened. Transfer to a paper bag (or place in a bowl and cover with clingfilm) and allow

(recipe continues)

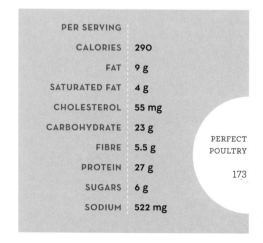

PER SERVING	
CALORIES	290
FAT	9 g
SATURATED FAT	4 g
CHOLESTEROL	55 mg
CARBOHYDRATE	23 g
FIBRE	5.5 g
PROTEIN	27 g
SUGARS	6 g
SODIUM	522 mg

to steam for 10 to 15 minutes. Use a table knife to scrape off the charred skins, being careful not to tear the peppers.

For the sauce: In a blender, combine the stemmed, roasted jalapeño pepper including the seeds, the tomatoes, onion, garlic, coriander and ¼ cup (50ml) water. Blend until smooth.

In a large, deep nonstick frying pan, heat the oil over medium heat. Add the puréed tomato mixture, cumin and salt. Simmer, uncovered, stirring occasionally, until slightly thickened and the colour turns deep red, 20 to 25 minutes.

Preheat the oven to 180°C/160°C fan/Gas 4.

Pour most of the sauce into the bottom of a 23 × 32cm baking dish (or pour some sauce into each of 5 individual 225g oval baking dishes).

For the filling: In a large nonstick frying pan, heat the oil over medium heat. Add the onion, garlic and coriander. Cook, stirring, until soft, about 2 minutes. Add the chicken, beans, stock, cumin, garlic powder, salt and black pepper to taste, and cook until the liquid has reduced, about 5 minutes.

Carefully stuff the filling into each pepper. Place the peppers seam side up on top of the sauce in the baking dish(es) and top each with cheese. Cover the dish tightly with foil. (You can stop here and refrigerate if you want to prepare this ahead.)

Bake until hot and bubbling, 20 to 30 minutes (or 30 to 40 minutes if the stuffed peppers were refrigerated). Serve hot with the remaining warm sauce on the side and garnished with coriander.

† If you can't find reduced-fat Colby-Jack cheese blend, a lighter cheddar will work well.

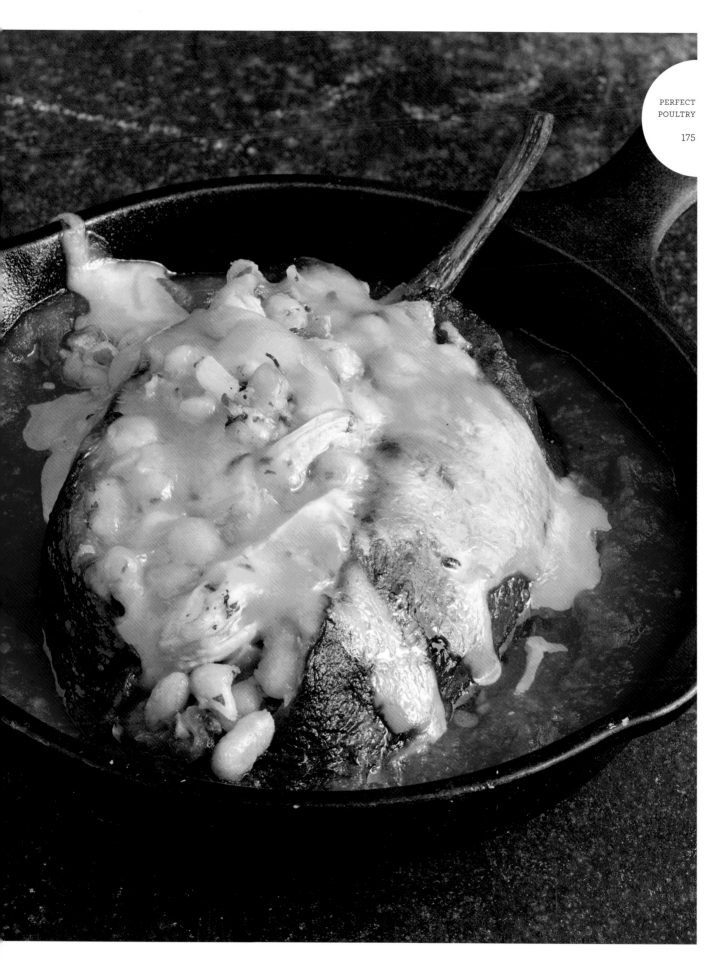

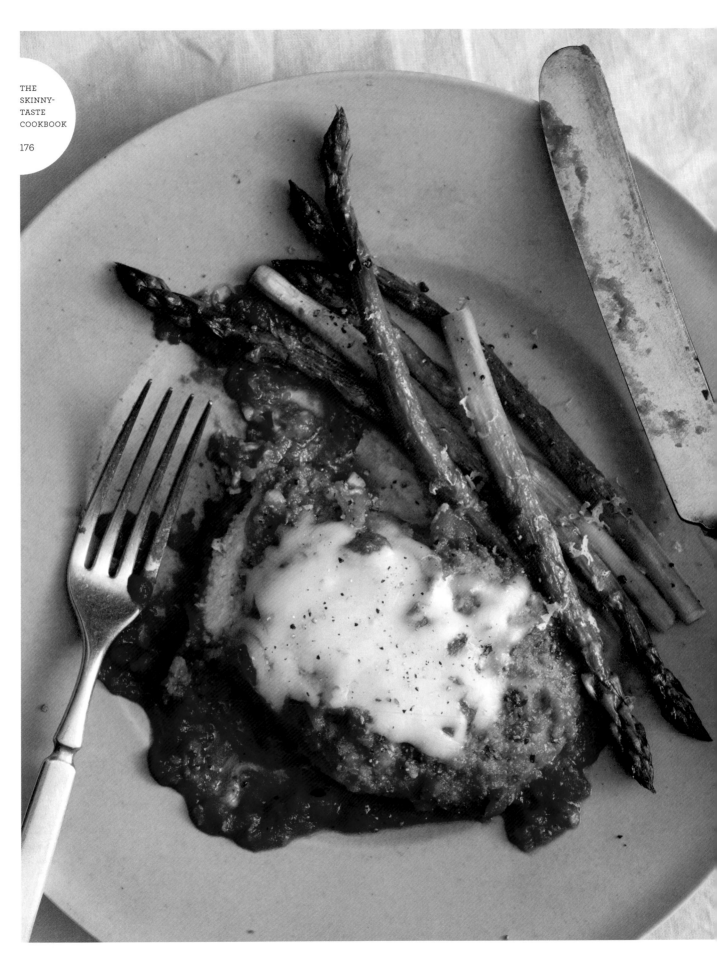

Skinny Chicken Parmesan

SERVES 6

Chicken Parmesan is one of the first dishes I learned to lighten up and one of my most popular recipes on *Skinnytaste*. If you're familiar with my blog, you'll notice some subtle differences. This iteration starts in the oven, and then finishes on the hob in a pan full of tomato sauce, so it's saucier than my previous version.

Cooking spray or oil mister

3 boneless, skinless chicken breasts (225g each), fat trimmed

¾ teaspoon sea salt

½ cup (40g) seasoned wholemeal bread crumbs, homemade (see page 110) or shop-bought

3 tablespoons grated Parmesan cheese

2 teaspoons melted unsalted butter

1 tablespoon olive oil

⅓ batch of Quickest Tomato Sauce (page 94) or shop-bought tomato sauce

9 tablespoons grated light mozzarella cheese

Preheat the oven to 220°C/200°C fan/Gas 8. Lightly spray a large baking sheet with oil.

Slice the chicken breasts in half horizontally to make 6 pieces. Season both sides with salt.

In a shallow bowl, combine the bread crumbs and Parmesan. In a small bowl, combine the butter and olive oil. Brush the butter and oil on both sides of the chicken, dredge the chicken in the bread-crumb mixture and put the chicken on the prepared baking sheet. Lightly spray oil on top of the chicken.

Bake until golden on the bottom, about 20 minutes. Turn the chicken over and bake until the centre is cooked through and the bottom is golden, 5 to 6 minutes.

Meanwhile, in a large, deep pan with a lid, cook the tomato sauce over medium heat until heated through, 2 to 3 minutes.

Place the baked chicken in the pan and top each piece with 1½ tablespoons of the mozzarella. Cover the pan and cook until the cheese melts, 3 to 4 minutes. Serve hot.

PERFECT PAIRINGS

Serve this over wholewheat pasta or along with **Lemon-Roasted Asparagus (page 278)**, pictured opposite. You can also serve it on a wholemeal baguette or bread to make it a skinny hero.

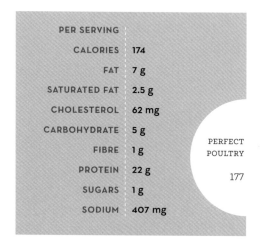

PER SERVING	
CALORIES	174
FAT	7 g
SATURATED FAT	2.5 g
CHOLESTEROL	62 mg
CARBOHYDRATE	5 g
FIBRE	1 g
PROTEIN	22 g
SUGARS	1 g
SODIUM	407 mg

PERFECT POULTRY

177

Asian Peanut Noodles with Chicken

SERVES 6

What's my Skinny secret to satisfy those noodle cravings while maintaining my waistline? For starters, I loaded up this dish with plenty of noodle-size vegetables. For the peanut sauce, I was able to cut the fat substantially by swapping the peanut butter for Better'n Peanut Butter. While nothing beats the taste of all-natural peanut butter spread over a slice of bread, I find Better'n Peanut Butter a suitable alternative when I'm cooking a dish that requires the same peanut taste without the fat. It's all-natural, with 85 per cent less fat and 40 per cent fewer calories. You can find it online, at Trader Joe's, and at natural foods stores.

PEANUT SAUCE

1 cup (225ml) low-salt chicken stock*

5 tablespoons Better'n Peanut Butter†

2 tablespoons honey

2 tablespoons soy sauce (or tamari* for gluten-free)

1 tablespoon Sriracha hot chilli sauce

1 tablespoon grated fresh ginger

2 garlic cloves, crushed

CHICKEN AND VEGETABLES

450g boneless, skinless chicken breast, cut into thin strips

Sea salt

Freshly ground black pepper

1 tablespoon Sriracha hot chilli sauce (or to taste)

1 tablespoon soy sauce (or tamari* for gluten-free)

Juice of ½ lime

4 garlic cloves, crushed

1 tablespoon grated fresh ginger

½ tablespoon sesame oil

¾ cup (90g) chopped spring onions

1¼ cups (200g) grated carrots

1¼ cups (115g) shredded green cabbage

225g rice noodles

2 tablespoons chopped unsalted roasted peanuts

6 lime wedges

6 sprigs of fresh coriander, for garnish

Read the label to be sure this product is gluten-free.

For the peanut sauce: In a small saucepan, combine the chicken stock, Better'n Peanut Butter, honey, soy sauce, Sriracha, ginger and garlic. Bring to a simmer over medium-low heat and cook, stirring occasionally, until the flavours blend and the sauce is slightly thickened, 8 to 10 minutes.

PER SERVING	
CALORIES	359
FAT	6 g
SATURATED FAT	1 g
CHOLESTEROL	48 mg
CARBOHYDRATE	53 g
FIBRE	4 g
PROTEIN	22 g
SUGARS	9 g
SODIUM	670 mg

(recipe continues)

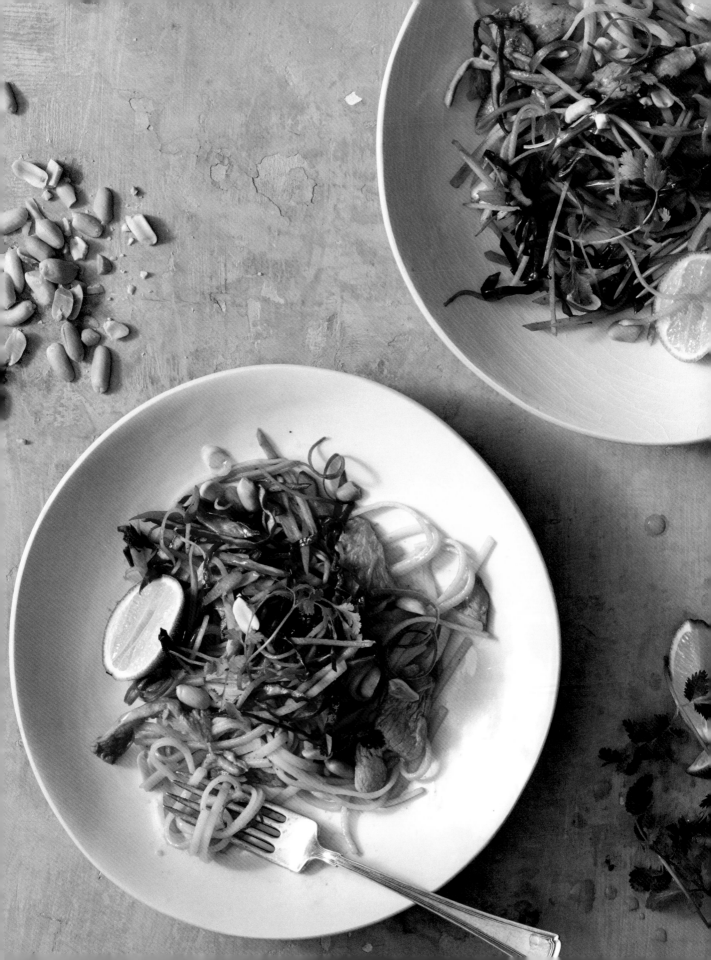

For the chicken: Season the chicken strips with ⅛ teaspoon of the salt and a pinch of black pepper, then transfer it to a large bowl and add the Sriracha, soy sauce, lime juice, 2 of the garlic cloves and the ginger.

Heat a large nonstick frying pan or wok over high heat. Add the sesame oil, then add the chicken. Cook, stirring, until cooked through, 2 to 3 minutes. Transfer to a plate. Add the remaining 2 garlic cloves, the spring onions, carrots and cabbage, and season with a pinch of salt. Cook, stirring, until the vegetables are crisp-tender, 1 to 2 minutes. Transfer to a plate.

Cook the noodles in a large pot of water according to packet instructions. Drain and put them in the hot wok. Add the chicken and peanut sauce and cook, tossing everything together, for 1 minute.

Divide the noodles and chicken evenly among the bowls. Top each with vegetables and 1 teaspoon peanuts. Serve with a lime wedge and a sprig of coriander, for garnish.

† If you can't find Better'n Peanut Butter, you can substitute this with a reduced-fat peanut butter.

Orecchiette with Sausage, Baby Kale and Pepper

SERVES 5

Weeknights are usually pretty hectic in my home. Madison keeps me super busy and wants my full, undivided attention, so I like to make meals as quick and simple as possible. Speed is what I love about this yummy pasta dish. In the same amount of time it takes to boil the water, the sausage and vegetables are cooked. Plus, this dish is a great way to incorporate healthy greens in your diet without having to do much prep work.

2¾ teaspoons sea salt

1 teaspoon olive oil

1 medium onion, chopped

1 medium red pepper, chopped

5 garlic cloves, chopped

Freshly ground black pepper

400g fresh sweet or hot Italian chicken sausages,* casings removed†

6 cups (240g) baby kale

275g wholewheat pasta such as orecchiette (use brown rice pasta for gluten-free)

¼ cup (25g) grated Pecorino Romano cheese, plus more for serving (optional)

¼ teaspoon crushed red chilli flakes (optional)

*Read the label to be sure this product is gluten-free.

Bring a large pot of water and 2 teaspoons of the salt to a boil.

Meanwhile, heat a large, deep nonstick frying pan over medium heat. Add the olive oil, onion, pepper, garlic, the remaining ¾ teaspoon salt and black pepper to taste. Cook, stirring, until soft, 4 to 5 minutes. Add the sausage and cook, using a wooden spoon to break the meat into small pieces as it browns, 6 to 8 minutes. Add the kale, cover and cook 2 to 3 minutes. Uncover, stir and cook until the kale is wilted, about 3 more minutes.

Add the pasta to the boiling water and cook to al dente according to the packet directions. Drain, reserving a cup of the pasta water, and add the cooked pasta to the pan. Add a third of the reserved pasta water. Increase the heat to medium-high, add

(recipe continues)

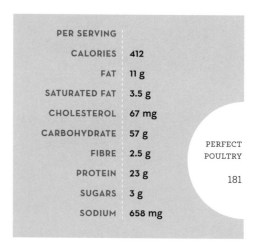

PER SERVING	
CALORIES	412
FAT	11 g
SATURATED FAT	3.5 g
CHOLESTEROL	67 mg
CARBOHYDRATE	57 g
FIBRE	2.5 g
PROTEIN	23 g
SUGARS	3 g
SODIUM	658 mg

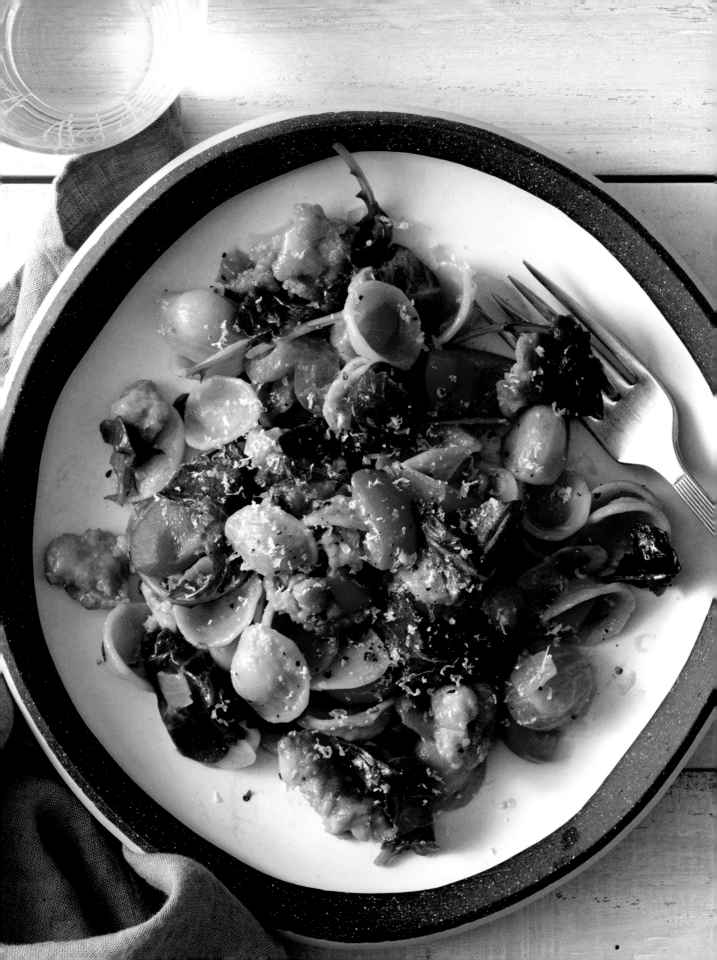

the Romano and chilli flakes (if using), and toss well. Cook for another 1 to 2 minutes, adding more of the reserved water, if needed. Transfer the pasta to a large bowl. Serve immediately with grated cheese, if desired.

✝ If you can't find Italian chicken sausages, another kind of chicken sausage or reduced-fat pork sausages will work well.

FOOD FACTS **kale, a super green**
Why should you love kale? Let us count the reasons. First, it's loaded with immune-boosting vitamin C, and it also chips in some vitamin A, vitamin K and calcium. Then there are all the phytochemicals: quercetin, kaempferol and sulphoraphane, which protect against a variety of diseases. And don't forget it's a source of alpha-linolenic acid, the plant form of omega-3 fatty acids.

Chicken Pasta Caprese

SERVES 5

Imagine a big bowl of pasta tossed with sweet tomatoes, lots of fresh basil, sautéed chicken breast and small chunks of mozzarella that start to melt when tossed with the hot pasta – good stuff! This is a summertime favourite in my home and a great way to use up all those glorious end-of-summer tomatoes. I personally love using unusual pasta shapes such as casarecce shown in the photo or gemelli, but penne would also work just fine.

450g skinless, boneless chicken breasts, cut into 1cm cubes

½ teaspoon dried basil

Sea salt

Freshly ground black pepper

Cooking spray or oil mister

250g pasta (use brown rice pasta for gluten-free)

4 teaspoons extra-virgin olive oil

6 garlic cloves, coarsely chopped

2½ cups (500g) halved baby plum tomatoes

¼ cup (15g) thinly sliced fresh basil

110g light mozzarella cheese, cut into cubes

Heat a large nonstick frying pan over high heat. Season the chicken with the dried basil, ¼ teaspoon of salt and black pepper to taste. Spray the pan with oil and add the chicken. Cook until the chicken is cooked through, about 3 minutes on each side. Transfer the chicken to a plate.

Cook the pasta to al dente in a pot of salted boiling water according to packet directions. Drain, reserving about ½ a cup (110ml) of the pasta water.

Meanwhile, increase the heat under the pan to high, add the olive oil and garlic and cook, stirring, until golden, being careful not to burn it, about 1 minute. Add the tomatoes, ⅛ teaspoon salt and black pepper to taste. Reduce the heat to medium-low. Cook, stirring, until the tomatoes become tender, 5 to 6 minutes.

Add the pasta to the tomatoes. If the pasta seems too dry, add some of the reserved pasta water. Add the chicken and toss well. Remove the pan from the heat, stir in the fresh basil and cheese and serve hot.

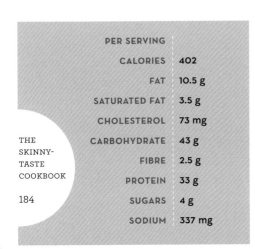

PER SERVING	
CALORIES	402
FAT	10.5 g
SATURATED FAT	3.5 g
CHOLESTEROL	73 mg
CARBOHYDRATE	43 g
FIBRE	2.5 g
PROTEIN	33 g
SUGARS	4 g
SODIUM	337 mg

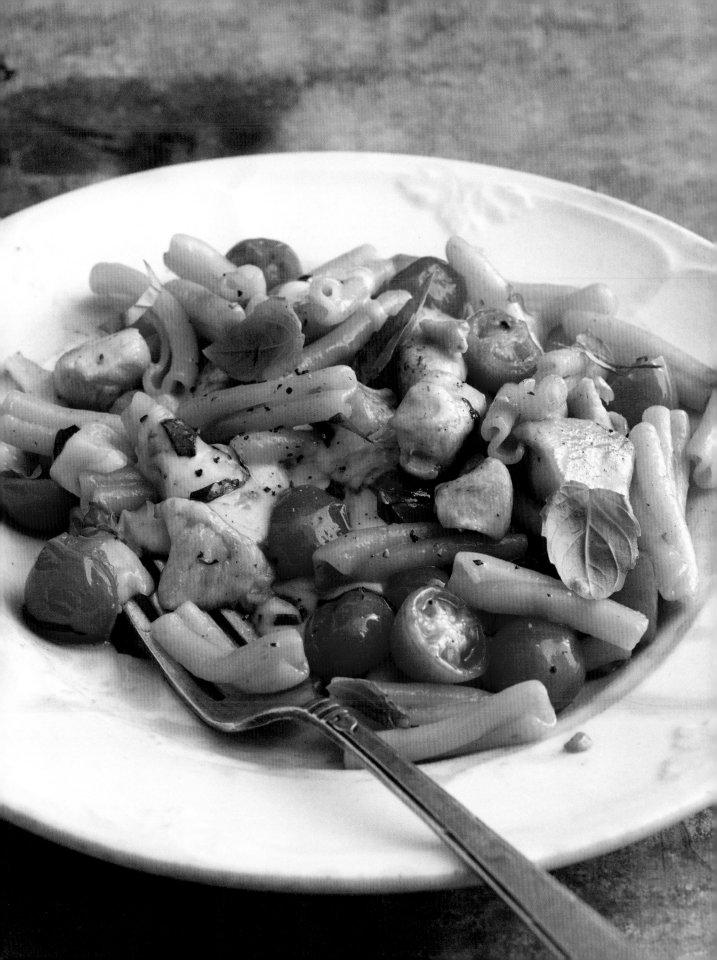

Cajun Chicken Pasta on the Lighter Side

SERVES 5

When I'm ragin' for Cajun, I love to make this colourful pasta dish loaded with yummy vegetables and sautéed chicken in a light, creamy sauce that has a bit of a kick! A few years back I was asked to remake this dish, which is popular at a chain restaurant. I love a challenge, so I was happy to tackle it, and it has since become one of the most popular dishes on *Skinnytaste* – it's that good!

⅓ cup (75ml) skimmed milk

1 tablespoon plain flour (or glutinous rice flour for gluten-free)

3 tablespoons light cream cheese

225g linguine (use brown rice pasta for gluten-free*)

Sea salt

450g boneless, skinless chicken breasts, sliced into strips

1¼ teaspoons Cajun seasoning (or more to taste)

1 teaspoon garlic powder

⅛ teaspoon freshly ground black pepper

Cooking spray or oil mister

1 tablespoon olive oil

1 medium red pepper, thinly sliced

1 medium yellow pepper, thinly sliced

½ medium red onion, sliced

3 garlic cloves, crushed

225g mushrooms, sliced

2 medium tomatoes, chopped

1 cup (225ml) low-salt chicken stock*

2 medium spring onions, chopped

Read the label to be sure this product is gluten-free.

In a blender, make a slurry by combining the milk, flour and cream cheese. Set aside.

Cook the pasta to al dente in a pot of salted water according to packet directions. Drain and set aside.

Meanwhile, heat a large, heavy nonstick frying pan over medium-high heat. Season the chicken with 1 teaspoon Cajun seasoning, ½ teaspoon of the garlic powder and ¼ teaspoon salt. Spray the pan with oil and add half of the chicken. Cook until cooked through, about 3 minutes on each side. Transfer to a plate and repeat with the remaining chicken.

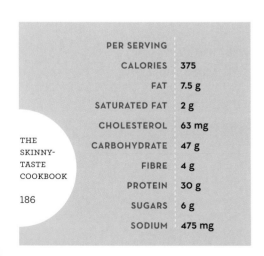

PER SERVING	
CALORIES	375
FAT	7.5 g
SATURATED FAT	2 g
CHOLESTEROL	63 mg
CARBOHYDRATE	47 g
FIBRE	4 g
PROTEIN	30 g
SUGARS	6 g
SODIUM	475 mg

Add the olive oil to the pan and reduce the heat to medium. Add the peppers, onion and garlic, cook, stirring, until almost tender, 3 to 4 minutes. Add the mushrooms and tomatoes and cook, stirring, until the vegetables are tender, 3 to 4 more minutes. Add the remaining ½ teaspoon garlic powder and season with ½ teaspoon salt and the black pepper. Reduce the heat to medium-low, add the chicken stock and the slurry and cook, stirring, until it begins to thicken, about 2 minutes.

Return the chicken strips to the pan. Adjust with ⅛ teaspoon salt and the remaining ¼ teaspoon Cajun seasoning, or more to taste, and cook until heated through, about 1 minute. Add the linguine and toss well to coat.

To serve, divide the pasta and chicken among the plates and sprinkle with the spring onions.

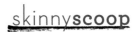

skinnyscoop

Have all your vegetables prepped and ingredients ready before you start cooking. That way, it will all come together in about the same amount of time it takes to cook the pasta.

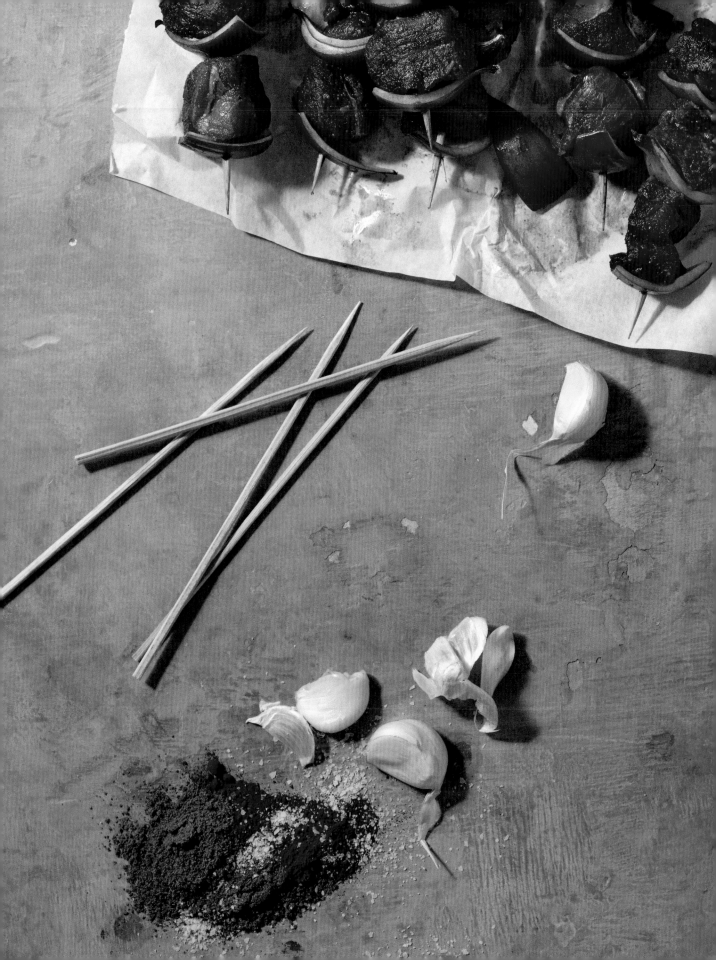

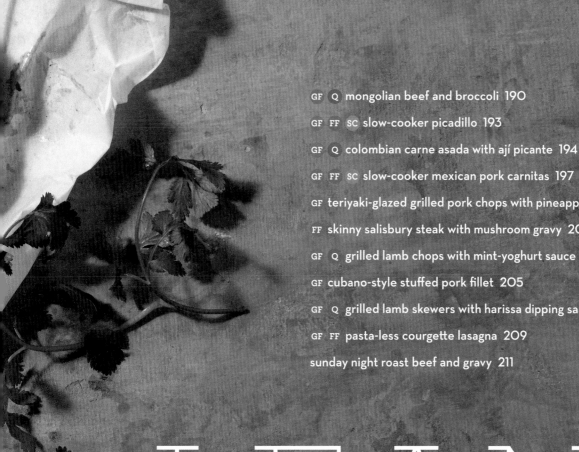

LEAN MEAT DISHES

Mongolian Beef and Broccoli

SERVES 4

Two dishes – Mongolian beef; beef and broccoli – combine in this easy and lighter alternative to a Chinese take away. It's made with lean strips of sirloin steak, broccoli florets and spring onions in a sweet and savoury light stir-fry sauce. Fortunately, nothing is quicker than stir-fry, perfect for weeknights.

2 teaspoons cornflour

3 tablespoons plus 2 teaspoons reduced-salt soy sauce (use tamari* for gluten-free)

2 teaspoons rice wine

4 teaspoons sesame oil

450g sirloin steak, trimmed of fat, thinly sliced against the grain

¼ teaspoon sea salt

4 cups (240g) broccoli florets

4 medium spring onions, cut into 2 to 3cm pieces; white and greens separated

1 tablespoon crushed garlic

½ teaspoon crushed fresh ginger

2 heaped tablespoons dark brown sugar

1 tablespoon oyster sauce*

PERFECT PAIRINGS
Serve this with ¾ cup (140g) cooked brown jasmine or basmati rice, or, if you have leftover brown rice, whip up **Vegetable Fried Brown Rice (page 273)**.

Read the label to be sure this product is gluten-free.

In a shallow glass container, whisk together the cornflour, 2 teaspoons of the soy sauce, the rice wine and 1 teaspoon of the sesame oil. Season the steak with salt, add to the marinade and turn to coat. Allow to sit at room temperature for 30 minutes.

Bring a large pot of water to a rolling boil. Add the broccoli and cook until bright green and crisp-tender, about 1 minute. Drain and run under cold water to stop the cooking.

Heat a large nonstick wok or frying pan over high heat. Add 1 teaspoon of the oil, then half of the beef. Cook for 30 seconds without disturbing, flip and cook another 30 seconds, moving the meat around until browned on all sides. Transfer to a plate and repeat with 1 teaspoon oil and the remaining beef.

Heat the remaining 1 teaspoon sesame oil in the wok and add the spring onion whites, garlic and ginger. Cook until fragrant, about 30 seconds. Add the broccoli, brown sugar, remaining 3 tablespoons soy sauce and the oyster sauce and cook, stirring, for 30 seconds. Add the beef and cook, stirring, 30 more seconds. Remove from the heat and stir in the spring onion greens.

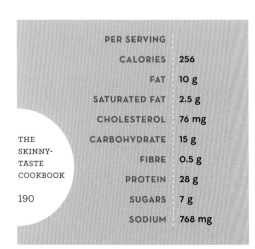

PER SERVING	
CALORIES	256
FAT	10 g
SATURATED FAT	2.5 g
CHOLESTEROL	76 mg
CARBOHYDRATE	15 g
FIBRE	0.5 g
PROTEIN	28 g
SUGARS	7 g
SODIUM	768 mg

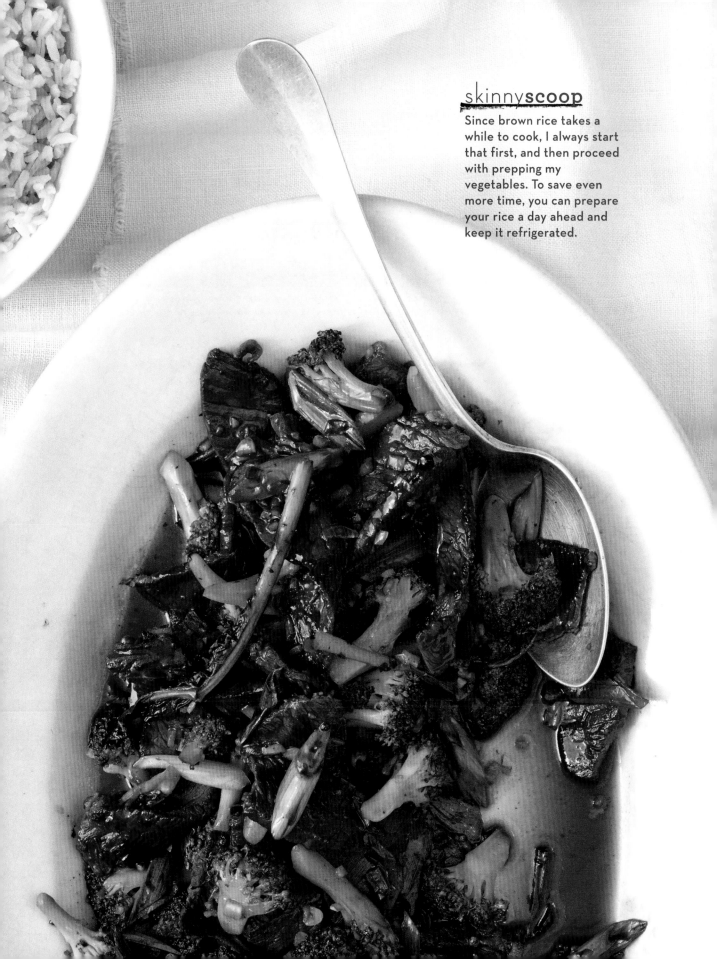

skinnyscoop

Since brown rice takes a while to cook, I always start that first, and then proceed with prepping my vegetables. To save even more time, you can prepare your rice a day ahead and keep it refrigerated.

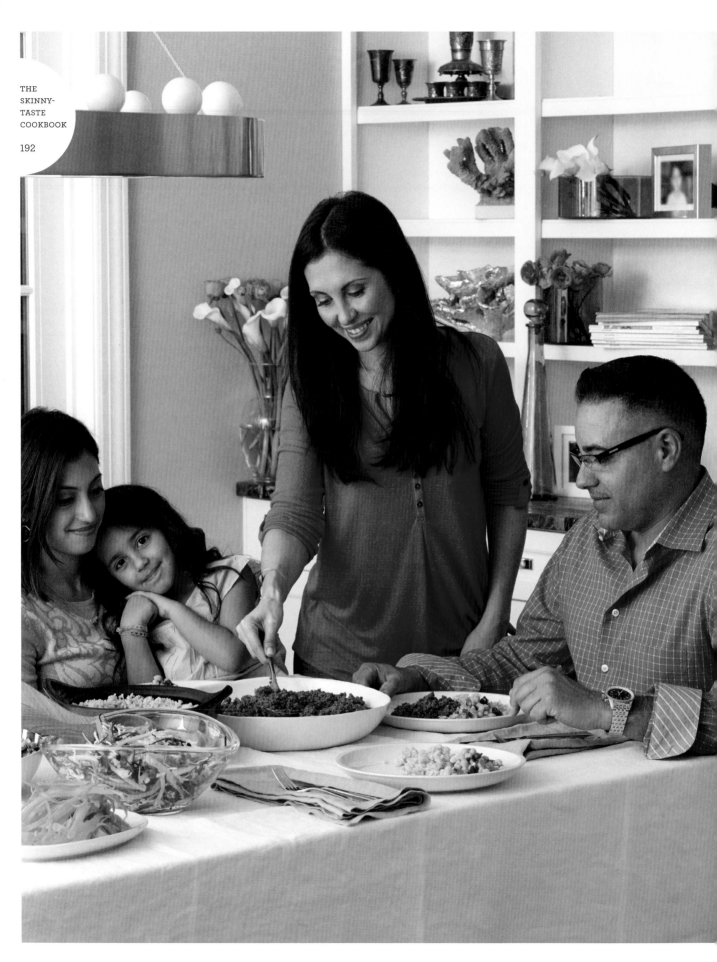

Slow-Cooker Picadillo

SERVES 10

At least once a month – if not more often – it's Picadillo Night at my house. My whole family loves it when I whip up this flavourful Cuban dish, and I love it because it's so easy and inexpensive. I grew up on this dish, which was one of Mom's specialities. Throughout the years, I've adapted her version by using leaner beef; and rather than making it on the hob, I find it convenient to make this in the slow cooker, which helps make the meat very tender. Some people also add raisins, but my family prefers it without them.

1.2kg lean beef mince

2 teaspoons sea salt

Freshly ground black pepper

1 cup (155g) finely chopped onion

1 cup (175g) chopped red pepper

3 garlic cloves, crushed

¼ cup (15g) finely chopped fresh coriander

1 small tomato, chopped

¼ cup (30g) stoned green olives or stoned pimento-stuffed Spanish olives

225g passata

1 tablespoon of the brine from the olives

1½ teaspoons ground cumin, plus more as needed

¼ teaspoon garlic powder

2 bay leaves

Set a large, deep frying pan over medium-high heat, add the beef and season it with the salt and a pinch of black pepper. Cook, using a wooden spoon to break the meat into small pieces as it browns, 4 to 5 minutes. Drain the liquid from the pan. Add the onion, pepper and garlic to the meat and cook until fragrant, 3 to 4 minutes.

Transfer the mixture to a slow cooker and add the coriander, tomato, olives, passata, brine, cumin, garlic powder, bay leaves and 1¼ cups (300ml) water. Cover and cook on high for 3 to 4 hours or on low for 6 to 8 hours.

To serve, taste for cumin and add more as needed. Discard the bay leaves. Serve a generous ladleful per person.

PERFECT PAIRINGS

Serve this over brown rice with a simple cabbage salad, like my **Confetti Slaw (page 285)**, pictured on page 192, or served with tortillas to make tacos. This also makes a great filling for stuffed peppers or empanadas.

PER SERVING	
CALORIES	207
FAT	8.5 g
SATURATED FAT	3.5 g
CHOLESTEROL	74 mg
CARBOHYDRATE	5 g
FIBRE	1 g
PROTEIN	28 g
SUGARS	3 g
SODIUM	477 mg

LEAN MEAT DISHES

Colombian Carne Asada with Ají Picante

SERVES 6

Carne asada is a marinated grilled steak dish that is a beloved staple in Colombia, where my mom was born. Whenever we get together for family barbecues, this is usually on the menu. The steaks are served with *ají picante*, a popular condiment that you can make as mild or as spicy as you like. It's a fantastic complement that adds a touch of heat, freshness and acidity, and it can be used in everything from soups and stews to steaks and empanadas.

STEAK

675g flank steak

1 teaspoon ground cumin

½ teaspoon dried oregano

½ teaspoon sea salt

Freshly ground black pepper

1 tablespoon olive oil

3 garlic cloves, crushed

3 spring onions, cut into 2 to 3cm lengths

¾ cup (175ml) light beer

AJÍ PICANTE

2 tablespoons fresh lime juice

½ tablespoon distilled white vinegar

¼ cup (30g) finely chopped spring onions

¼ cup (15g) finely chopped fresh coriander (stems and leaves)

¼ cup (50g) seeded and finely chopped tomato

1 tablespoon finely chopped fresh jalapeño, serrano or other green chilli

¼ teaspoon plus ⅛ teaspoon sea salt

Cooking spray or oil mister

skinny

I never throw away the stems of the coriander! They add so much flavour and texture to the *ají* sauce.

For the steak: Using a sharp knife, lightly score the steak about 2.5mm deep on both sides in a crisscross pattern at 1cm intervals. Put the steak in a shallow glass baking dish.

In a small bowl, combine the cumin, oregano, salt and a few turns of black pepper. Rub the olive oil and garlic over both sides of the steak, and then rub in the spice mix. Add the spring onions and beer, turn the steak over a few times to coat both sides, cover the dish, and refrigerate for at least 3 hours, turning occasionally, or as long as overnight.

For the ají picante: In a medium jar or container with a fitted lid, combine ¼ cup (50ml) water, the lime juice, vinegar, spring onions, coriander, tomato, jalapeño and salt. Refrigerate until ready to use and for up to 2 days.

(recipe continues)

PER SERVING	
CALORIES	208
FAT	9.5 g
SATURATED FAT	3 g
CHOLESTEROL	78 mg
CARBOHYDRATE	3 g
FIBRE	0.5 g
PROTEIN	25 g
SUGARS	1 g
SODIUM	233 mg

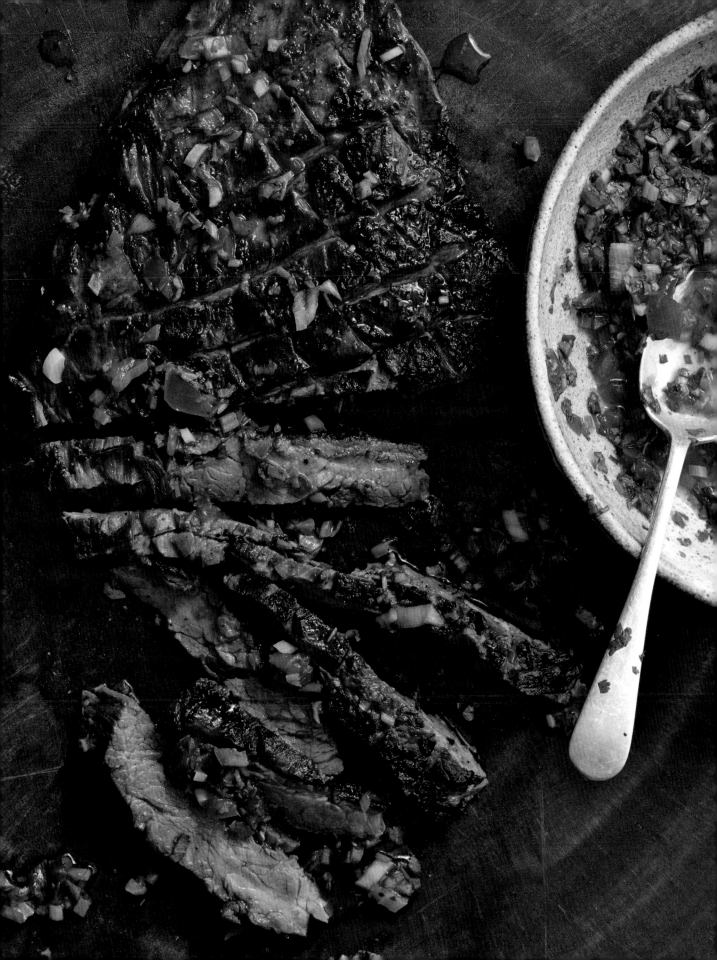

Typically, my family serves this with small potatoes or grilled arepas, which are Colombian corn cakes; but you can serve it with grilled corn on the cob, rice or on top of a bed of salad leaves to make a steak salad. Or try it with **Grilled Mexican Corn Salad (page 289)**.

Preheat a barbecue or grill pan to high.

Lightly oil the grate. Remove the steaks from the marinade, discarding the marinade, and grill to desired doneness, 3 to 4 minutes per side for medium-rare, turning the steaks a quarter-turn after 1½ minutes to form crisscross grill marks, if desired. Transfer the steaks to a chopping board and allow to rest 5 minutes. Thinly slice the steaks across the grain. Transfer to a platter and serve with *ají picante* on the side.

Steak Out!

You can have your meat and it eat, too – you just have to pick the leanest and healthiest types. Here's how.

CHECK THE CUT: There are plenty of lean cuts of meat (those containing less than 10 grams of total fat and 4.5 grams or less saturated fat per 100 gram serving), but in general, sirloin steaks are your best bet. Fillet and flank steak are also good choices. And, of course, you can always consult with the butcher.

Slow-Cooker Mexican Pork Carnitas

SERVES 10

Taco night is a weekly event in my home, and this spicy pork makes the perfect filling. Pork shoulder is often sold with the bone in. To save time, I have my butcher remove the bone for me, but you can leave it in and increase the cooking time to 10 hours. This makes enough for several dinners, so it's super economical and can be used so many different ways, from tacos to salads, or even served over rice.

900g boneless pork shoulder joint, trimmed

½ teaspoon sea salt

DRY ADOBO RUB

1¼ teaspoons ground cumin

½ teaspoon garlic powder

½ teaspoon dried oregano

½ teaspoon plus ¼ teaspoon sea salt

¼ teaspoon ground black pepper

6 garlic cloves, crushed

½ cup (120ml) low-salt chicken stock*

2 bay leaves

2 chipotle chillies in adobo sauce, chopped (or more if you like it spicy)†

¼ teaspoon ground cumin

Read the label to be sure this product is gluten-free.

Season the pork all over with the salt. Set a large nonstick pan over medium-high heat, add the pork and brown on all sides for about 10 minutes. Remove from the heat.

For the dry arobo rub: In a small bowl, combine 1 teaspoon of the cumin, the garlic powder, oregano, ½ teaspoon of the salt and the black pepper.

Using a sharp paring knife, insert the knife into the pork about 2 to 3cm deep and insert the crushed garlic, rubbing any excess over the pork. Rub the pork all over with the dry adobo rub.

Pour the chicken stock into the slow cooker and add the bay leaves, chipotle chillies and pork. Cover and cook on low for 8 hours. After 8 hours, transfer the pork to a large dish. Discard the bay leaves. Shred the pork using two forks and return it to the slow cooker with the juices. Add the remaining ¼ teaspoon cumin and the ¼ teaspoon salt. Serve.

† If you can't find chipotle chillies in adobo sauce, chipotle paste would work well as an alternative.

PERFECT PAIRINGS
Serve this pork on warmed tortillas and top with some **Confetti Slaw (page 285)**. We also like to serve it over coriander lime rice (combine ¾ cup (140g) cooked brown rice with a squeeze of lime juice and 1 tablespoon chopped fresh coriander).

PER SERVING	
CALORIES	112
FAT	3 g
SATURATED FAT	1 g
CHOLESTEROL	50 mg
CARBOHYDRATE	1 g
FIBRE	0 g
PROTEIN	19 g
SUGARS	0 g
SODIUM	213 mg

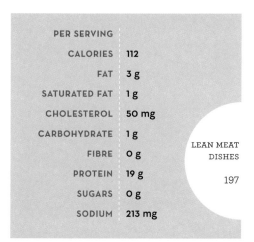

LEAN MEAT DISHES

197

Teriyaki-Glazed Grilled Pork Chops with Pineapple Salsa

SERVES 5

The homemade pineapple-teriyaki glaze is really the star of this dish. It's so good you may even want to double the recipe and keep it in your refrigerator – it's great on everything from burgers to salmon and steak! I love pork chops, but lean chops can sometimes be tricky because they dry out if not cooked properly. Marinating them in pineapple juice, which is acidic, and cooking them on the grill for about 6 minutes on each side yields perfectly juicy chops. If pork isn't your thing, you can replace it with skinless chicken breasts or lean sirloin steaks instead.

PORK CHOPS

¼ cup (50ml) pineapple juice

4 teaspoons reduced-salt soy sauce (or tamari* for gluten-free)

1 large garlic clove, crushed

½ teaspoon grated fresh ginger

5 boneless pork loin chops (110g each), trimmed of fat

TERIYAKI SAUCE

1 teaspoon cornflour

3 tablespoons reduced-salt soy sauce (or tamari* for gluten-free)

¼ cup (50ml) pineapple juice

2 tablespoons dark brown sugar

½ teaspoon grated fresh ginger

1 small garlic clove, crushed

PINEAPPLE SALSA

1⅓ cups (255g) fresh pineapple, cut into 1cm cubes

1 jalapeño or other green chilli, finely chopped

2 tablespoons finely chopped red onion

1 tablespoon finely chopped fresh coriander

Cooking spray or oil mister

Read the label to be sure this product is gluten-free.

For the pork chops: In a small bowl, combine the pineapple juice, soy sauce, garlic and ginger. Put the pork chops in a container and pour the marinade over them. Allow to sit for about 30 minutes.

For the teriyaki sauce: In a small bowl, whisk together the cornflour and 3 tablespoons cold water until dissolved. In a small saucepan, combine the soy sauce, pineapple juice, brown sugar, ginger and garlic. Bring to a boil over medium-low heat and cook until reduced and thickened, about 4 minutes. Add the cornflour

(recipe continues)

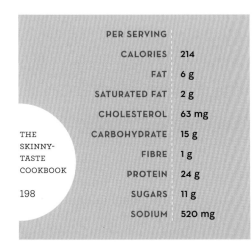

PER SERVING	
CALORIES	214
FAT	6 g
SATURATED FAT	2 g
CHOLESTEROL	63 mg
CARBOHYDRATE	15 g
FIBRE	1 g
PROTEIN	24 g
SUGARS	11 g
SODIUM	520 mg

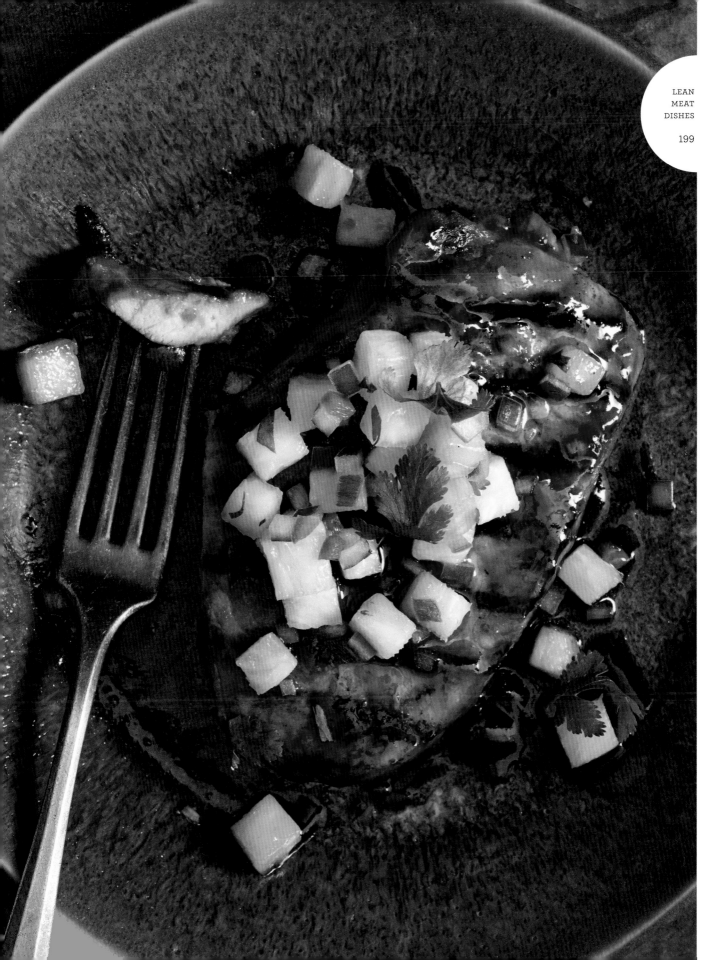

Try this with stir-fried vegetables, **Roasted Sesame Green Beans (page 272)**, or a side of **Vegetable Fried Brown Rice (page 273)**.

skinny**scoop**

When it comes to fruit, I always prefer fresh, but if you're pressed for time, you can use pre-cut to make the salsa. Look for pineapple that is packed in pineapple juice; you can use the juice from the tin to make the marinade.

mixture and cook until thickened, about 2 more minutes. Remove the pan from the heat and set aside to cool.

For the pineapple salsa: In a small bowl, combine the pineapple, jalapeño, red onion and coriander. Set aside.

Preheat a barbecue to medium-high (or preheat a grill pan over medium-high heat).

Remove the chops from the marinade, discarding the marinade. Oil the grill grates or spray a grill pan with oil. Grill the chops until no longer pink, 6 to 7 minutes per side. Spoon 1 tablespoon of the teriyaki sauce over each chop in the final 30 seconds of cooking time.

To serve, put a chop on each dish and top each with pineapple salsa.

Skinny Salisbury Steak with Mushroom Gravy

SERVES 8

The name 'Salisbury steak' reminds me of frozen TV dinners from way back when, but these are nothing like those tasteless meat patties. This dish is moist and flavourful, with a delicious mushroom gravy that is wonderful over Cheesy Cauliflower 'Mash'.

1½ teaspoons olive oil

¾ cup (115g) finely chopped onion

450g lean beef mince

450g lean turkey breast mince

½ cup (50g) fine dried bread crumbs

1 large egg

1 large egg white

2 cups (450ml) beef stock

¼ teaspoon plus ⅛ teaspoon sea salt

⅛ teaspoon freshly ground black pepper, plus more for seasoning

2 tablespoons plain flour

2 tablespoons tomato paste

1 teaspoon red wine vinegar

2 teaspoons Worcestershire sauce

½ teaspoon mustard powder

225g sliced mushrooms

2 tablespoons chopped fresh parsley, for garnish

Heat a large, deep nonstick frying pan over medium heat. Add the oil and onion and cook, stirring, until golden, about 5 minutes.

In a large bowl, combine half of the cooked onion, the beef, turkey, bread crumbs, whole egg, egg white, an eighth of the beef stock, ¼ teaspoon of the salt and the black pepper. Form into 8 oval patties that are about 2cm thick.

In a bowl, whisk together the flour and remaining beef stock. Stir in ¼ cup (50ml) water, the remaining cooked onion, tomato paste, vinegar, Worcestershire sauce and mustard powder.

Wipe down the pan and heat over medium-high heat. Working in batches so you don't overcrowd the pan, cook the patties until browned, 2 to 3 minutes per side. Transfer to a plate.

Add the mushrooms to the pan, season with the remaining ⅛ teaspoon salt and black pepper to taste and cook, stirring, until slightly browned, 2 to 3 minutes. Return the patties to the pan and pour in the sauce. Reduce the heat to low, cover and simmer, stirring occasionally, until the meat is tender, 25 minutes. Serve hot with parsley sprinkled on top.

PERFECT PAIRINGS
Try this with **Cheesy Cauliflower 'Mash' (page 269)** and some steamed sweetcorn or peas on the side.

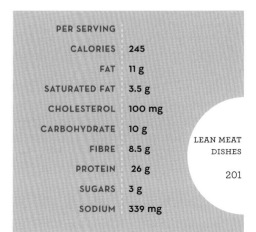

PER SERVING	
CALORIES	245
FAT	11 g
SATURATED FAT	3.5 g
CHOLESTEROL	100 mg
CARBOHYDRATE	10 g
FIBRE	8.5 g
PROTEIN	26 g
SUGARS	3 g
SODIUM	339 mg

LEAN MEAT DISHES

Grilled Lamb Chops with Mint-Yoghurt Sauce

SERVES 4

Lamb loin chops are perfect for weeknight meals because they take less than 15 minutes to cook. They're also a lot less expensive than lamb cutlets and they're much leaner if trimmed – it's a win-win! Mint and lamb are a perfect combination, so this yoghurt sauce makes a great complement to the meat. I like to marinate the chops for a few hours prior to cooking and prepare the yoghurt sauce ahead of time to let the flavours settle. Don't worry if you don't have the time – it will still taste great.

MINT-YOGHURT SAUCE

¾ cup (185g) fat-free Greek yoghurt

1 teaspoon extra-virgin olive oil

1 teaspoon fresh lemon juice

2 tablespoons finely chopped fresh mint

1½ tablespoons finely chopped fresh chives

½ teaspoon sea salt

Freshly ground black pepper

LAMB CHOPS

8 lamb loin chops (100g each), fat trimmed

1 teaspoon sea salt

½ teaspoon freshly ground black pepper

2 tablespoons fresh lemon juice

4 garlic cloves, crushed

1 tablespoon fresh rosemary

½ teaspoon dried oregano

Cooking spray or oil mister

PERFECT PAIRINGS
This pairs perfectly with the **Roasted Winter Beetroot and Red Potatoes (page 279).**

For the mint-yoghurt sauce: In a medium bowl, combine the yoghurt, olive oil, lemon juice, mint, chives, salt and black pepper to taste. Cover and refrigerate for a few hours to let the flavours develop.

For the lamb chops: Season both sides of the lamb chops with the salt and black pepper to taste. Place the chops in a large bowl and pour the lemon juice over them. Add the garlic, rosemary and oregano. Cover with clingfilm and marinate at room temperature for 1 hour, or as long as overnight in the refrigerator.

Preheat a barbecue to medium-high (or preheat a grill pan over medium-high heat). Oil the grill grates or spray the grill pan with oil. Grill the chops until a thermometer inserted in the side of each chop registers 63°C for medium-rare or higher to your taste, 4 to 6 minutes on each side.

Serve the lamb chops with the mint-yoghurt sauce on the side.

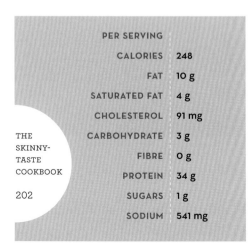

PER SERVING	
CALORIES	248
FAT	10 g
SATURATED FAT	4 g
CHOLESTEROL	91 mg
CARBOHYDRATE	3 g
FIBRE	0 g
PROTEIN	34 g
SUGARS	1 g
SODIUM	541 mg

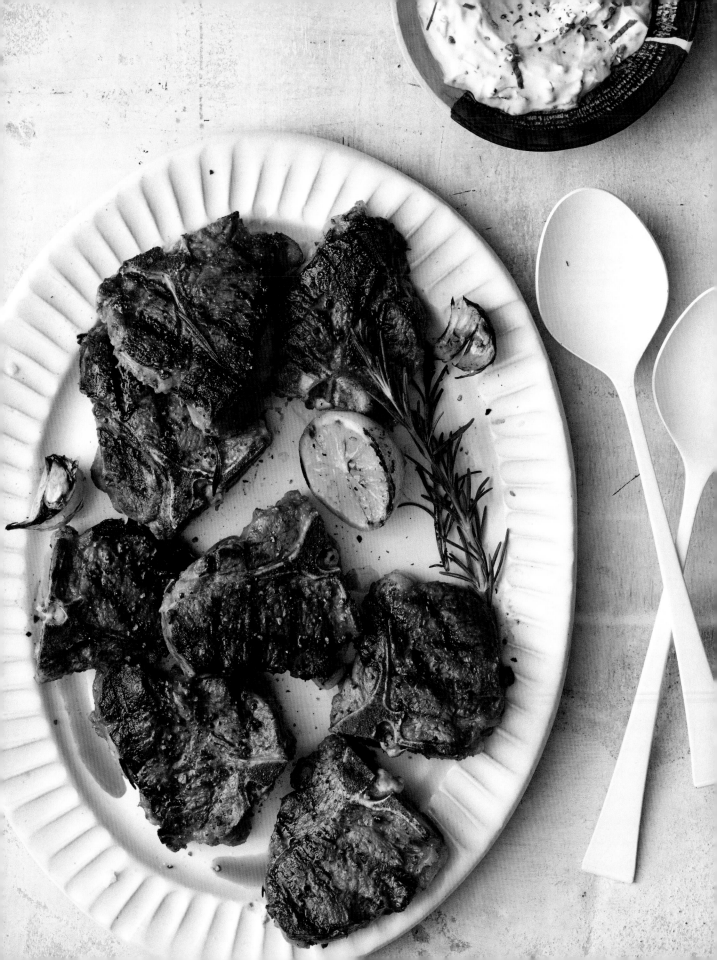

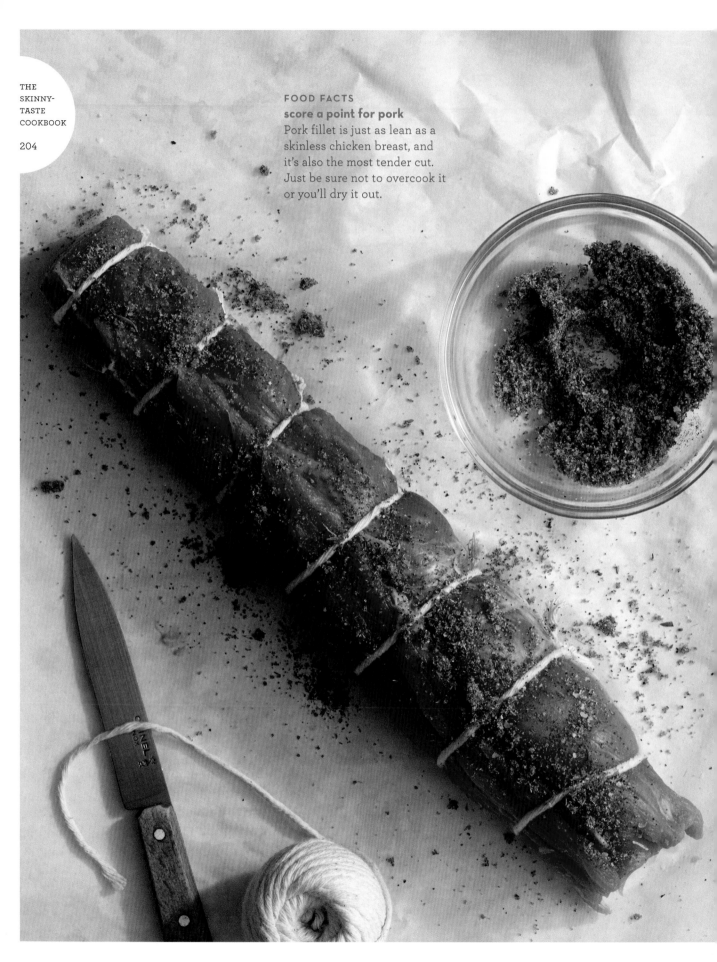

FOOD FACTS
score a point for pork
Pork fillet is just as lean as a
skinless chicken breast, and
it's also the most tender cut.
Just be sure not to overcook it
or you'll dry it out.

Cubano-Style Stuffed Pork Fillet

SERVES 4

 GF

When I was in my early twenties I discovered a Cuban café in Queens called El Sitio that made the *best* Cubano (grilled pork, ham and cheese) sandwiches! Although it's been years since my last visit, a craving for that sandwich still arises. Inspired by that sandwich, this pork dish is my Cubano skinny solution.

PORK

450g pork fillet

1 tablespoon American mustard

50g thinly sliced ham*

50g lighter Swiss cheese, sliced

2 thin slices dill pickle, about 10cm long, patted dry

1 teaspoon olive oil

DRY RUB

1 teaspoon dark brown sugar

¾ teaspoon sea salt

1 teaspoon garlic powder

½ teaspoon chilli powder*

½ teaspoon ground cumin

¼ teaspoon dried oregano

⅛ teaspoon freshly ground black pepper

Read the label to be sure this product is gluten-free.

Preheat the oven to 220°C/200°C fan/Gas 7.

For the pork: Cut a lengthwise slit down the centre of the fillet to within 1cm of the bottom and open the fillet so it lies flat. On each half, make another lengthwise slit down the centre to within 1cm of the bottom and open it up. Wrap with clingfilm. Pound with a mallet until 5mm thick. Remove the clingfilm and spread the mustard on one side. Layer the ham on the mustard and lay the Swiss cheese and pickles along the centre of the pork. Starting with a long side, roll the pork up Swiss-roll style. Tie the pork at 4 to 5cm intervals with kitchen string. Rub with the olive oil.

For the dry rub: In a medium bowl, combine the brown sugar, salt, garlic powder, chilli powder, cumin, oregano and black pepper. Rub the mixture over the pork, discarding any excess. Put the pork in a shallow baking dish.

Roast until a thermometer inserted in the pork registers 71°C, about 35 minutes. Transfer to a chopping board. Allow to rest 10 minutes before removing the string and slicing into 8 pieces.

PERFECT PAIRINGS
The Latina in me likes to serve this with rice, but a great big salad on the side is also perfect. Try **My House Salad, Made with Love (page 267)**.

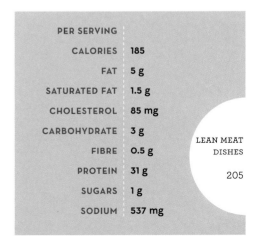

PER SERVING	
CALORIES	185
FAT	5 g
SATURATED FAT	1.5 g
CHOLESTEROL	85 mg
CARBOHYDRATE	3 g
FIBRE	0.5 g
PROTEIN	31 g
SUGARS	1 g
SODIUM	537 mg

LEAN MEAT DISHES

Grilled Lamb Skewers with Harissa Dipping Sauce

MAKES 12 SKEWERS · SERVES 6

If I'm throwing a backyard party, I like to grill all kinds of different skewers and let everyone dig in. There's something fun and casual about forgoing forks and eating food right off a stick. These lamb skewers are a favourite for their exotic flavours and spicy harissa dipping sauce. Harissa is a traditional accompaniment to Moroccan and North African food. In a pinch, you can purchase jarred harissa, but making it yourself gives you complete control over how spicy you want it. Leftovers can be refrigerated and used on everything from eggs and burgers to couscous and soups.

LAMB

675g trimmed boneless leg of lamb, cut into 2 to 3cm cubes

½ tablespoon olive oil

3 garlic cloves, crushed

1 tablespoon finely chopped fresh coriander

2¼ teaspoons ground cumin

½ teaspoon sweet paprika

¾ teaspoon sea salt

12 wooden skewers, soaked in water for 30 minutes

1 medium red onion, quartered and layers separated

HARISSA

1 tablespoon olive oil

2 large garlic cloves, peeled

350g roasted red peppers in water, jarred, drained

1 teaspoon fresh lemon juice

1½ teaspoons sea salt

1 teaspoon crushed red chilli flakes (or to taste)

½ teaspoon ground coriander

½ teaspoon ground cumin

½ teaspoon sweet paprika

PERFECT PAIRINGS
Serve this with a Persian salad (see recipe in **Naked Persian Turkey Burgers [page 156]**) or try this with my **Quinoa Tabbouleh (page 287)**.

For the lamb: Place the lamb in a bowl and rub it with the olive oil, garlic and coriander. In a small bowl, combine the cumin, paprika and salt and rub the mixture on the lamb. Marinate for 3 to 4 hours. Thread the lamb onto the skewers, 3 to 4 per skewer, with onion slices in between.

For the harissa: In a small pan, heat the oil over medium heat. Add the garlic and cook, stirring, until golden and fragrant, 1 to 2 minutes. Transfer the garlic to a blender and add the roasted red peppers, lemon juice, salt, chilli flakes, coriander, cumin and paprika. Blend until smooth.

Preheat a barbecue to high (or preheat a grill pan over high heat).

Grill the skewers 3 to 4 minutes per side. Transfer to a platter and serve with the harissa on the side.

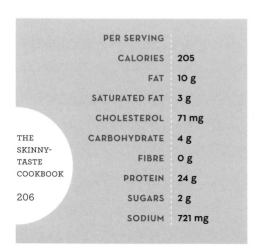

PER SERVING	
CALORIES	205
FAT	10 g
SATURATED FAT	3 g
CHOLESTEROL	71 mg
CARBOHYDRATE	4 g
FIBRE	0 g
PROTEIN	24 g
SUGARS	2 g
SODIUM	721 mg

skinny**scoop**

If you're not a fan of lamb, replace it with chicken breast or beef. To make a speedy harissa, I use jarred roasted peppers packed in water. If you want to roast the peppers yourself, use 2 red peppers, seeded and peeled after roasting (see page 233).

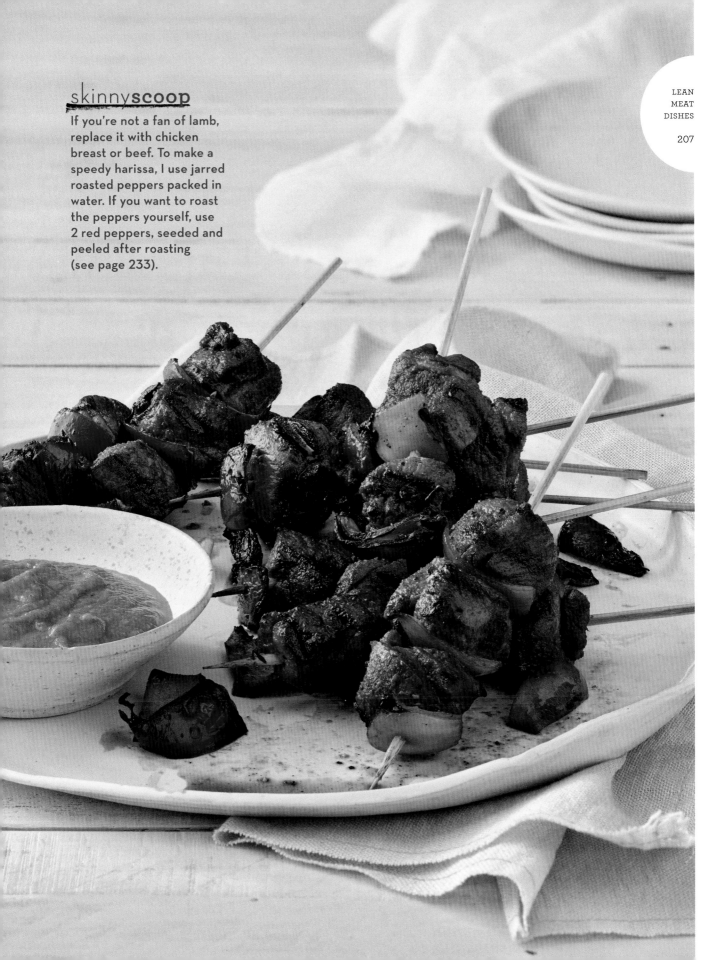

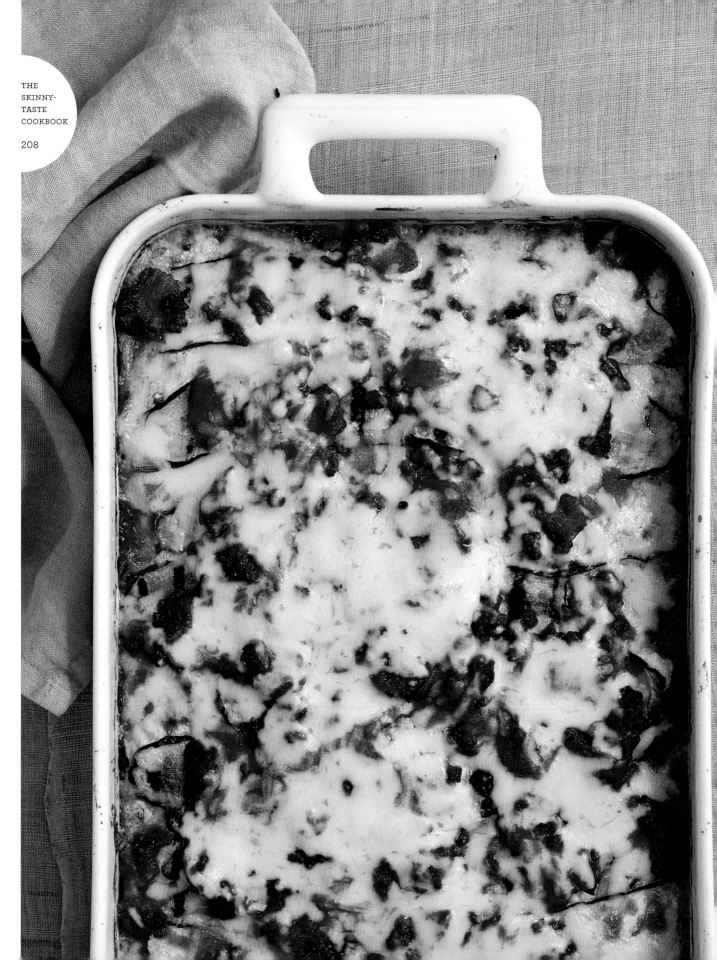

Pasta-less Courgette Lasagna

SERVES 8

Thinly sliced courgette ribbons replace pasta in this delicious, low-carb dish. This lasagna totally satisfies my cravings for cheesy and indulgent Italian comfort food. It's perfect in the summer when I have tons of garden-fresh courgette and herbs, but I also love making it during the colder months when I want something hot and comforting. Although it takes a little longer than most of my recipes, it's totally worth it!

450g lean beef mince

1¼ teaspoons sea salt

1 teaspoon olive oil

½ large onion, chopped

3 garlic cloves, crushed

2 x 400g tins chopped tomatoes

2 tablespoons chopped fresh basil

Freshly ground black pepper

3 medium courgettes

Cooking spray or oil mister

1½ cups (375g) low-fat ricotta cheese

¼ cup (25g) grated Parmesan cheese

1 large egg

4 cups (450g) grated light mozzarella cheese

Heat a large, deep nonstick frying pan over high heat. Add the meat, season with ½ teaspoon of the salt and cook, using a wooden spoon to break the meat into small pieces as it browns, 4 to 5 minutes. Drain the meat in a colander and wipe the pan with kitchen paper.

Put the pan over medium heat. Add the olive oil and onion and cook, stirring, until soft, 3 to 4 minutes. Add the garlic and cook 1 minute. Return the meat to the pan, add the tomatoes, basil, ¼ teaspoon of the salt and the black pepper to taste. Reduce the heat to low, cover and simmer, stirring occasionally, 25 minutes. Remove the lid and simmer uncovered 10 minutes, until thickened.

Meanwhile, slice the courgette lengthwise with a mandoline into 2.5mm-thick slices (you should have at least 30 to 35 long courgette ribbons). Lightly salt the courgette with the remaining ½ teaspoon salt and set aside for 15 minutes. Blot the courgette with kitchen paper.

(recipe continues)

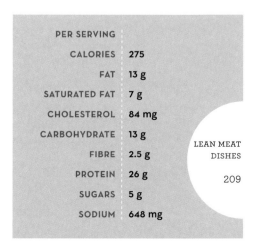

PER SERVING	
CALORIES	275
FAT	13 g
SATURATED FAT	7 g
CHOLESTEROL	84 mg
CARBOHYDRATE	13 g
FIBRE	2.5 g
PROTEIN	26 g
SUGARS	5 g
SODIUM	648 mg

LEAN MEAT DISHES

Preheat a barbecue to medium heat (or preheat a grill pan over medium heat).

Oil the grill grates or spray the grill pan with cooking spray to avoid sticking. Grill the courgette until cooked and slightly browned, 2 to 3 minutes on each side. Transfer to a plate lined with kitchen paper and press to absorb excess moisture.

Preheat the oven to 190°C/170°C fan/Gas 5.

In a medium bowl, combine the ricotta, Parmesan and egg.

Spread a good spoonful of the meat sauce in the bottom of a 23 × 32 × 6cm baking dish. Make a layer of the courgette over the sauce to cover the bottom of the dish. Spread a third of the ricotta mixture over the courgette and sprinkle with a quarter of the mozzarella. Make another layer of courgette, top with a third meat sauce, a third ricotta mixture, a quarter mozzarella. Repeat the layers with the remaining ingredients for a total of 3 layers. Finish the lasagna by topping with the remaining courgette and meat sauce. Cover the dish with foil.

Bake for 30 minutes, remove the foil and bake 20 minutes uncovered. Add the remaining mozzarella and bake uncovered until bubbling and the cheese is melted, 10 more minutes. Allow to stand for 5 to 10 minutes before cutting into 8 pieces.

Sunday Night Roast Beef and Gravy

SERVES 10

When it comes to roast beef, I have pretty big shoes to fill – my mom's was the best. The key to making perfect roast beef is to use a meat thermometer, so there's no guessing if it's cooked to your liking. I like mine a little on the rare side, so I take it out when the thermometer reads 57°C.

1.2kg beef roasting joint, all fat trimmed off

Cooking spray or oil mister

3 garlic cloves, sliced into very thin slivers

¼ teaspoon sea salt, plus more as needed

1 tablespoon Dijon mustard

½ teaspoon dried rosemary

¼ teaspoon freshly ground black pepper, plus more as needed

2 tablespoons plain flour

2 cups (450ml) low-salt beef stock

Remove the beef from the refrigerator about 1 hour before cooking to reach room temperature.

Preheat the oven to its highest setting. Lightly spray a roasting pan with oil.

Using a sharp knife, pierce holes in the beef about 1cm deep and insert slivers of garlic in each. Season with ¼ teaspoon of the salt, rub the mustard all over the beef and sprinkle with the rosemary and pepper. Put the beef in the roasting pan.

Roast for 20 minutes. Reduce the oven temperature to 130°C/110°C fan/Gas ½ and roast until a thermometer registers 57°C for rare, 60°C for medium-rare, 65°C for medium and 68° to 71°C for well-done, about 1 hour 15 minutes or longer. Remove the roast from the oven and allow to rest 10 to 15 minutes. (The temperature will rise about an additional 5°C as it sits.)

In a small saucepan, whisk together the flour and beef stock. Bring to a boil over medium heat and cook, whisking occasionally, until thickened, about 1 minute. Pour the pan drippings into the gravy and continue to cook, whisking, for 1 minute. Add a pinch of salt and black pepper to taste, if needed.

Using a good sharp carving knife, thinly slice the roast and serve with gravy.

PERFECT PAIRING
This dish works well with **Cheesy Cauliflower 'Mash' (page 269)** and sautéed vegetables on the side. Try any leftovers in **Roast Beef Sandwiches with Creamy Horseradish Spread (page 81)** or in a **Roast Beef and Watercress Pasta Salad (page 144)**.

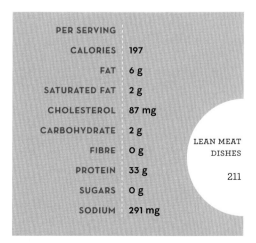

PER SERVING	
CALORIES	197
FAT	6 g
SATURATED FAT	2 g
CHOLESTEROL	87 mg
CARBOHYDRATE	2 g
FIBRE	0 g
PROTEIN	33 g
SUGARS	0 g
SODIUM	291 mg

LEAN MEAT DISHES

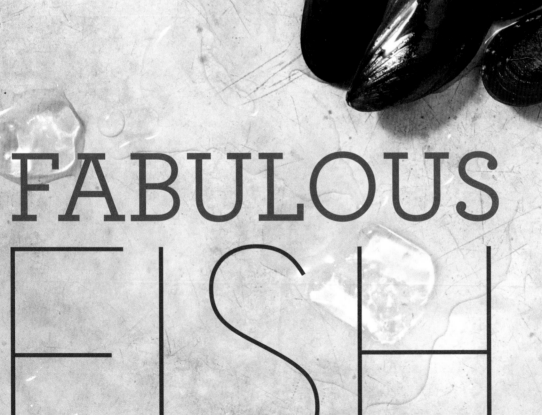

FABULOUS FISH

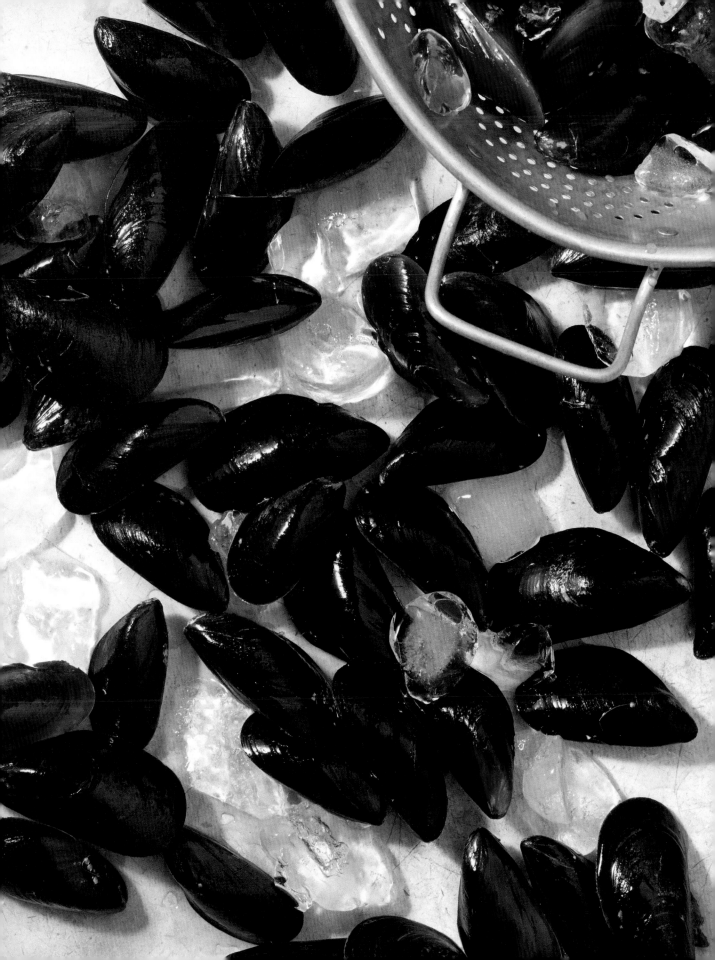

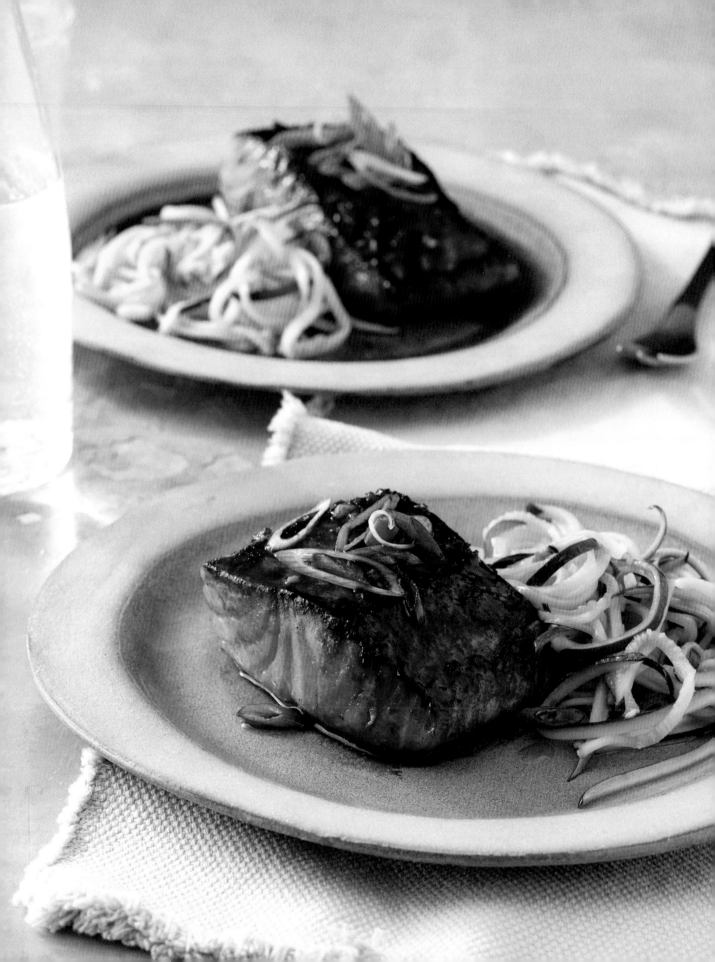

Sweet 'n' Spicy Sriracha-Glazed Salmon

SERVES 4

This is one of my favourite ways to prepare salmon. The marinade in this recipe is the perfect combination of spicy, sweet and savoury – in fact, I also love to use it with steaks or chicken. The Sriracha sauce is a must, and you can find it in the Asian section of most supermarkets.

¼ cup (50ml) reduced-salt soy sauce (or tamari* for gluten-free)

2 tablespoons honey

1 tablespoon rice vinegar

1 tablespoon Sriracha hot chilli sauce (or to taste)

1 tablespoon grated fresh ginger

1 tablespoon crushed garlic

450g wild salmon fillet, cut into 4 pieces

1½ teaspoons sesame oil

2 tablespoons finely chopped spring onions, for garnish

Read the label to be sure this product is gluten-free.

In a ziplock plastic bag, combine the soy sauce, honey, vinegar, Sriracha, ginger and garlic. Add the salmon, toss to coat evenly and refrigerate for at least 1 hour, or up to 8 hours, turning the fish once.

Remove the salmon from the bag, reserving the marinade. Heat a large sauté pan over medium-high heat and add the sesame oil. Rotate the pan to coat the bottom evenly and add the salmon. Cook until one side of the fish is browned, about 2 minutes. Flip the salmon and cook until the other side browns, 2 more minutes. Reduce the heat to low and pour in the reserved marinade. Cover and cook until the fish is cooked through, 4 to 5 minutes.

To serve, place a piece of salmon on each plate and sprinkle with the spring onions.

PERFECT PAIRINGS
This is perfect served over brown rice with **Roasted Sesame Green Beans (page 272)**. For a fantastic, quick, low-carb option, I make courgette noodles. Use a spiralizer or mandoline fitted with a julienne blade to cut the courgette into spaghetti-like strands, then sauté them with a little sesame oil and garlic for 2 minutes.

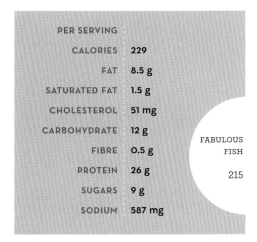

PER SERVING	
CALORIES	229
FAT	8.5 g
SATURATED FAT	1.5 g
CHOLESTEROL	51 mg
CARBOHYDRATE	12 g
FIBRE	0.5 g
PROTEIN	26 g
SUGARS	9 g
SODIUM	587 mg

Easy Tenderstem Broccoli Halibut Bake

SERVES 4

A meal that takes 20 minutes to make – start to finish – sounds pretty appetizing, right? This simple cooking method is a favourite of mine for fish: I basically sauté some vegetables, season my fish, layer it all in a baking dish, bake and voilà, dinner is ready! Halibut is a great choice for picky palates because it has a very mild taste, but you can use any fresh white fish that's available in your area.

Cooking spray or oil mister

170g tenderstem broccoli

3 teaspoons extra-virgin olive oil

Sea salt

¾ cup (150g) halved cherry tomatoes

2 garlic cloves, crushed

Pinch of crushed red chilli flakes

4 halibut fillets (about 110g each)

Freshly ground black pepper

2 tablespoons fresh lemon juice

1 teaspoon chopped fresh oregano

2 tablespoons freshly grated Parmesan cheese

skinny**scoop**

When you buy fish, ask your fishmonger what's freshest. I always use my nose to test its freshness. It shouldn't smell fishy; it should smell like the ocean. If you press the flesh of the meat with your finger (or ask the fishmonger to do so), the meat should spring back. If your finger leaves an indent, leave it at the store.

Preheat the oven to 230°C/210°C fan/Gas 8. Lightly spray a 23 × 32cm baking dish with oil.

Trim 2 to 3cm off the stems of the broccoli and halve the stalks lengthwise. Heat a large nonstick frying pan over medium heat. Add 2 teaspoons of the olive oil, then add the broccoli. Season with ⅛ teaspoon salt and cook, stirring occasionally, until crisp-tender, about 4 minutes. Add the tomatoes and a pinch of salt and cook for 1 minute. Add the garlic and chilli flakes and cook for 1 more minute.

Season the fish with ¼ teaspoon salt and black pepper, to taste. Put the fish in the prepared baking dish and drizzle with the remaining 1 teaspoon oil and the lemon juice, and sprinkle with the oregano.

Bake until the fish is partly cooked, about 5 minutes. Remove the baking dish from the oven, top the fish with the broccoli and Parmesan, and return the dish to the oven. Bake until the fish is cooked through and opaque, about 10 more minutes. Serve hot.

PER SERVING	
CALORIES	166
FAT	6 g
SATURATED FAT	1.5 g
CHOLESTEROL	58 mg
CARBOHYDRATE	4 g
FIBRE	1.5 g
PROTEIN	23 g
SUGARS	1 g
SODIUM	228 mg

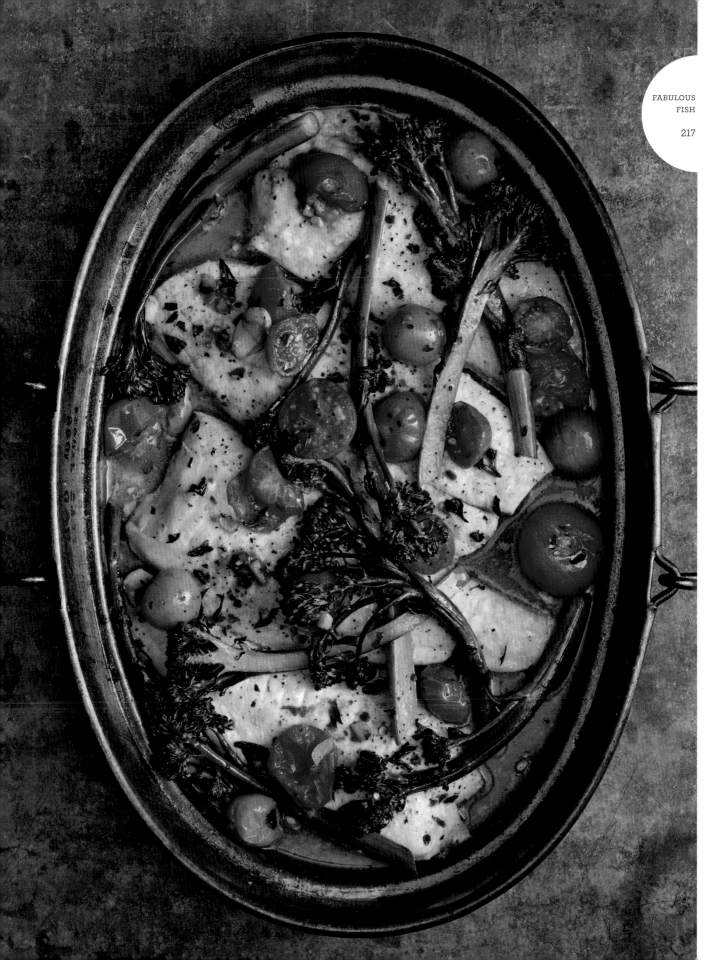

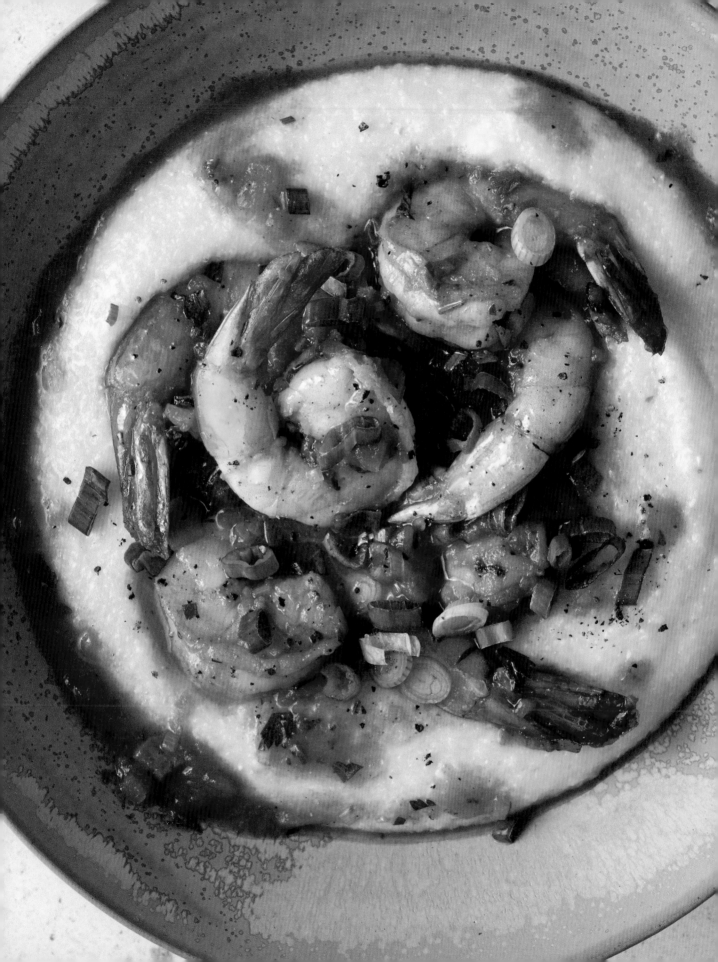

Kiss My (Prawns and) Grits

SERVES 4

The first time I had prawns and grits was at the Sou'Wester restaurant at the stunning Mandarin Oriental hotel in DC, and it was love at first bite. It reminded me of creamy Italian polenta, only with a Southern twist. To give grits a lighter touch while keeping them creamy – with that wonderful cheese flavour (because, after all, that's what makes them so darn delicious) – I slowly simmer the grits in both skimmed milk and chicken stock. At the very end, I stir in some Havarti and Pecorino cheese (a naturally low-fat cheese that packs a lot of flavour). If you can't find quick-cooking grits, you can use fine cornmeal or polenta.

GRITS

2 cups (450ml) reduced-salt chicken stock*

1¼ cups (300ml) skimmed milk

1 teaspoon sea salt

1 cup (150g) quick-cooking grits, fine cornmeal or polenta (not instant)

Knob of unsalted butter

25g Havarti cheese, grated†

1 tablespoon grated Pecorino Romano cheese

PRAWNS

24 peeled and deveined jumbo prawns

1 teaspoon Old Bay seasoning

1½ teaspoons olive oil

50g lean smoked ham, finely chopped

¼ cup (30g) finely chopped shallots

½ cup (100g) tinned chopped tomatoes, drained

⅔ cup low-salt chicken stock*

1 bay leaf

Freshly ground black pepper

1 tablespoon chopped fresh parsley

1 lemon wedge

3 tablespoons sliced spring onions, for garnish

Read the label to be sure this product is gluten-free.

For the grits: In a medium pot, combine ¼ cup (50ml) water, the chicken stock, milk and salt and bring to a boil over medium heat. Slowly stir in the grits. Return to a boil, reduce the heat to the lowest setting, cover with a fitted lid and simmer, stirring every 5 minutes or so to prevent the grits from sticking to the bottom, adding more water if necessary, until smooth, 28 to 30 minutes. Stir in the butter and cheeses, remove the pan from the heat and keep warm.

(recipe continues)

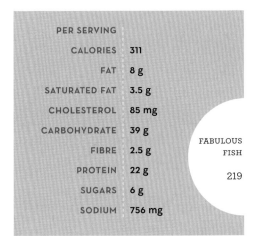

PER SERVING	
CALORIES	311
FAT	8 g
SATURATED FAT	3.5 g
CHOLESTEROL	85 mg
CARBOHYDRATE	39 g
FIBRE	2.5 g
PROTEIN	22 g
SUGARS	6 g
SODIUM	756 mg

FABULOUS FISH

219

For the prawns: Sprinkle the prawns with the Old Bay. Heat a large sauté pan over high heat. Add 1 teaspoon of the olive oil and the prawns and cook until browned, about 1 minute. Flip the prawns and cook 1 more minute or until opaque. Transfer the prawns to a plate.

Reduce the heat to medium-low and add the remaining ½ teaspoon oil and the ham. Cook until slightly browned, 3 to 4 minutes. Add the shallots and cook, stirring, until golden, 2 to 3 minutes. Add the drained tomatoes, chicken stock, bay leaf and black pepper to taste. Increase the heat to medium and simmer until the sauce thickens and reduces slightly, 8 to 10 minutes. Remove the pan from the heat, add the prawns and parsley and finish with a squeeze of lemon juice. Stir well and discard the bay leaf.

Divide the grits among 4 plates and spoon the prawns and sauce over the top of each. Sprinkle with the spring onions and serve.

† If you can't find Havarti cheese, Tilsit makes a good alternative.

Pan-Fried Lemon Sole with Tomatoes and Capers

SERVES 4

When my mom prepared fish when I was a kid, she would breadcrumb and fry it nine times out of ten, probably because my father liked it that way. For those of you who think that's the only way fish tastes good, I'm here to tell you there are better ways! Poaching fish in a flavourful tomato broth with white wine, lemon and capers is my favourite method. It becomes juicy and flavourful, and is ready in less than 15 minutes. Even my youngest loves to eat fish this way – I just tell her it's chicken (wink, wink!).

2 teaspoons extra-virgin olive oil

2 garlic cloves, crushed

2½ cups (500g) chopped fresh tomatoes or no-salt-added tinned chopped tomatoes

¼ cup (50ml) dry white wine

1 teaspoon herbes de Provence (or dried thyme)

1⅛ teaspoons sea salt

Freshly ground black pepper

1 teaspoon fresh lemon juice

3 tablespoons capers, drained

4 fillets lemon sole (140g each)

Heat a large, deep nonstick frying pan over medium heat. Add the oil and garlic and cook, stirring, until golden, about 1 minute. Add the tomatoes, wine, herbes de Provence, ¾ teaspoon of the salt and black pepper to taste. Cook until the wine reduces, 2 to 3 minutes. Add the lemon juice and capers. Lay the fish on top, season with the remaining ⅛ teaspoon salt and a pinch of black pepper and cover; reduce the heat to medium-low and cook until the fish is opaque and flakes easily, about 10 minutes.

To serve, put a piece of fish on each plate and spoon the sauce on top.

PERFECT PAIRING
Summer Giant Couscous (page 288) or **Lemon Roasted Asparagus (page 278)** would make the perfect side dish.

skinny**scoop**

Lemon sole is a flaky white fish found in the Atlantic. Despite its name, it does not taste like lemons at all, but it has a mild flavour with delicate, white flesh. If you can't find it, use any white fish, including plaice or cod. Fresh tomatoes or tinned tomatoes both work fine. If you want to add a little heat, you can add a pinch of crushed red chilli flakes.

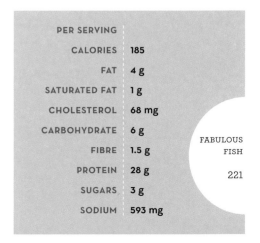

PER SERVING	
CALORIES	185
FAT	4 g
SATURATED FAT	1 g
CHOLESTEROL	68 mg
CARBOHYDRATE	6 g
FIBRE	1.5 g
PROTEIN	28 g
SUGARS	3 g
SODIUM	593 mg

FABULOUS FISH

221

Mahi Mahi Fish Tacos with Spicy Avocado Cream

SERVES 5

Fish tacos are the perfect summer dish, whether you're whipping them up for a quick weeknight dinner with the family or having some friends over for a casual meal. But rather than the battered, deep-fried versions you find at taco stands, these delicious ones are gently poached in a flavourful combination of tomatoes, green chillies, cumin, garlic and lime juice. I serve it with warmed corn tortillas, cabbage infused with coriander and lime and a spicy avocado cream sauce.

SLAW

2 cups (150g) shredded red cabbage

1 tablespoon roughly chopped fresh coriander

2 tablespoons fresh lime juice

⅛ teaspoon sea salt

AVOCADO CREAM

2 tablespoons light soured cream

½ tablespoon fresh lime juice

½ medium avocado, chopped

½ small jalapeño or other green chilli, seeded

1 tablespoon chopped fresh coriander

⅛ teaspoon sea salt

Freshly ground black pepper

FISH

1 teaspoon olive oil

1 small onion, chopped

4 garlic cloves, crushed

275g tinned chopped tomatoes, drained

1 tablespoon chopped fresh coriander

½ teaspoon ground cumin

½ teaspoon sea salt

Freshly ground black pepper

450g mahi mahi fillet

½ lime

10 extra-thin corn tortillas

For the slaw: In a large bowl, combine the cabbage, coriander, lime juice and salt. Toss well and set aside.

For the avocado cream: In a blender, combine 2 tablespoons water, the soured cream, lime juice, avocado, jalapeño, coriander, salt and black pepper to taste. Blend until smooth.

(recipe continues)

PER SERVING	
CALORIES	298
FAT	13 g
SATURATED FAT	4 g
CHOLESTEROL	47 mg
CARBOHYDRATE	23 g
FIBRE	5 g
PROTEIN	20 g
SUGARS	5 g
SODIUM	577 mg

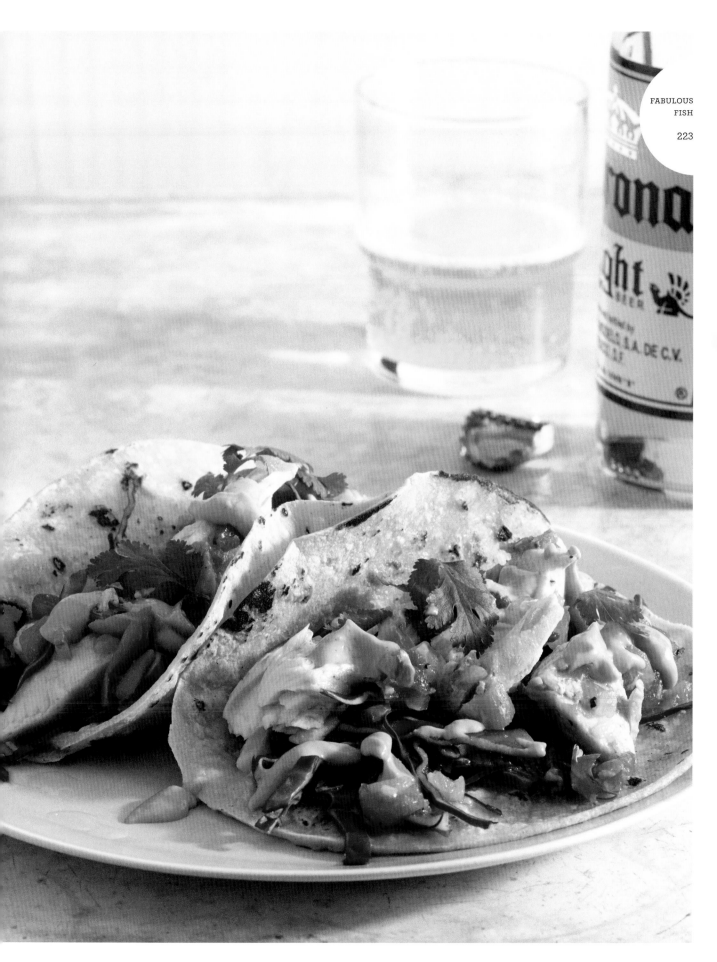

skinnyscoop

I prefer the mild, sweet flavour of mahi mahi for my fish tacos, but you can always substitute halibut, tilapia or your favourite fish.

For the fish: In a large nonstick frying pan, heat the olive oil over medium-high heat. Add the onion and cook, stirring, until translucent, 2 to 3 minutes. Add the garlic and cook until fragrant, about 1 minute. Add the tomatoes, coriander, cumin, salt and black pepper to taste. Cook for 1 minute. If it seems too dry, add about 3 tablespoons water. Reduce the heat to medium and put the mahi mahi in the pan. Cover and cook until the fish is opaque in the centre and flakes easily, 6 to 7 minutes. Using a wooden spoon, break up the fish and mix it into the tomatoes. Squeeze the lime over the fish.

To serve, heat the tortillas in a hot frying pan set over high heat, 30 to 40 seconds on each side. Fill each tortilla with fish, top with about 3 tablespoons slaw and drizzle with 1 tablespoon avocado cream.

Coriander-Lime Prawns

SERVES 6

I find it hard to believe that there are people who don't like coriander (Julia Child hated it!). The herb is a staple in my kitchen, and I love the flavour it adds to just about anything. If you're one of those people who detest coriander, you can simply leave it out or replace it with another fresh herb, such as chives or parsley. Prawns are another one of my kitchen staples – I always keep some stashed in my freezer for those nights when I don't plan ahead. It's the perfect go-to 'skinny' protein when I need a quick, light meal.

675g peeled and deveined jumbo prawns

¼ teaspoon plus ⅛ teaspoon ground cumin

¼ teaspoon sea salt

Freshly ground black pepper

2 teaspoons extra-virgin olive oil

5 garlic cloves, crushed

2 tablespoons lime juice (from 1 medium lime)

3 to 4 tablespoons chopped fresh coriander

Season the prawns with the cumin, salt and black pepper to taste.

Heat a large nonstick frying pan over medium-high heat. Add 1 teaspoon of the oil to the pan, then add half of the prawns. Cook them undisturbed for about 2 minutes. Turn the prawns over and cook until opaque throughout, about 1 minute. Transfer to a plate. Add the remaining 1 teaspoon oil and the remaining prawns to the pan and cook, undisturbed, for about 2 minutes. Turn the prawns over, add the garlic and cook until the prawns are opaque throughout, about 1 minute. Return the first batch of prawns to the pan, mix well so that the garlic is evenly incorporated and remove the pan from the heat.

Squeeze the lime juice over all the prawns. Add the coriander, toss well and serve.

FOOD FACTS **coriander: why you should learn to love it**
People all over the world have been using coriander for more than 3,000 years to boost health and ward off diseases, from diabetes to depression to high blood pressure. According to studies, the plant's powers likely come from its antioxidants (including flavonoids and polyphenols) and its essential oils.

PERFECT PAIRING
I usually serve this over rice or turn it into a big salad with sliced avocado. It's also delicious as weeknight prawn tacos: simply serve it with warmed corn tortillas and shredded cabbage.

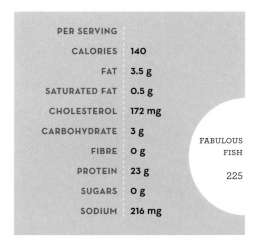

PER SERVING	
CALORIES	140
FAT	3.5 g
SATURATED FAT	0.5 g
CHOLESTEROL	172 mg
CARBOHYDRATE	3 g
FIBRE	0 g
PROTEIN	23 g
SUGARS	0 g
SODIUM	216 mg

FABULOUS FISH

225

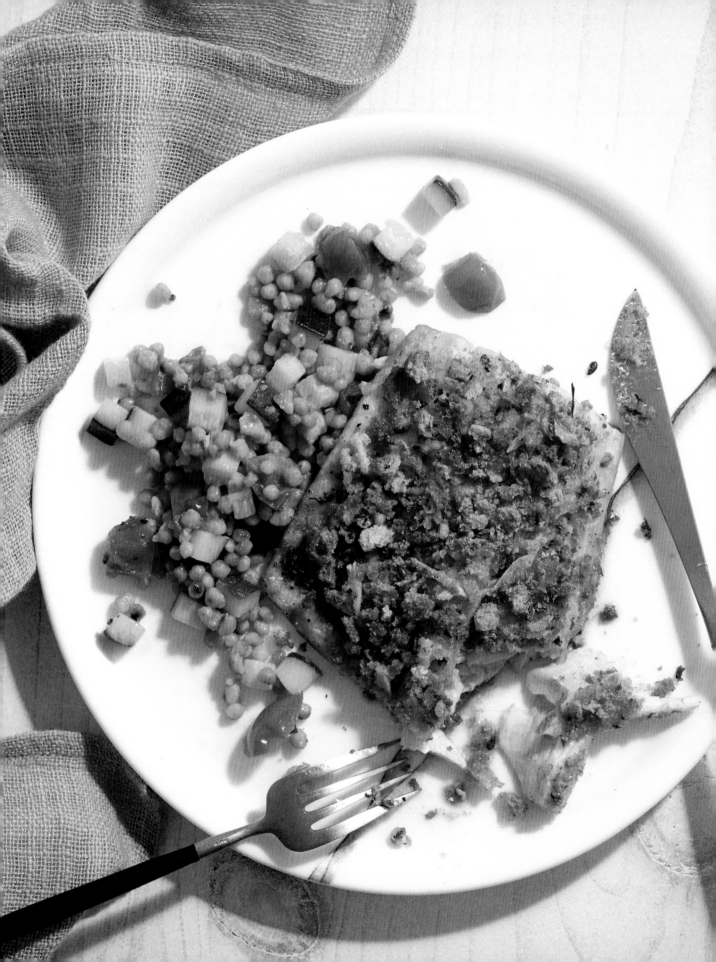

Sea Bass with Garlic Crumb Topping

SERVES 4

This is my favourite foolproof method for preparing fish that is sure to please even the pickiest of fish eaters. But the real trick to making the best-tasting fish dishes is, of course, buying the fish fresh, preferably caught the same day. Sea bass is a great option for people who are picky because it's a mild-tasting fish, with a thick, meaty flesh and a large firm flake.

4 skin-on sea bass fillets (140g each)

¼ teaspoon sea salt

Freshly ground black pepper

¼ cup (50ml) white wine

1 tablespoon olive oil

Knob of unsalted butter, melted

2 garlic cloves, crushed

2 tablespoons seasoned wholemeal bread crumbs, homemade (page 110) or shop-bought

Preheat the oven to 190°C/170°C fan/Gas 5.

Put the fish in a 23 × 32cm baking dish and season with the salt and black pepper. Drizzle the white wine, olive oil and melted butter over the fish, then top with the crushed garlic and bread crumbs.

Bake until the fish is opaque in the centre and flakes easily, 12 to 15 minutes. Remove from the oven and set the oven to grill. Grill until the crumb topping is golden in colour, watching closely so it doesn't burn, 1 to 2 minutes.

PERFECT PAIRINGS
This is wonderful with **Summer Giant Couscous (page 288),** but if you're feeding a larger crowd, you can make this with **Tricolour Summer Penne (page 239).**

skinny**scoop**

If sea bass is not in season or available, you can substitute it with halibut or cod.

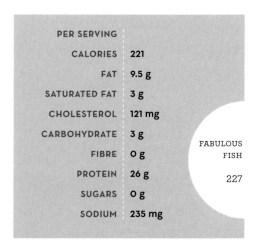

PER SERVING	
CALORIES	**221**
FAT	**9.5 g**
SATURATED FAT	**3 g**
CHOLESTEROL	**121 mg**
CARBOHYDRATE	**3 g**
FIBRE	**0 g**
PROTEIN	**26 g**
SUGARS	**0 g**
SODIUM	**235 mg**

FABULOUS
FISH

227

Garlicky Lemon Prawns and Tenderstem Broccoli Stir-Fry

SERVES 4

Stir-frying is my favourite way to get a quick, healthy meal on the table in minutes! This one is made with lots of garlic – but don't worry, it doesn't overpower the dish. Instead, it creates a fragrant, tangy sauce that's delicious with the prawns. Tenderstem broccoli is sweet and tender and takes just a few minutes to cook, which makes it perfect for quick stir-fries. You can swap the tenderstem broccoli for other fast-cooking vegetables, such as asparagus, broccoli florets or sugar snap peas.

170g tenderstem broccoli

½ cup (120ml) low-salt chicken stock*

2 tablespoons reduced-salt soy sauce (or tamari* for gluten-free)

2 teaspoons cornflour

1 tablespoon rapeseed oil

450g peeled and deveined large prawns

8 garlic cloves, chopped

3 tablespoons fresh lemon juice

Freshly ground black pepper

PERFECT PAIRING
Forget take aways. Try this stir-fry with **Vegetable Fried Brown Rice (page 273)** to make your own Asian-inspired dinner.

skinny**scoop**

If you buy prawns with the shells on for this recipe, buy an extra 100g so that you end up with 450g of peeled prawns.

Read the label to be sure this product is gluten-free.

Trim 2 to 3cm off the stems of the broccoli and thinly slice it lengthwise.

In a small bowl, combine the chicken stock and soy sauce. In a separate small bowl, whisk together the cornflour and 2 tablespoons water.

Heat a large wok over high heat. Add ½ tablespoon of the oil, then add the prawns. Cook, stirring, until opaque throughout, 1½ to 2 minutes. Transfer to a plate.

Add the remaining ½ tablespoon oil to the wok, reduce the heat to medium and add the garlic and broccoli. Cook, stirring, until the garlic is golden and the broccoli is tender crisp, about 3 to 4 minutes. Increase the heat to high and add the soy sauce mixture. Bring to a boil and cook about 1½ minutes. Add the lemon juice, cornflour mixture and black pepper to taste. Bring to a simmer, add the prawns and stir well to coat. Serve hot.

PER SERVING	
CALORIES	188
FAT	5.5 g
SATURATED FAT	0.5 g
CHOLESTEROL	172 mg
CARBOHYDRATE	9 g
FIBRE	1.5 g
PROTEIN	28 g
SUGARS	1 g
SODIUM	525 mg

FOOD FACTS *prawns, quite a catch!*

Prawns deliver big nutrition benefits. A serving (75 grams) offers more than 11 grams of protein for just 60 calories and less than 1 gram of fat. They are also rich in the mineral selenium and contain heart-healthy omega-3 fats. And a study in *The American Journal of Clinical Nutrition* found that even though prawns are high in dietary cholesterol, the shellfish can be included in a heart-healthy diet because the dietary cholesterol doesn't affect blood cholesterol levels.

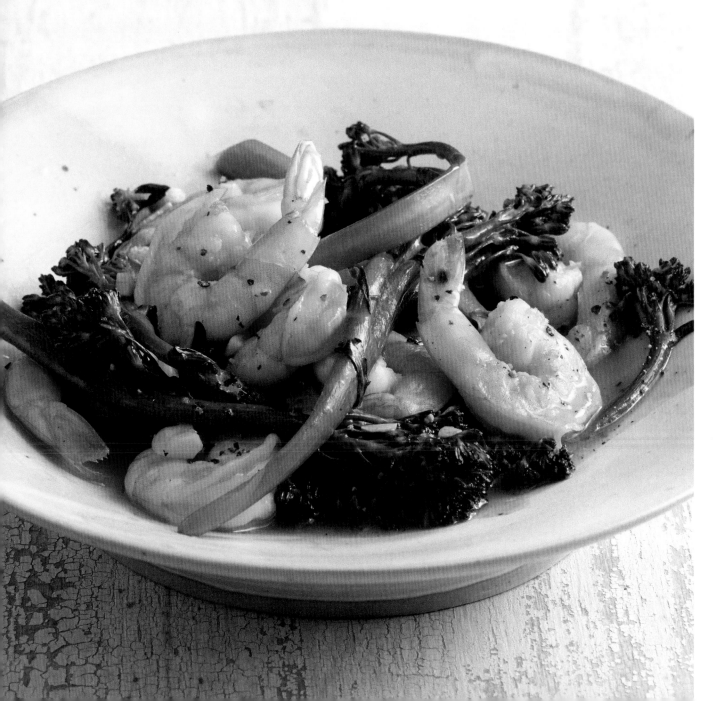

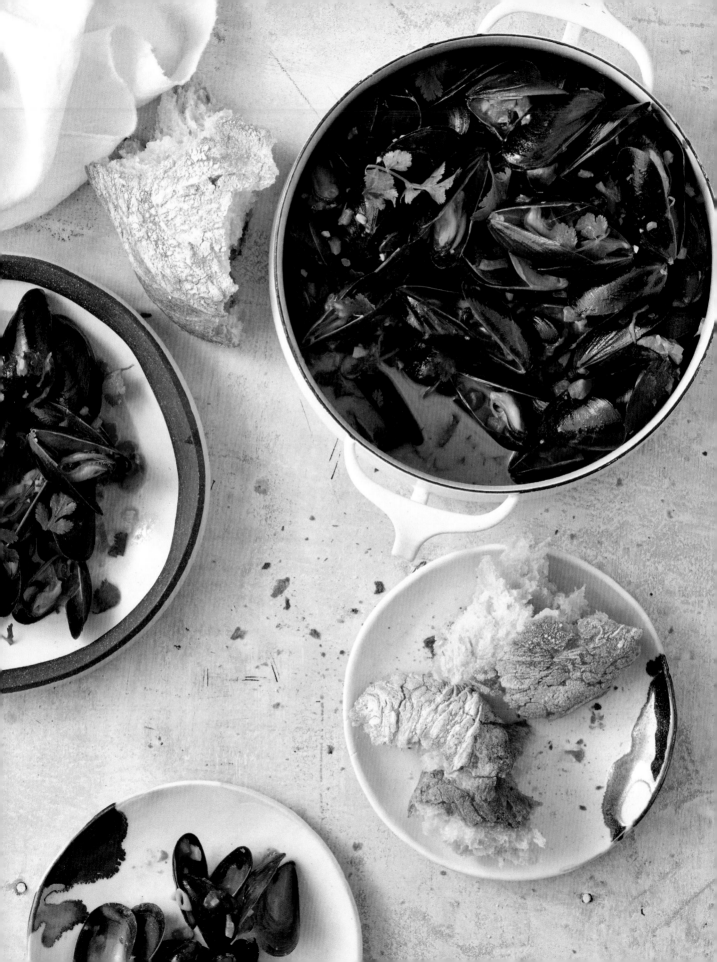

Thai Coconut Mussels

SERVES 5

On the weekends I re-energize. I get more rest, play with my kids, visit the farmers' market and recharge my body with delicious dishes like these aromatic mussels simmered in coconut milk with tomatoes, spring onions and ginger. My husband and I love the flavours of Thai cuisine and these mussels, which are inexpensive and take just minutes to prepare, are an ideal source of lean protein.

1 teaspoon coconut oil

½ cup (85g) finely chopped red pepper

3 medium spring onions, thinly sliced

4 garlic cloves, crushed

1 tablespoon chopped fresh ginger

400g tin chopped tomatoes

400g tin light coconut milk

1 to 2 fresh red chillies, finely chopped (or ½ to ¾ teaspoon crushed red chilli flakes)

½ cup (25g) roughly chopped fresh coriander

½ teaspoon sea salt

1.3kg mussels, scrubbed and debearded (about 60 medium)

½ lime

In a large pot, heat the coconut oil over medium-low heat. Add the pepper and spring onions and cook, stirring, until soft, 1 to 2 minutes. Add the garlic and ginger and cook until fragrant, about 1 minute. Add the tomatoes, coconut milk, chillies, half of the coriander and salt. Cover and simmer for 10 minutes to blend the flavours.

Add the mussels, cover and cook until the mussels open, 5 to 7 minutes. Squeeze the lime over the mussels and top with the remaining coriander. Divide the mussels and broth equally among 5 bowls and serve.

PERFECT PAIRINGS
To help soak up every last drop of this delicious broth, I serve the mussels over brown rice or with a crusty piece of bread.

skinny**scoop**

When purchasing mussels, look for uncracked, tightly closed shells or shells that close when lightly tapped. Scrub them with a stiff brush under cold running water to remove any sand. The shells will remain closed until you cook them; discard any shells that don't open. To debeard, use your fingers to firmly pull out the hairy filaments.

PER SERVING	
CALORIES	302
FAT	12.5 g
SATURATED FAT	5.5 g
CHOLESTEROL	54 mg
CARBOHYDRATE	21 g
FIBRE	1.5 g
PROTEIN	33 g
SUGARS	5 g
SODIUM	918 mg

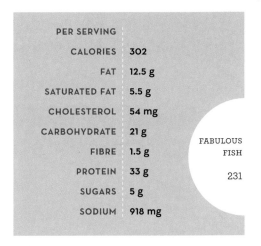

FABULOUS FISH

Spanish Seafood Stew

SERVES 4

This dish was inspired by paella, one of my favourite Spanish dishes, but it's made without the rice, and in a fraction of the time, making it a perfect weeknight dinner option. There's no need to make your own fish stock, as the anchovies add great depth of flavour, not to mention omega-3 fats. And don't worry; the dish won't taste like anchovies. Any combination of fish and shellfish can be used. If you want to get a little fancy, try it with scallops and lobster tails. A crusty piece of bread is a must to soak up all that wonderful saffron-infused broth!

450g firm white fish fillet (such as halibut, cod or sea bass), cut into 4 pieces

20 medium prawns, peeled and deveined

¼ teaspoon sea salt

Freshly ground black pepper

1 teaspoon extra-virgin olive oil

45g dried chorizo, cut into 5mm-thick slices

1 small onion, finely chopped

3 garlic cloves, crushed

2 anchovy fillets, rinsed

1 medium tomato, finely chopped

1 teaspoon smoked paprika

2 cups (450ml) low-salt chicken stock

2 tablespoons tomato paste

3 bay leaves

About ¼ teaspoon saffron

155g frozen peas

1 large roasted red pepper, jarred or homemade (see page 233), cut into 1cm-wide slices

12 clams, scrubbed

12 mussels, scrubbed and debearded

1 tablespoon finely chopped fresh parsley

4 (25g) slices crusty wholemeal French bread

Season the fish and prawns with the salt and black pepper. Heat a large, deep nonstick frying pan over medium heat. Add the oil, chorizo and prawns and cook, stirring occasionally, until the prawns are browned on both sides, about 3 minutes. Transfer the prawns to a plate, leaving the chorizo in the pan.

Add the onion and cook, stirring, until soft, about 5 minutes. Add the garlic and anchovies and cook, stirring, until the mixture is very fragrant, about 1 minute. Add the tomato and paprika and cook, stirring occasionally, 2 to 3 minutes. Add the chicken stock, tomato paste, bay leaves and saffron, increase the heat to high and bring to a boil. Add the peas and roasted pepper, cover, reduce the heat to low and simmer until the flavours combine, about 10 minutes. Add the fish, cover, and leave to cook for

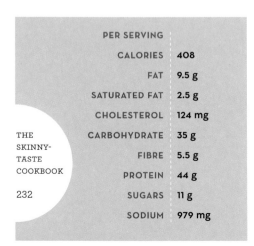

PER SERVING	
CALORIES	408
FAT	9.5 g
SATURATED FAT	2.5 g
CHOLESTEROL	124 mg
CARBOHYDRATE	35 g
FIBRE	5.5 g
PROTEIN	44 g
SUGARS	11 g
SODIUM	979 mg

4 minutes. Add the clams and mussels, cover and leave to cook until the clams and mussels have opened, about 5 to 7 minutes. Return the prawns to the pan, cover and cook until the fish is opaque throughout and flakes easily, 1 minute. Remove the pan from the heat. Discard any unopened shells and the bay leaves. Garnish with the parsley.

Ladle the fish and shellfish, along with the broth and vegetables, into 4 large bowls and serve with a crusty slice of bread.

FOOD FACTS **brain food**
Mussels are a stellar source of vitamin B12, which is essential for normal brain function. Just 75g of the shellfish provide 1,000 per cent of the US recommended daily allowance for B12.

Roasting Peppers

To roast peppers, place them directly over the burners of a gas hob on a medium-low flame, turning them frequently, until the skin has turned completely black and has started to blister. If you don't have a gas hob, you can roast them in the oven: preheat the oven to 200°C/180°C fan/Gas 6. Line a baking sheet with foil. Lay the peppers on their sides on the baking sheet and roast for 20 minutes. Using tongs, turn the peppers over, then place back in the oven for another 20 to 24 minutes, or until the skin is charred and soft and the peppers look slightly collapsed. Transfer the peppers to a bowl, cover tightly with clingfilm and allow to steam for 10 minutes. Uncover the bowl and peel off the skins. Core or seed the peppers, then chop the flesh.

Skinny Prawns, Chicken and Sausage Gumbo

SERVES 6

This makeover of a Cajun classic has so much flavour and comfort in every bite that you won't even miss all the fat of the original. My lightening techniques include simmering the 'Holy Trinity' of Cajun cuisine – onions, celery and peppers – to get them nicely caramelized, and then making a lighter roux with olive oil in place of butter and far less flour. Also, a key ingredient is Applegate's Organic Andouille Sausage. Made from turkey and chicken, it's leaner than traditional pork andouille, and it really adds great flavour and just the right amount of heat.

1 tablespoon rapeseed oil

1 cup (155g) chopped onion

½ cup (85g) chopped green pepper

¼ cup (35g) chopped celery

¼ cup (15g) chopped fresh parsley

6 bone-in, skinless chicken drumsticks (75g each)

1¼ teaspoons sea salt

Freshly ground black pepper

2 tablespoons plain flour

170g Applegate's chicken and turkey andouille sausage, thinly sliced†

1 cup (200g) chopped tomatoes

1 cup (100g) frozen sliced okra

1 bay leaf

350g peeled and deveined large prawns

¼ cup (30g) chopped spring onions

3 cups (555g) cooked brown rice

Heat a large, deep nonstick frying pan over medium heat. Add the oil, onion, pepper and celery. Cook until the vegetables are softened, 3 to 4 minutes. Add the parsley and cook for 1 more minute. Push the vegetables to the edges of the pan, add the chicken and season with 1 teaspoon of the salt and black pepper to taste. Cook until browned, 2 to 3 minutes per side. Sprinkle the flour over the chicken and vegetables. Add 3 cups (675ml) water, the sausage, tomato, okra, bay leaf, the remaining ¼ teaspoon salt and black pepper to taste. Cover, reduce the heat to low and simmer until the chicken is tender and cooked through, 30 to 35 minutes.

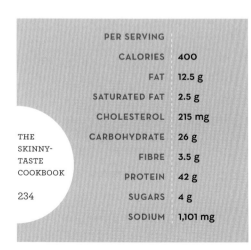

PER SERVING	
CALORIES	400
FAT	12.5 g
SATURATED FAT	2.5 g
CHOLESTEROL	215 mg
CARBOHYDRATE	26 g
FIBRE	3.5 g
PROTEIN	42 g
SUGARS	4 g
SODIUM	1,101 mg

Increase the heat to medium-high, uncover the pot and add the prawns. Cook until the prawns are opaque throughout, about 3 minutes. Remove the bay leaf and sprinkle with the spring onions.

To serve, put 1 drumstick and the gumbo into 6 shallow bowls and top each with some brown rice.

✝ If you can't find Applegate's sausage, another kind of chicken or turkey sausage will work well.

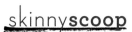

skinnyscoop

Bones add flavour and help make a rich broth, so when I make this, I always use skinless chicken on the bone.

Fishing for Heart Health

Talk about a real catch: fish are high in protein, low in saturated fat and a good source of heart-healthy omega-3 fatty acids. That's why the British Dietetic Association recommends eating fish, particularly fatty fish, at least two times (two servings) a week. Next time you go fishing, whether it's in the ocean or at the market, seek out these top 15 omega-3 winners:

Atlantic salmon (farmed or wild)	Fresh tuna	Rockfish
Blue crab	Halibut	Scallops
Canned white or light tuna	Lobster	Prawns
Coho salmon (farmed or wild)	Oysters	Swordfish
Flounder or sole	Rainbow trout (farmed or wild)	Wild catfish

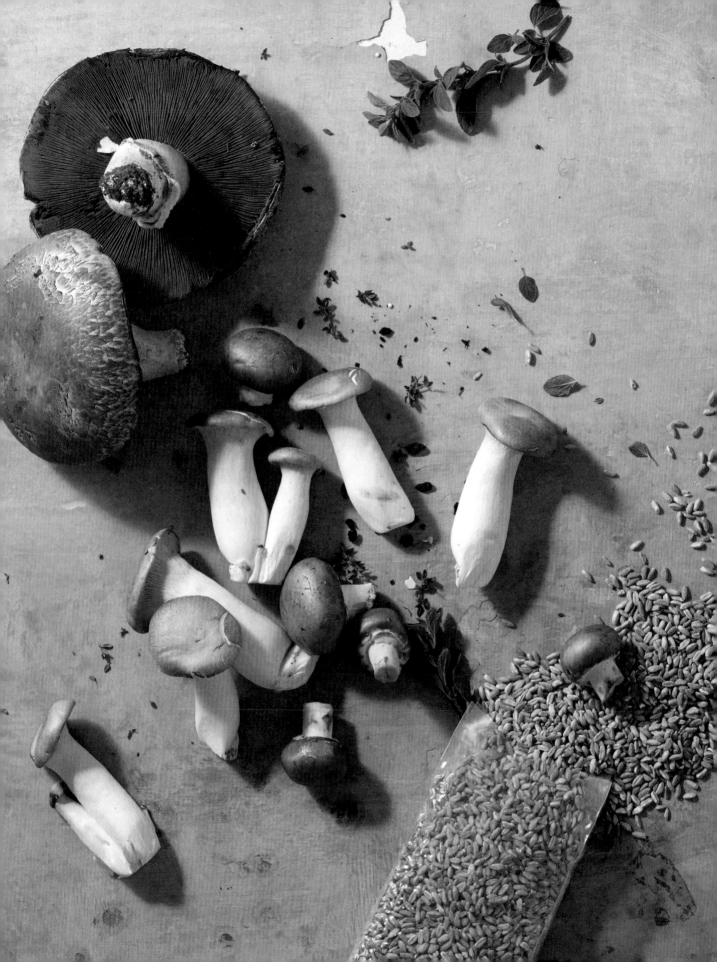

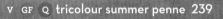

MEATLESS MAINS

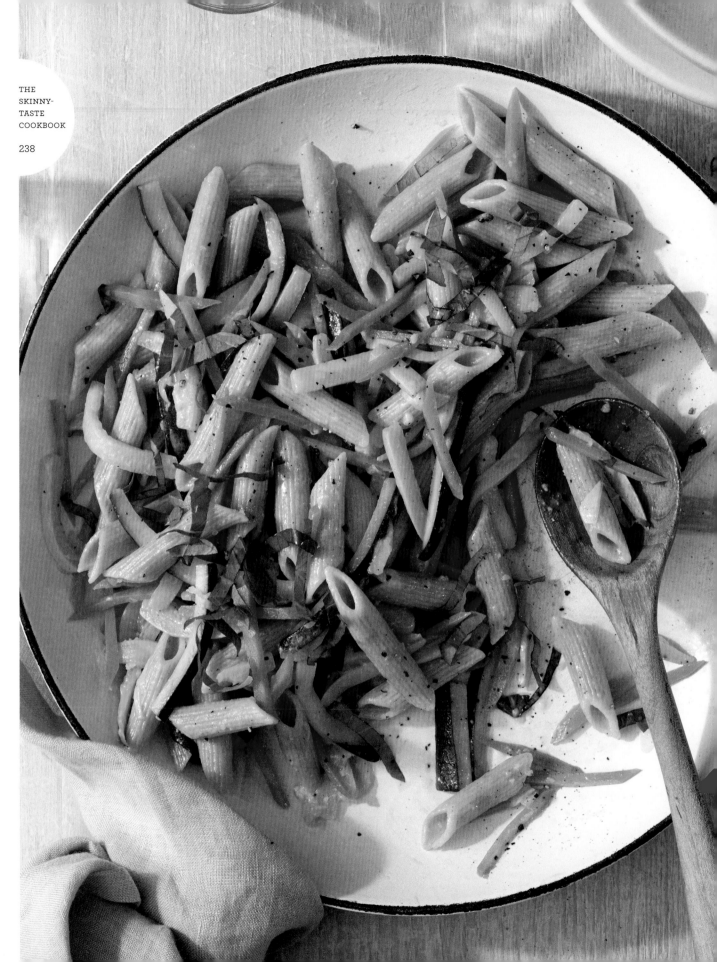

Tricolour Summer Penne

SERVES 4

Lots of wonderfully fresh vegetables are showcased in this quick pasta dish. Courgettes, yellow squash and carrots, all loaded with disease-fighting antioxidants, are cut into matchsticks and tossed with pasta, garlic and oil. I can't think of a better way to use up the summer's bounty. Once you have the veggies prepped, this dish takes less than 15 minutes to cook.

Sea salt

225g penne pasta (use brown rice* or quinoa pasta for gluten-free)

1 courgette, seeded and cut into 5mm-thick matchsticks

1 yellow squash, seeded and cut into 5mm-thick matchsticks

1¼ cups (200g) grated carrots

1 tablespoon olive oil

4 garlic cloves, thinly sliced

¼ cup (25g) grated Pecorino Romano cheese

Freshly ground black pepper

2 tablespoons thinly sliced fresh basil

*Read the label to be sure this product is gluten-free.

Cook the pasta to al dente in a pot of salted boiling water according to packet directions, adding the courgette, squash and carrots to the water in the last 2 minutes of cooking. Reserving ½ cup (110ml) of the cooking water, drain the pasta.

Heat a large nonstick frying pan over medium heat. Add the oil and the garlic and cook, stirring, until golden, 2 to 3 minutes. Quickly add the drained pasta and vegetables, ¼ cup (50ml) of the reserved pasta water, the Pecorino Romano, ½ teaspoon salt and black pepper to taste. Cook, tossing everything together well, for about 1 minute, adding the remaining pasta water if the mixture seems dry. Remove the pan from the heat, toss with the fresh basil and serve hot.

skinnyscoop

The quickest way to cut courgettes into matchsticks is to start by using a mandoline to slice the vegetables lengthwise 5mm thick. Then use a knife to cut them crosswise into matchsticks about 5mm × 5mm thick. If you don't own a mandoline, you could also do this with a sharp knife.

PER SERVING	
CALORIES	290
FAT	6.5 g
SATURATED FAT	1.5 g
CHOLESTEROL	6 mg
CARBOHYDRATE	50 g
FIBRE	2 g
PROTEIN	13 g
SUGARS	4 g
SODIUM	266 mg

MEATLESS
MAINS

239

Crustless Swiss Chard Pie

SERVES 6

I'm a lover of all things green – spinach, kale, escarole, collards, you name it! But one green I downright adore is Swiss chard. It's ridiculously healthy and has a buttery flavour that stands up to sautéing, braising and steaming. Unfortunately, not everyone in my home shares my sentiment, so when I want to prepare chard, I really need to get creative to showcase it in a way that even the pickiest of eaters will enjoy. This savoury crustless pie does just that.

Cooking spray or oil mister

1 small bunch Swiss chard, washed well

15g unsalted butter

1 large onion, cut into thin half moons

½ teaspoon sea salt, plus more as needed

Freshly ground black pepper

½ cup (60g) grated lighter Swiss cheese

2 tablespoons grated Parmesan cheese

½ cup (75g) wholemeal flour

1 teaspoon baking powder

⅔ cup (150ml) skimmed milk

1 teaspoon olive oil

2 large eggs, beaten

PERFECT PAIRINGS
This pie is perfect for brunch, lunch or as a side or a main for dinner. As a main dish, you can pair it with a salad on the side such as **My House Salad, Made with Love (page 267)**.

Preheat the oven to 200°C/180°C fan/Gas 6. Lightly spray a 23cm pie plate or dish with oil.

Separate the stems from the leaves of the chard. Finely chop the stems. Roll up the leaves and slice them into thin ribbons.

In a 25cm frying pan, melt half of the butter over low heat. Add the onion and a pinch each of salt and black pepper. Cook, stirring occasionally, until translucent, 8 to 10 minutes. Increase the heat to medium and cook until the onions caramelize, 8 to 10 more minutes. Transfer to a large bowl.

Increase the heat to medium-high, add the remaining butter and the chard stems. Cook, stirring, until tender, 3 to 4 minutes. Add the chard leaves and cook until wilted, 2 to 3 minutes. Season with ¼ teaspoon of the salt and black pepper to taste and add them to the bowl of onions. Add the cheeses and toss well.

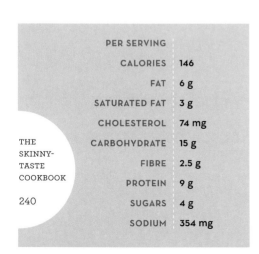

PER SERVING	
CALORIES	146
FAT	6 g
SATURATED FAT	3 g
CHOLESTEROL	74 mg
CARBOHYDRATE	15 g
FIBRE	2.5 g
PROTEIN	9 g
SUGARS	4 g
SODIUM	354 mg

Sift the flour and baking powder into a medium bowl. Whisk in the milk, olive oil, eggs and the remaining ¼ teaspoon salt. Pour into the bowl of Swiss chard and mix well. Pour the mixture into the prepared pie dish.

Bake until a knife inserted in the centre of the pie comes out clean, 27 to 30 minutes. Let it stand at least 5 minutes before serving. Slice into 6 wedges.

FOOD FACTS **super chard**
Chard is famous for its nutrient density and mildly bitter and briny flavour, which hints at its ancestor, the sea beetroot. Small, young leaves are delicious raw, while sautéing subdues the stronger flavour found in mature leaves (talk to your doctor before adding it to your diet if you use a blood thinner).

Quinoa-Stuffed Peppers

SERVES 4

I LOVE stuffed peppers. I stuff them with just about anything – beef, turkey and even my leftover Slow-Cooker Santa Fe Chicken (page 73). On nights when I want to go meatless, these Italian-inspired quinoa-stuffed peppers are simple to make, packed with protein and delicious! For extra flavour, I like to cook my quinoa in stock, or water with a little salt, a garlic clove and a sprig of parsley. This recipe can easily be doubled and frozen if you want to make an extra batch of meals for the month.

FILLING

½ cup (100g) quinoa

1 cup (225ml) low-salt vegetable stock*

1 teaspoon extra-virgin olive oil

2 garlic cloves, chopped

¾ cup (150g) tinned chopped tomatoes

¼ teaspoon sea salt

Freshly ground black pepper

3 tablespoons grated Pecorino Romano cheese

½ cup (25g) chopped baby spinach

2 tablespoons chopped fresh basil

¼ cup (25g) grated light mozzarella cheese

PEPPERS

2 large red peppers

4 tablespoons tinned chopped tomatoes

2 teaspoons grated Pecorino Romano cheese

¼ cup (25g) grated light mozzarella cheese

⅓ cup (75ml) low-salt vegetable stock

Read the label to be sure this product is gluten-free.

Rinse the quinoa under running water for about 2 minutes. Put the quinoa in a medium saucepan, add the vegetable stock and bring to a rolling boil. Reduce the heat to low, cover and cook until the liquid is absorbed, about 15 minutes. Remove the pan from the heat and allow to stand, covered, for 5 minutes. Fluff with a fork.

Preheat the oven to 180°C/160°C fan/Gas 4.

Heat a medium saucepan over medium heat. Add the oil and garlic and cook, stirring, until golden, about 1 minute. Add the tomatoes, salt and black pepper to taste and cook, stirring, for 5 minutes to develop the flavours. Remove the pan from the heat, add the cooked quinoa, Romano, spinach, basil and mozzarella.

(recipe continues)

PER SERVING	
CALORIES	183
FAT	6 g
SATURATED FAT	2 g
CHOLESTEROL	11 mg
CARBOHYDRATE	25 g
FIBRE	5 g
PROTEIN	8 g
SUGARS	6 g
SODIUM	411 mg

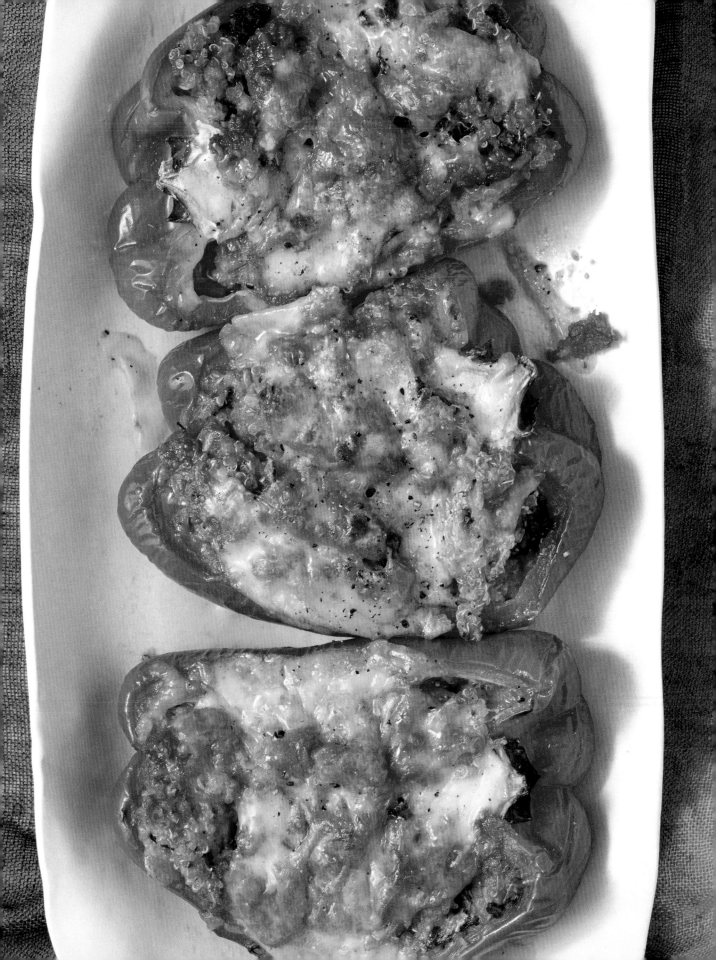

PERFECT PAIRINGS
One serving is very filling, but
if you want to serve this with
a side dish, I recommend **My
House Salad, Made with Love
(page 267)**.

For the peppers: Halve the peppers lengthwise and remove the core, seeds and stem. Place the peppers cut side up in a baking dish. Fill each pepper with the filling. Top each with 1 tablespoon tomatoes, ½ teaspoon Romano and 1 tablespoon mozzarella. Pour the stock into the bottom of the dish. Cover tightly with foil.

Bake until the peppers are soft, about 50 minutes. Remove them from the oven and allow to cool for 5 minutes before serving.

The Power of Protein

Strong, shiny nails? Sexy, sculpted shoulders? A leaner, meaner body? This powerhouse nutrient, which is found in every cell, tissue and organ in your body, can help you build muscle, burn calories and boost immunity. So how much is enough? The average healthy adult should get at least 0.8 grams of protein for every kilogram (2.2 pounds) of body weight. For a 63kg (10 stone) woman, that's 50 grams of protein each day.

To pump up your protein intake, eat a diet rich in meat, poultry, fish, dairy, eggs, legumes and nuts. If you are a vegetarian and worrying about how to get enough protein in your diet, here's a list of protein-rich meat-free options:

Tofu (170g) – 15 grams

Shelled edamame (½ cup/80g) – 8 grams

Lentils (½ cup/100g cooked) – 9 grams

Peanut butter (2 tablespoons) – 9 grams

Black beans (½ cup/85g cooked) – 8 grams

Kidney beans (½ cup/90g cooked) – 8 grams

Split peas (½ cup/100g cooked) – 8 grams

Chickpeas (½ cup/80g cooked) – 7 grams

Chia seeds (25g) – 5 grams

Peanuts (2 tablespoons) – 5 grams

Sesame seeds (25g) – 5 grams

Quinoa (½ cup/90g cooked) – 4 grams

Creamy Carrot Farrotto

SERVES 4

If you like creamy risotto as much as I do, then you'll love this creamy 'farrotto', a healthier version that's made with pearled farro, a whole grain with a wonderful nutty flavour. This dish was inspired by an unforgettable carrot risotto that I enjoyed a few years ago at a quaint restaurant in Carmel, California. This version is a whole lot easier to make than the original, too, because you don't have to stand over it the whole time as you do when you use Arborio rice.

SALAD

1 medium carrot, peeled into ribbons

2 tablespoons fresh lemon juice

1 teaspoon extra-virgin olive oil

⅛ teaspoon sea salt

Freshly ground black pepper

1½ cups (65g) rocket

CARROT PURÉE

1 tablespoon olive oil

½ cup (55g) finely chopped shallots

3 garlic cloves, crushed

1½ cups (235g) chopped carrots

2 cups (450ml) low-salt vegetable stock

½ teaspoon sea salt

⅛ teaspoon freshly ground black pepper

FARROTTO

1¼ cups (280g) semi-pearled farro, rinsed

3 cups (675ml) low-salt vegetable stock, plus more if needed

½ teaspoon sea salt

¼ cup (25g) grated Parmesan cheese, plus 2 tablespoons freshly shaved, for garnish

For the salad: In a medium bowl, combine the carrot ribbons, lemon juice, olive oil, salt and a pinch of black pepper to taste. Refrigerate until ready to serve.

For the carrot purée: In a large deep nonstick frying pan, heat the oil over medium heat. Add the shallots and garlic and cook, stirring, until soft, 3 to 4 minutes. Add the carrots and vegetable stock and season with the salt and black pepper. Bring to a boil. Reduce the heat to medium-low, cover and simmer until the carrots are soft, about 30 minutes. Remove the pan from the heat and allow to cool slightly.

(recipe continues)

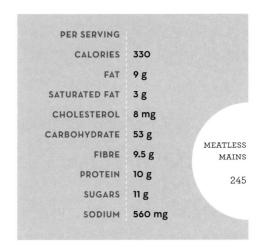

PER SERVING	
CALORIES	330
FAT	9 g
SATURATED FAT	3 g
CHOLESTEROL	8 mg
CARBOHYDRATE	53 g
FIBRE	9.5 g
PROTEIN	10 g
SUGARS	11 g
SODIUM	560 mg

MEATLESS
MAINS

245

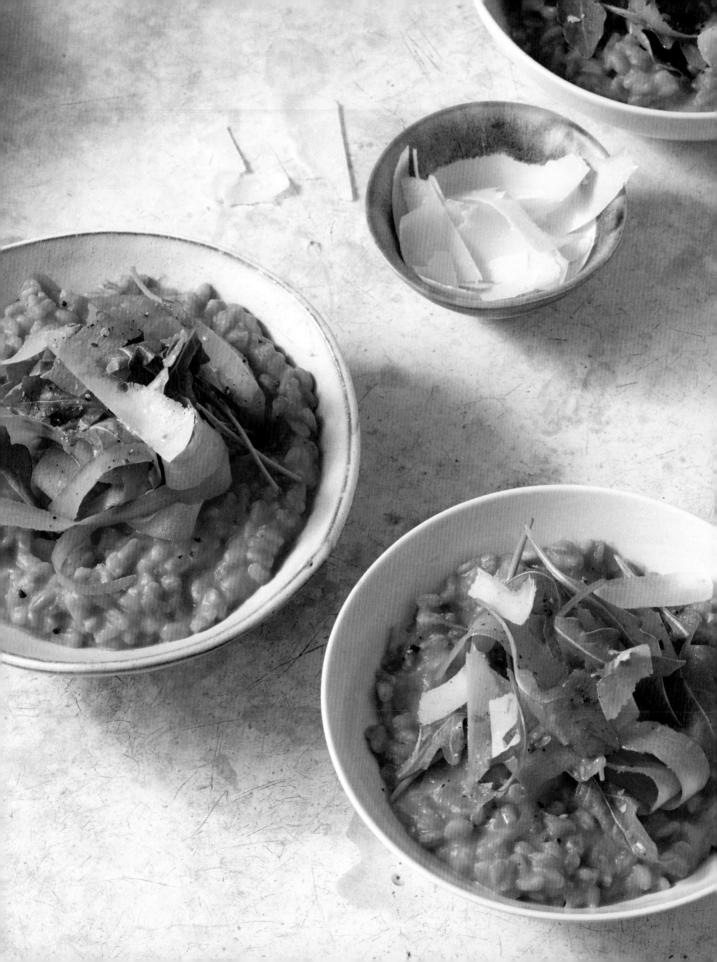

Purée the carrots in a blender or with a hand blender (be careful to keep the lid slightly ajar to release steam, and cover with a kitchen towel to catch any splatters). Set aside.

For the farrotto: In a large saucepan, combine the farro, vegetable stock and salt. Bring to a low boil over medium-low heat and cook until the farro is al dente, 15 to 20 minutes or according to packet directions. Drain and return the farro to the pan.

Add the carrot purée to the farro and cook over medium-low heat, stirring occasionally, until creamy, 4 to 6 minutes, adding more vegetable stock if needed. Stir in the grated Parmesan.

To serve, toss the rocket with the carrot ribbons. Divide the farrotto among 4 plates, sprinkle with the shaved Parmesan and top with the carrots and rocket.

FOOD FACTS **fabulous farro**

Farro (also called emmer wheat) is a grain that's starting to gain popularity. It was a staple crop in ancient Rome, and was widely used in other countries up until the twentieth century, at which point it was replaced by other forms of wheat that are easier to harvest and hull. Farro is now making a comeback, thanks to its taste, firm and chewy texture and nutrition profile. A study from scientists in Turkey found that farro had higher levels of antioxidants than other forms of wheat.

Butternut Squash Lasagna Rolls

SERVES 9

I have such fond memories of helping my mom make lasagna as a kid. I was in charge of layering the pasta, sauce, ricotta and mozzarella. Today, my lasagna is a bit lighter than my mom's. Rather than making it in a large tray, I prefer to make rolls – which I load up with vegetables – for better portion control. And here I swap tomato sauce for a wonderfully savoury butternut squash sauce with shallots, garlic and Parmesan cheese.

BUTTERNUT SQUASH

450g peeled butternut squash, diced

1 teaspoon sea salt

LASAGNA ROLLS

1 teaspoon olive oil

¼ cup (30g) finely chopped shallots

2 cloves garlic, crushed

½ teaspoon sea salt

⅛ teaspoon freshly ground black pepper

½ cup (50g) plus 2½ tablespoons freshly grated Parmesan cheese

275g frozen chopped spinach, cooked according to packet directions, cooled and squeezed dry

1¾ cups (425g) low-fat ricotta cheese

1 large egg

9 lasagna sheets, wheat- or gluten-free,* cooked

75g grated light mozzarella cheese

Read the label to be sure this product is gluten-free.

Preheat the oven to 180°C/160°C fan/Gas 4.

For the butternut squash: Place the squash in a large pot with enough water to cover the squash by 5cm. Add the salt and bring to a boil. Cover and cook over medium-low heat until soft, about 12 to 14 minutes. Remove the butternut squash with a slotted spoon and place it in a blender with ¼ cup (50ml) of the liquid it was cooked in. Reserve an additional 1 cup (225ml) of liquid and set aside. Purée the squash.

For the lasagna rolls: In a medium nonstick frying pan, add the oil and sauté the shallots and garlic over medium-low heat until soft and golden, about 4 to 5 minutes. Add the puréed butternut squash, the ¼ teaspoon salt and a pinch of black

(recipe continues)

PER SERVING	
CALORIES	234
FAT	5 g
SATURATED FAT	2.5 g
CHOLESTEROL	32 mg
CARBOHYDRATE	29 g
FIBRE	3 g
PROTEIN	17 g
SUGARS	3 g
SODIUM	449 mg

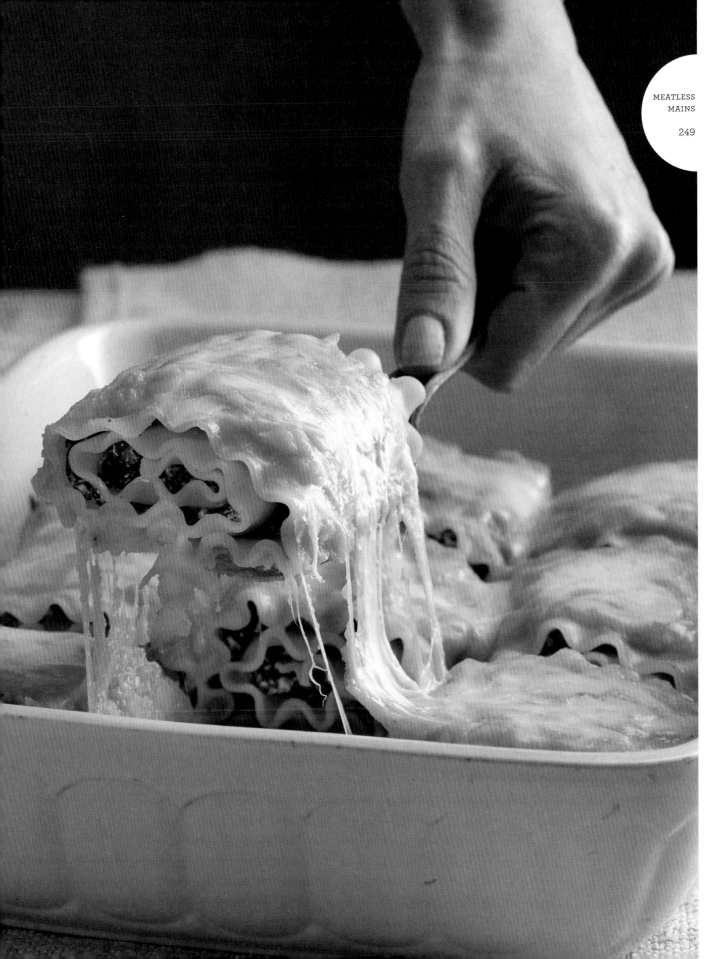

I always dish this up with **My House Salad, Made with Love (page 267)**.

skinny**scoop**

For best freezing results, freeze the lasagna rolls after you bake them in a freezer-safe ziplock bag or container. To reheat put the frozen lasagna rolls in a baking dish. Cover with foil and bake at 190°C/170°C fan/Gas 5 for 45 to 50 minutes.

pepper, adding about a half to three-quarters of the reserved liquid to thin out the sauce until smooth. Stir in 2½ tablespoons of the Parmesan cheese and set aside.

In a medium bowl, combine the spinach, ricotta, the remaining Parmesan, egg, ¼ teaspoon salt and the black pepper.

Ladle a couple of spoons of the butternut sauce into the bottom of a 23 × 32cm baking dish.

Put a piece of greaseproof paper on a work surface and lay the cooked lasagna sheets out on it. Make sure the sheets are dry. Spread the ricotta mixture over each sheet. Carefully roll them up and put them seam side down in the baking dish. Ladle the remaining sauce over the lasagna rolls and top each with 1 tablespoon mozzarella. Tightly cover the dish with foil.

Bake until the inside is heated through and the cheese is melted, about 40 minutes.

Black Bean Burrito Bowls

SERVES 5

When you consider my family's heritage – I'm half Colombian and my husband is half Puerto Rican – you can imagine how much we love rice and beans in my house. The funny thing is, as a kid I never cared much for beans. My mom always joked that I should have been Italian. But in my twenties, I grew to love beans and to appreciate all the varieties and different ways to prepare them. Black beans are one of my favourites, and when I have the time, I make a big pot from scratch using dried beans that I soak overnight and cook in my pressure cooker. It takes time and planning. On a busy weeknight, I'm not above using tinned beans – if they're prepared correctly, they're wonderful.

RICE

¼ teaspoon sea salt

1¼ cups (250g) long-grain brown rice

1 teaspoon olive oil

Juice of ½ lime (or more to taste)

3 tablespoons chopped fresh coriander

SALSA

½ cup (100g) fresh or frozen sweetcorn kernels

2 tablespoons chopped red onion

1½ tablespoons fresh lime juice

⅛ teaspoon sea salt

1 small tomato, chopped

1 small jalapeño or other green chilli, seeded and finely chopped (for hotter salsa, leave the seeds)

1 small garlic clove, crushed

2 tablespoons chopped fresh coriander

BEANS

2 teaspoons olive oil

⅔ cup (100g) chopped onion

2 garlic cloves, crushed

2 spring onions, chopped

2 tablespoons chopped red pepper

3 tablespoons chopped fresh coriander

1 teaspoon red wine vinegar

1 (400g) tin black beans*

1 bay leaf

½ teaspoon ground cumin

¼ teaspoon dried oregano

¼ teaspoon sea salt

Freshly ground black pepper

TOPPINGS

10 tablespoons grated reduced-fat cheddar-Jack cheese blend†

1 avocado, thinly sliced

1⅔ cups (70g) finely shredded romaine lettuce

Read the label to be sure this product is gluten-free.

For the rice: In a pot of salted boiling water, cook the rice according to the packet directions. Transfer the rice to a large bowl and add the olive oil, lime juice and coriander. Toss well and set aside.

(recipe continues)

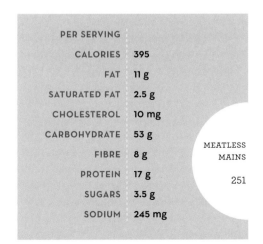

PER SERVING	
CALORIES	395
FAT	11 g
SATURATED FAT	2.5 g
CHOLESTEROL	10 mg
CARBOHYDRATE	53 g
FIBRE	8 g
PROTEIN	17 g
SUGARS	3.5 g
SODIUM	245 mg

MEATLESS MAINS

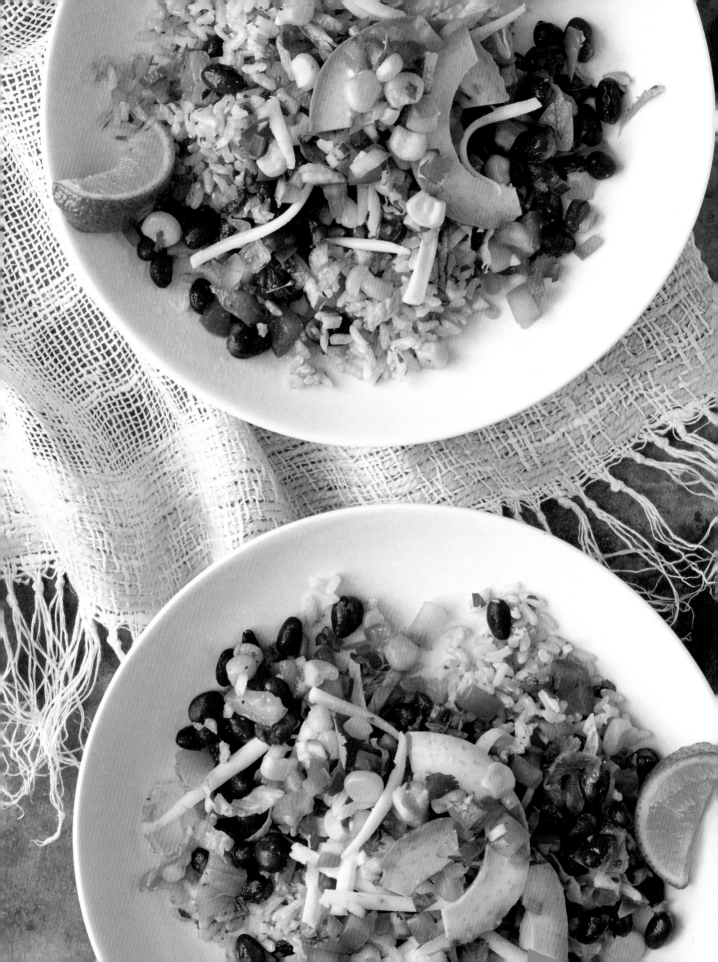

For the salsa: Cook the sweetcorn in a small pan of boiling water for 5 minutes. Drain and set aside to cool.

In a medium bowl, combine the red onion, lime juice and the salt. Allow to sit for 5 minutes. Add the cooled corn, tomato, jalapeño, garlic and coriander.

For the beans: Heat a medium pot over medium heat. Add the olive oil, onion, garlic, spring onions, pepper and coriander. Cook, stirring, until the vegetables are soft, 3 to 5 minutes. Add ½ cup (110ml) water, the vinegar, beans, bay leaf, cumin, oregano, salt and black pepper to taste. Bring to a boil. Reduce the heat to low, cover and simmer, stirring occasionally, for 15 minutes to blend the flavours. Remove the bay leaf.

For the toppings: To serve, divide the rice equally among 5 bowls. Top each bowl with black beans, 2 tablespoons grated cheese, salsa, avocado slices and romaine lettuce.

† If you can't find reduced-fat cheddar-Jack cheese blend, a lighter cheddar will work well.

Cheesy Baked Penne with Aubergine

SERVES 8

One of my favourite dishes to make for my family is this baked pasta dish, with all its cheesy goodness and hidden bits of sweet aubergine. Picky eaters of all ages – and devout meat eaters, too – love this.

Olive oil spray or oil mister

1 cup (225g) low-fat ricotta cheese

2 cups (225g) grated light mozzarella cheese

½ cup (45g) grated Pecorino Romano cheese

¼ cup (7g) chopped fresh parsley

1 tablespoon olive oil

4 garlic cloves, roughly chopped

1 aubergine, cut into 2 to 3cm cubes

2 teaspoons sea salt

Freshly ground black pepper

3½ cups (875g) tinned chopped tomatoes

2 tablespoons chopped fresh basil

350g penne rigate pasta, wheat- or gluten-free*

skinny**scoop**

To freeze, let the pasta cool and then divide it into portions. Wrap the portions in clingfilm and place them in a large freezer bag. The day before eating, transfer a piece to the refrigerator to thaw overnight.

Read the label to be sure this product is gluten-free.

Preheat the oven to 190°C/170°C fan/Gas 5. Spray a 23 × 32cm baking dish with olive oil.

In a medium bowl, combine the ricotta, half of the mozzarella, 6 tablespoons of the Romano and the parsley.

In a large, deep pan, heat the olive oil over medium heat. Add the garlic and cook, stirring, until golden, about 1 minute. Add the aubergine, ¾ teaspoon of the salt and black pepper and cook until golden, 4 to 5 minutes. Add the tomatoes, basil, ¼ teaspoon of the salt and black pepper. Reduce the heat to low and cook until the aubergine is tender, about 5 minutes.

Add the remaining 1 teaspoon salt to a large pot of boiling water. Add the pasta and cook to 4 minutes less than al dente. Drain. Put half of the pasta into the prepared dish and top with one-third of the sauce. Spoon the ricotta mixture on top. Cover with the remaining pasta and sauce. Top with the remaining mozzarella and 2 tablespoons Romano. Cover with foil.

Bake for 20 minutes. Remove the foil and bake until the mozzarella is melted and the edges are lightly browned, 6 to 7 minutes.

THE SKINNY-TASTE COOKBOOK

254

PER SERVING	
CALORIES	325
FAT	9 g
SATURATED FAT	0 g
CHOLESTEROL	20 mg
CARBOHYDRATE	44 g
FIBRE	4.5 g
PROTEIN	18 g
SUGARS	6 g
SODIUM	716 mg

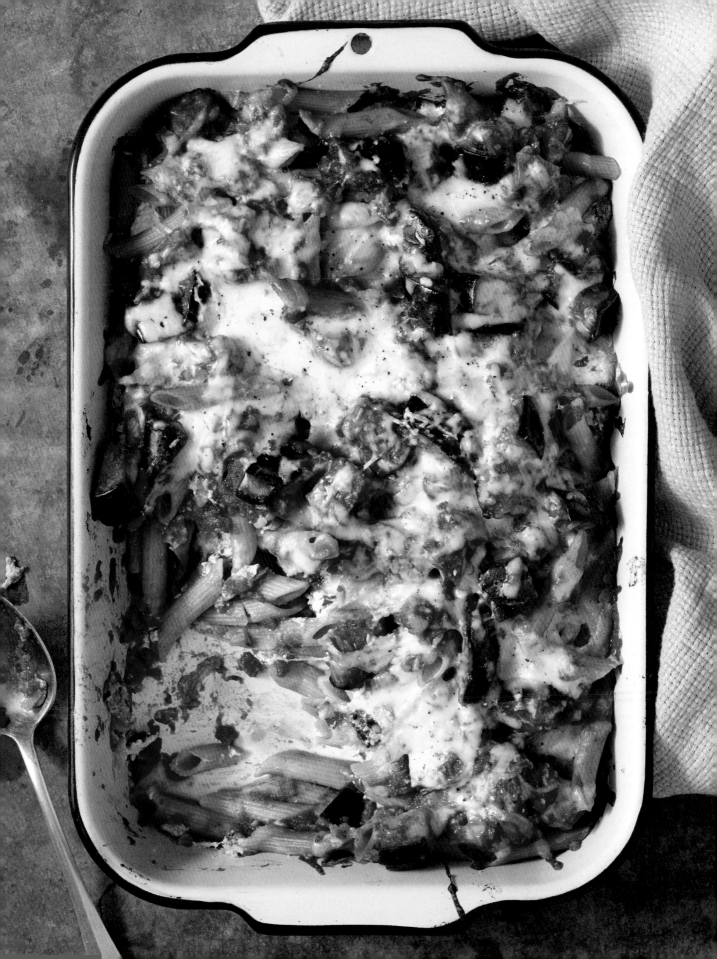

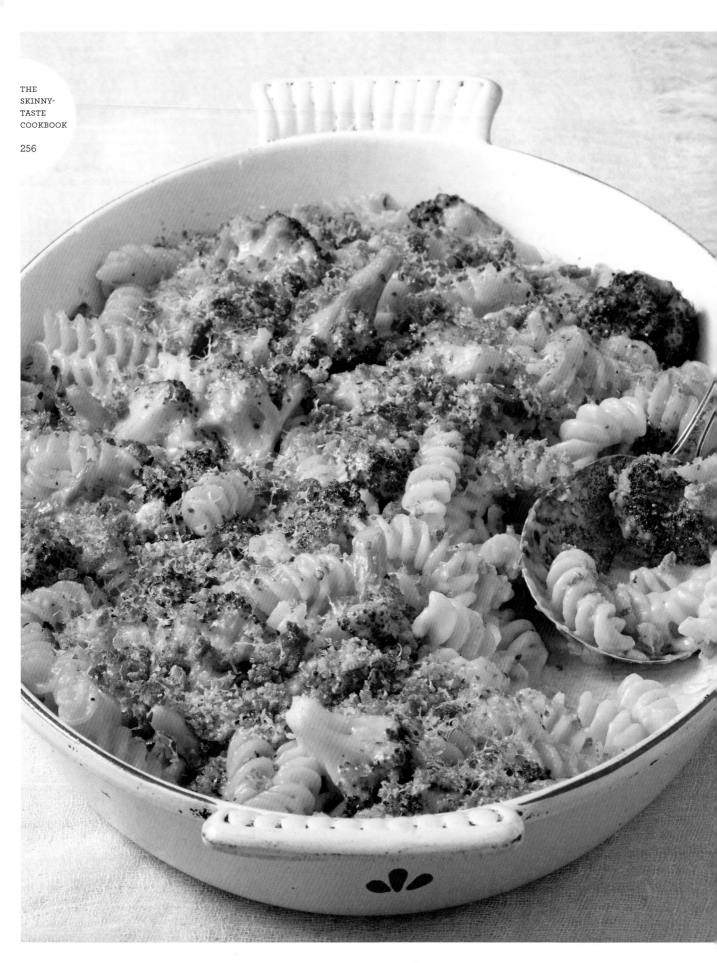

Skinny Broccoli Mac and Cheese

SERVES 8

Mac and cheese is the ultimate comfort food. Eliminating it from my diet was not an option, so early on I decided I would figure out a way to make it work. My secret weapon was to add some greens – broccoli, in particular, because broccoli and cheese are a match made in heaven. I also developed a lighter cheese sauce to further ease the calorie guilt. I love that extra crunch you get from toasted bread crumbs, so I sprinkle a little on top just before I bake it.

Cooking spray or oil mister

Sea salt

350g broccoli florets

350g fusilli pasta

25g unsalted butter

⅓ cup (50g) finely chopped onion

¼ cup (30g) plain flour

2 cups (450ml) skimmed milk

1 cup (225ml) low-salt chicken stock (or vegetable stock)

Freshly ground black pepper

2 cups (225g) grated lighter cheddar cheese

¼ cup (20g) seasoned wholemeal bread crumbs, homemade (see page 110) or shop-bought

2 tablespoons grated Parmesan cheese

Preheat the oven to 190°C/170°C fan/Gas 5. Spray a 23 × 32cm baking dish with oil.

Cook the broccoli and pasta to 3 minutes less than al dente in a large pot of salted boiling water according to packet directions. Drain and set aside.

In a large nonstick frying pan, melt the butter over medium-low heat. Add the onion and cook, stirring, until soft, about 2 minutes. Add the flour and cook, stirring, 1 minute. Whisk in the milk and stock, increase the heat to medium-high and continue whisking until the mixture boils. Cook until the sauce is smooth and thick, 7 to 8 minutes. Season with ¼ teaspoon salt and black pepper to taste. Remove the pan from the heat and stir in the cheddar until melted. Add the pasta and broccoli and stir well. Pour into the prepared dish and top with the bread crumbs and Parmesan. Spray with oil.

Bake for 18 to 20 minutes. Turn the oven to grill and cook until the bread crumbs are golden, keeping an eye on them so they do not burn, about 2 minutes.

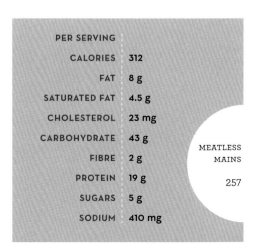

PER SERVING	
CALORIES	312
FAT	8 g
SATURATED FAT	4.5 g
CHOLESTEROL	23 mg
CARBOHYDRATE	43 g
FIBRE	2 g
PROTEIN	19 g
SUGARS	5 g
SODIUM	410 mg

MEATLESS MAINS

Spinach Falafel Lettuce Wraps

SERVES 4

My challenge: to create a healthier falafel that is quick and easy, skipping the deep-frying and soaking the chickpeas overnight. With a few smart swaps, I created my ideal falafels – using tinned chickpeas, spinach, lots of fresh herbs and spices and quinoa to bind them – that are light but packed with protein and a cinch to make. Also, instead of serving them in pitta bread, I wrap the patties in crisp lettuce leaves.

TZATZIKI

¾ cup (185g) fat-free Greek yoghurt

¾ cup (130g) peeled, seeded and grated cucumber

¼ teaspoon sea salt

1 small garlic clove, crushed

1 tablespoon finely chopped fresh dill

1 tablespoon finely chopped fresh chives

1 teaspoon fresh lemon juice

Freshly ground black pepper

FALAFEL

1 cup (45g) baby spinach

½ cup (60g) chopped spring onions

½ cup (15g) chopped fresh parsley

⅓ cup (20g) chopped fresh coriander

4 garlic cloves, crushed

½ tablespoon ground cumin

1 teaspoon ground coriander

¾ teaspoon sea salt

1 (425g) tin chickpeas,* rinsed and drained

⅓ cup (60g) cooked quinoa

1 large egg, beaten

1 teaspoon olive oil

Cooking spray or oil mister

4 large outer iceberg lettuce leaves

1 cup (200g) chopped tomatoes

¼ cup (40g) grated carrots

¼ cup (15g) shredded red cabbage

¼ cup (55g) hummus

8 teaspoons harissa, homemade (see page 206) or shop-bought

Read the label to be sure this product is gluten-free.

For the tzatziki: Spoon the yoghurt into a colander lined with a few sheets of kitchen paper and allow to drain for 10 minutes. Lightly sprinkle the cucumber with ⅛ teaspoon of the salt and set aside for 10 minutes to release some of its liquid. Using kitchen paper, squeeze the excess moisture from the cucumber.

In a medium bowl, combine the yoghurt, cucumber, garlic, dill, chives, lemon juice, the remaining ⅛ teaspoon salt and a pinch of black pepper. Refrigerate until ready to serve.

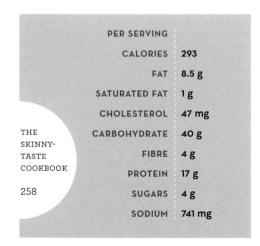

PER SERVING	
CALORIES	293
FAT	8.5 g
SATURATED FAT	1 g
CHOLESTEROL	47 mg
CARBOHYDRATE	40 g
FIBRE	4 g
PROTEIN	17 g
SUGARS	4 g
SODIUM	741 mg

For the falafel: In a food processor, combine the spinach, spring onions, parsley, coriander, garlic, cumin, ground coriander and salt and process until smooth. Add the chickpeas and pulse 12 to 15 times, until coarsely mashed. Fold in the quinoa and egg. Form the mixture into 12 small flattened patties and refrigerate for 15 to 20 minutes.

Heat a large nonstick griddle or frying pan over medium-high heat. Add the oil, swirling to coat the bottom of the pan. Put the patties in the pan and cook until golden brown, 4 to 5 minutes. Lightly spray the tops with oil, flip and cook until the second side is golden brown, 4 to 5 minutes.

To serve, put a lettuce leaf on each plate, spread each with tzatziki and top each with 3 falafel patties, an equal amount of diced tomato, carrots, cabbage and hummus, and 1 tablespoon harissa. Roll it up like a wrap and eat immediately.

PERFECT PAIRINGS
If you'd like to make a falafel platter, serve the patties with **Quinoa Tabbouleh (page 287)** and some hummus on the side.

skinnyscoop

Quinoa has been called the 'miracle grain' because it's nutritious, satisfying and easy to prepare. Best of all, you can cook it and keep it in the fridge for up to 5 days, which makes it easy to throw together a weeknight meal. You can keep it in the freezer for up to 2 months, too!

Chickpea and Potato Curry

SERVES 6

When I worked in Manhattan, my good friend Tricia and I would have Indian for lunch once a week. It's probably what I miss most about working in the city. Often – but not intentionally – I found myself having a vegetarian meal, usually some type of curry. Whenever I make a pot of this rich, hearty dish of chickpeas, peas and potatoes, the scent of the Indian spices brings me back to those memorable lunches.

1½ cups (300g) brown basmati rice

1 tablespoon coconut oil or rapeseed oil

½ medium onion, finely chopped

5 garlic cloves, crushed

½ teaspoon ground cumin

1½ teaspoons garam masala*

2 teaspoons curry powder*

1 (425g) tin chopped tomatoes

1 (400g) tin chickpeas,* drained

1½ cups (235g) frozen green peas

2 medium all-purpose potatoes, peeled and cut into 2 to 3cm cubes

¼ cup (15g) plus 2 tablespoons chopped fresh coriander

1 fresh chilli, chopped (optional)

1⅛ teaspoons sea salt

PERFECT PAIRINGS

I serve this stew over brown basmati rice topped with fresh coriander. Or you could pick up some Indian flatbread such as naan or roti, which are perfect for soaking up the sauce. This would also be wonderful with **Turmeric-Roasted Cauliflower (page 270)**.

Read the labels to be sure these products are gluten-free.

Cook the rice according to packet directions. Set aside.

Heat a large nonstick deep frying pan over medium heat. Add the oil, onion and garlic and cook, stirring, until soft, 2 to 3 minutes. Add the cumin, garam masala and curry powder and cook for 1 more minute. Add 1¼ cups (300ml) water, the tomatoes, chickpeas, green peas, potatoes, 2 tablespoons of the coriander and the chilli (if using). Season with the salt, cover, reduce the heat to low and simmer until the potatoes are firm-tender, about 30 minutes.

To serve, divide the rice among 6 bowls. Divide the curry over the rice and top with the remaining coriander.

PER SERVING	
CALORIES	369
FAT	6 g
SATURATED FAT	2 g
CHOLESTEROL	0 mg
PROTEIN	12 g
CARBOHYDRATE	71 g
FIBRE	7 g
SUGARS	6 g
SODIUM	531 mg

Spicy Black Bean Burgers with Chipotle Mayo

SERVES 4

One bite of this spicy burger, and you'll understand why all the adult carnivores in my home are big fans of it. When we want to go meatless, these burgers, which are loaded with fibre and protein, totally hit the spot. They're also very economical because they're made with tinned beans, which are so inexpensive. And, they're pretty simple to make and have one small trick: the patties need to be frozen before you cook them so they keep their shape. You can even double the recipe and freeze burgers so you have them ready to go whenever you need a quick, healthy, last-minute dinner.

SPICY CHIPOTLE MAYO

3½ tablespoons light mayonnaise (I prefer Hellmann's Light)

1 tablespoon chopped chipotle chilli in adobo sauce†

BLACK BEAN BURGERS

1 (400g) tin black beans, rinsed and drained

½ red pepper, roughly chopped

½ cup (60g) roughly chopped spring onions

3 tablespoons roughly chopped fresh coriander

3 garlic cloves

½ cup (50g) rolled oats

1 large egg

1 teaspoon cayenne pepper hot sauce

1 tablespoon ground cumin

¼ teaspoon sea salt

Cooking spray or oil mister

4 wholemeal rolls

1 medium avocado, thinly sliced

For the spicy chipotle mayo: In a small bowl, combine the mayonnaise and chipotle. Set aside.

For the black bean burgers: Dry the beans well after rinsing (any extra moisture will keep the burgers from holding together well). Put the beans in a medium bowl and mash them with a fork or potato masher until thick and pasty.

(recipe continues)

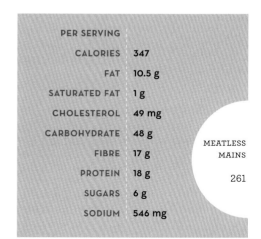

PER SERVING	
CALORIES	347
FAT	10.5 g
SATURATED FAT	1 g
CHOLESTEROL	49 mg
CARBOHYDRATE	48 g
FIBRE	17 g
PROTEIN	18 g
SUGARS	6 g
SODIUM	546 mg

MEATLESS MAINS

Try these with **Seasoned Sweet Potato Wedges (page 277)** for a healthier spin on the classic burger-and-fries.

In a food processor, combine the pepper, spring onions, coriander and garlic and pulse until finely chopped. Add the oats, egg, hot sauce, cumin and salt and pulse a few times, until mixed well. Fold the mixture into the mashed beans. Form the mixture into 4 patties (using slightly oiled or wet hands helps) and put them on a baking sheet lined with greaseproof paper. (If the mixture is too wet, refrigerate it for 30 minutes or add another tablespoon of oats.) Freeze for at least 2 hours before cooking.

To cook, heat a nonstick frying pan over medium heat. Lightly spray the pan with oil and cook the frozen burgers until browned, about 7 minutes per side. (Alternatively, preheat a barbecue to medium, lightly spray a sheet of foil with oil, put the burgers on the foil and cook until browned, 7 to 8 minutes per side.)

To serve, place the burgers on the buns and top with the spicy chipotle mayo and avocado slices.

✝ If you can't find chipotle chilli in adobo sauce, chipotle paste would work well as an alternative.

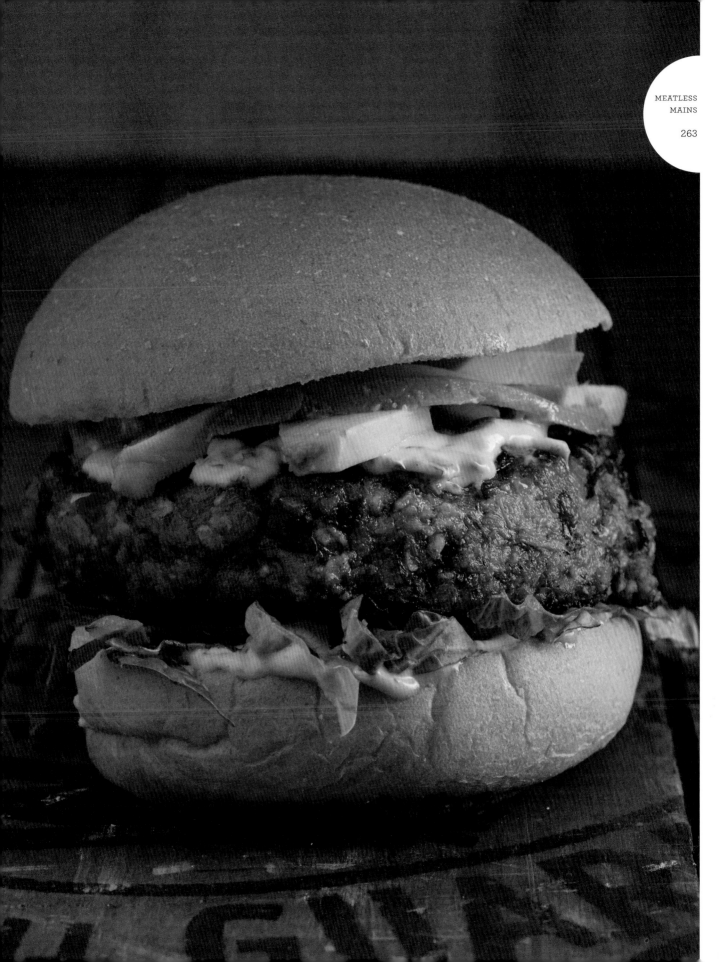

VEGGIE-LICIOUS
SIDES

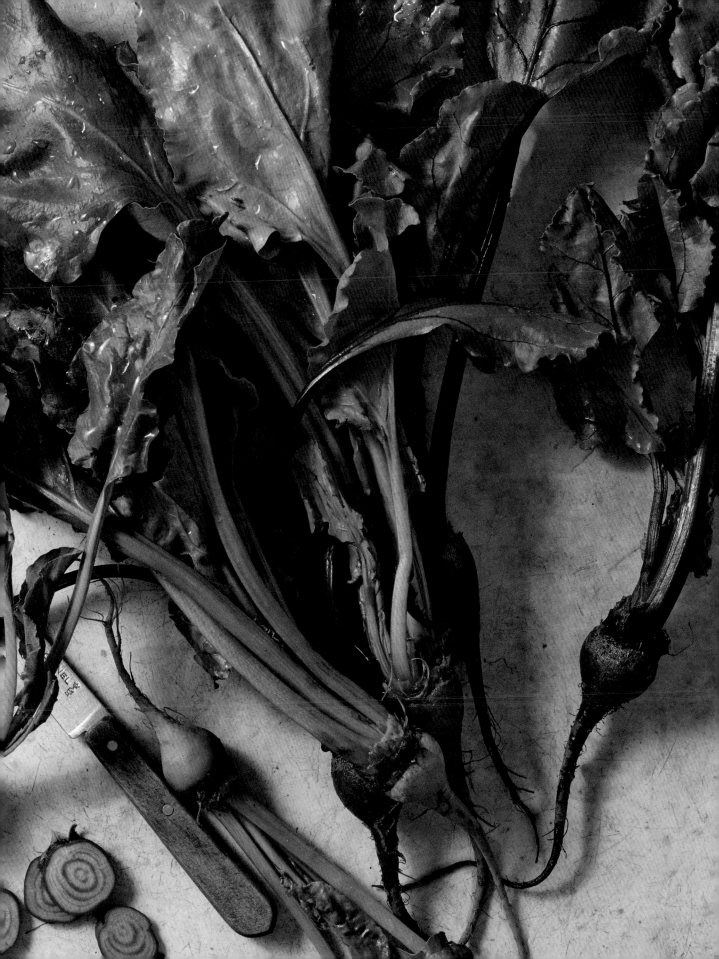

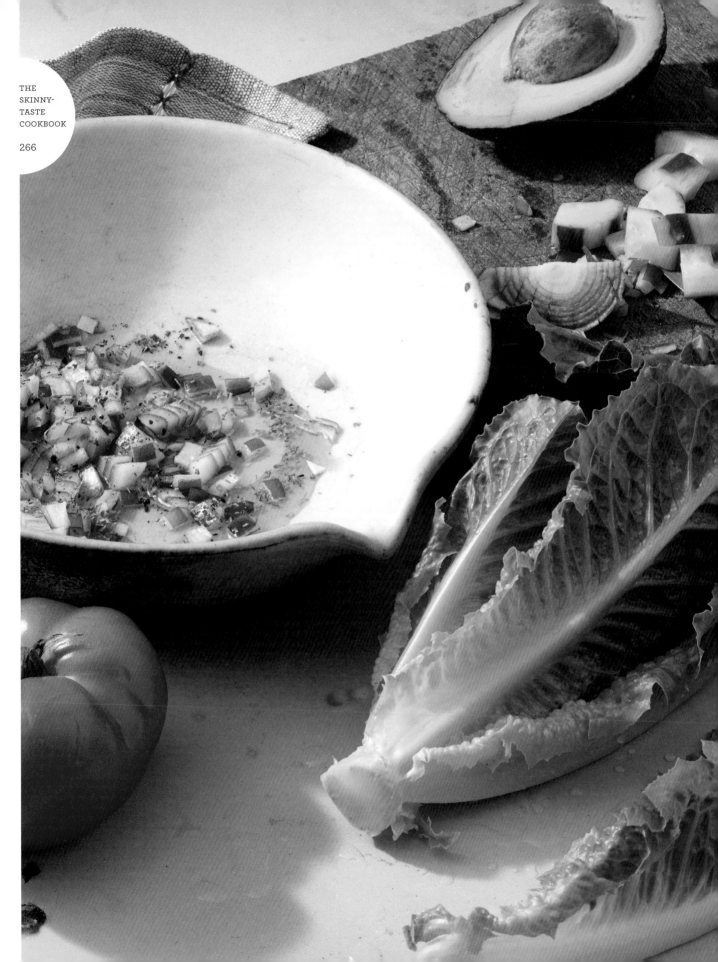

My House Salad, Made with Love

SERVES 4

This everyday salad is *my* special house salad. What makes it great isn't the ingredients but the love that goes into making it. I picked this up from my mother-in-law, who taught me how to make a truly tasty salad. She doesn't just combine all the ingredients at once with a quick toss. It's a process.

3 tablespoons roughly chopped red onion

1 tablespoon plus 1 teaspoon extra-virgin olive oil

1½ tablespoons apple cider vinegar

½ teaspoon sea salt

Freshly ground black pepper

1 cup (200g) chopped tomato

⅛ teaspoon garlic powder

⅛ teaspoon dried oregano

1 cucumber, peeled and cut into 2 to 3cm pieces

1 medium avocado, chopped

3 cups (150g) chopped romaine lettuce

In a large bowl, combine the red onion with 1 tablespoon of the olive oil, 1 tablespoon of the vinegar, ¼ teaspoon of the salt and black pepper to taste. Allow to sit until the onion flavour mellows, 5 minutes.

Add the tomato, garlic powder, oregano, the remaining ¼ teaspoon salt and a pinch of pepper, and allow to sit for at least another 5 minutes. Add the cucumber and toss.

When ready to serve, toss in the avocado and lettuce, the remaining 1 teaspoon olive oil and the remaining ½ tablespoon vinegar.

skinny**scoop**

Letting the chopped tomato sit a while with the onions and salt allows the juices to release and helps create a lighter dressing (a tasty way to cut back on oil).

PER SERVING	
CALORIES	117
FAT	10 g
SATURATED FAT	1.5 g
CHOLESTEROL	0 mg
CARBOHYDRATE	7 g
FIBRE	4 g
PROTEIN	2 g
SUGARS	3 g
SODIUM	148 mg

VEGGIE-LICIOUS SIDES

Squashta (Spaghetti Squash)

SERVES 5

I didn't grow up eating spaghetti squash. In fact, the first time I tried it was just a few years ago at a dinner at a friend's house. She served it as a side dish, roasted with a little olive oil, salt and pepper. I thought it was great, and I have since played around with it in many different ways. Here are two basic ways to prepare it – a roasted method I often use when I'm not in a rush and a quick microwave technique I rely on when I have only 15 minutes. How you top it is completely up to you!

1 medium spaghetti squash (about 1kg)

Sea salt and freshly ground black pepper

skinny**scoop**

To serve, drizzle the squash with a little extra-virgin olive oil and sprinkle with grated Pecorino Romano. Top it with Quickest Tomato Sauce (page 94), or toss with some pesto. It's wonderfully versatile!

To roast in the oven: Preheat the oven to 200°C/180°C fan/ Gas 6.

Halve the squash lengthwise and scoop out the seeds and fibres with a spoon. Season with a pinch of salt and black pepper and put the squash halves on a baking sheet, cut side down. Bake until the skin gives easily under pressure and the inside is tender, 50 minutes to 1 hour. Remove from the oven and allow to cool for 10 minutes. Using a fork, scrape out the squash flesh – it will separate into spaghetti-like strands.

To quickly cook in the microwave: Using a sharp knife, poke holes all over the squash. Cook it in the microwave for 6 minutes on high. Turn the squash and cook until the shell is tender, 6 to 8 minutes. Remove it from the microwave and allow to cool for 8 to 10 minutes. Halve the squash lengthwise. (There should be no resistance, but if there is, microwave it for a few more minutes.) Remove the seeds and use a fork to scrape out the spaghetti-like strands of squash. Season with a pinch of salt and black pepper.

PER SERVING	
CALORIES	71
FAT	1.5 g
SATURATED FAT	0 g
CHOLESTEROL	0 mg
CARBOHYDRATE	16 g
FIBRE	3.5 g
PROTEIN	1 g
SUGARS	6 g
SODIUM	53 mg

Cheesy Cauliflower 'Mash'

SERVES 5

I love mashed potatoes just as much as the next girl, but I try to limit my carbs to just a few servings a day. That means if I have toast for breakfast and a sandwich for lunch, I try to skip the starches at dinner. To the rescue: mashed cauliflower, which is a lighter – but just as tasty – replacement for mashed potatoes. Adding cheese and fresh herbs makes them only better!

1 large head cauliflower, cut into florets

4 garlic cloves, crushed

⅓ cup (75ml) buttermilk

1 tablespoon unsalted butter

¾ teaspoon sea salt

Freshly ground black pepper

1 tablespoon finely chopped fresh chives

⅓ cup (40g) grated lighter cheddar cheese

Bring a large pot of water to a boil. Add the cauliflower and garlic and cook until the cauliflower is soft, 15 to 20 minutes. Drain and return the vegetables to the pot. Add the buttermilk, butter, salt and black pepper to taste. Using a hand blender or a regular blender, purée the cauliflower. Stir in the chives and cheddar and serve hot.

PERFECT PAIRINGS
This is a great side dish to have with **Sunday Night Roast Beef and Gravy (page 211)**, **Skinny Salisbury Steak with Mushroom Gravy (page 201)**, roasted turkey breast, meatloaf or any dish you'd normally serve with mashed potatoes.

PER SERVING	
CALORIES	76
FAT	2 g
SATURATED FAT	1 g
CHOLESTEROL	6 mg
CARBOHYDRATE	10 g
FIBRE	3.5 g
PROTEIN	6 g
SUGARS	4 g
SODIUM	281 mg

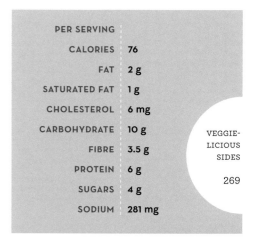

VEGGIE-LICIOUS SIDES

269

Turmeric-Roasted Cauliflower

SERVES 5

Once you've tasted roasted cauliflower, you'll never want to make it any other way – the vegetable becomes tender with slightly browned edges and a nutty taste that is pure yumminess. The garlic, cumin and fresh coriander give this side dish a fragrant finish with a warm, earthy tone. You'll also get a nice, vibrant colour from the turmeric, which has been shown to have powerful curative properties.

6 heaped cups (675ml) cauliflower florets

3 garlic cloves, crushed

¼ cup (50ml) olive oil

1 teaspoon turmeric

1 teaspoon ground cumin

¼ teaspoon crushed red chilli flakes

½ teaspoon sea salt

2 tablespoons chopped fresh coriander (optional)

PERFECT PAIRINGS
Try this as a side dish to chicken or lamb, or my **Chickpea and Potato Curry (page 260)**.

Preheat the oven to 230°C/210°C fan/Gas 8.

Cut the cauliflower florets into 2 to 3cm pieces and combine with the garlic in a large bowl. Drizzle with the olive oil and toss to coat.

In a small bowl, combine the turmeric, cumin, chilli flakes and salt. Sprinkle over the cauliflower and toss to coat. Spread the cauliflower out on a large baking tray.

Bake, stirring occasionally, until browned on the edges and tender, 23 to 27 minutes. Remove from the oven, sprinkle with the coriander (if using) and serve hot.

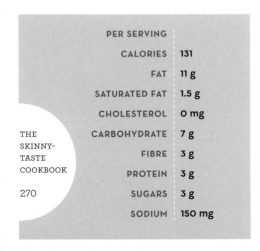

PER SERVING	
CALORIES	131
FAT	11 g
SATURATED FAT	1.5 g
CHOLESTEROL	0 mg
CARBOHYDRATE	7 g
FIBRE	3 g
PROTEIN	3 g
SUGARS	3 g
SODIUM	150 mg

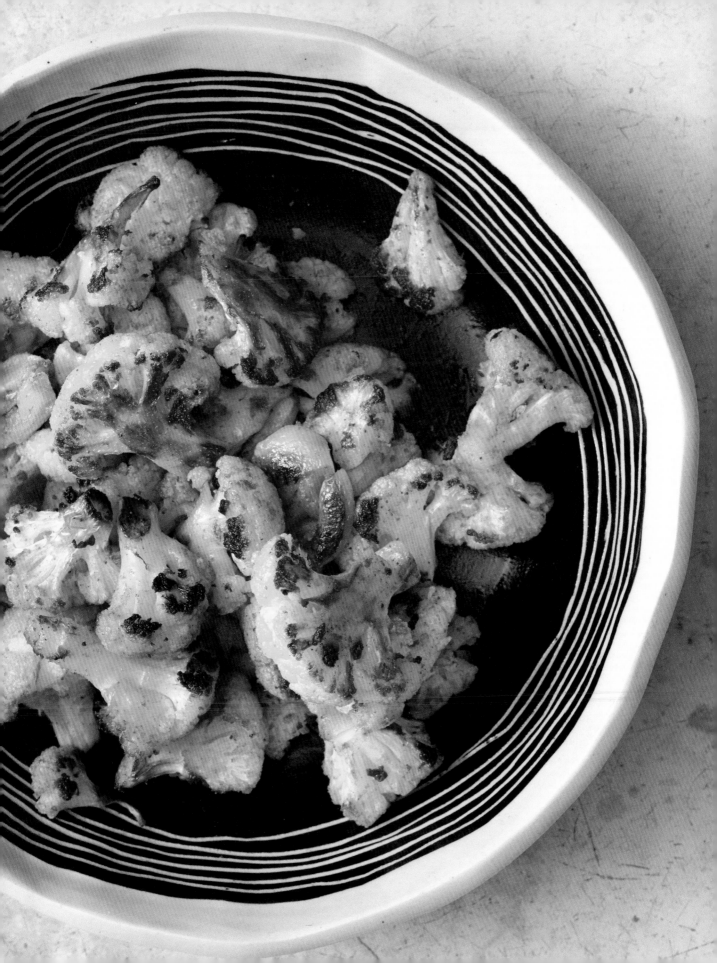

Roasted Sesame Green Beans

SERVES 4

In my opinion, green beans should never be mushy. They should be tender, but still crisp and slightly browned on the edges. The easiest way to achieve this is to roast or sauté them. To give them an Asian flair, I toss them with sesame oil and the popular Japanese condiment called *furikake* – a combination of sesame seeds, red shiso and nori – that will take these string beans to a whole other level!

350g green beans, trimmed

2 teaspoons sesame oil

¼ teaspoon garlic powder

1½ tablespoons furikake

⅛ teaspoon crushed red chilli flakes

Sea salt

skinny**scoop**

If you don't have furikake, you can replace it with sesame seeds and salt.

Adjust an oven rack in the lower third of the oven and preheat to 220°C/200°C fan/Gas 7. Line a large baking sheet with foil.

Arrange the green beans on the baking sheet and drizzle them with the sesame oil. Shake to coat evenly, then season with the garlic powder, furikake, chilli flakes and a pinch of sea salt. Toss well.

Bake until browned on the bottom, about 10 minutes. Shake the pan or stir the beans and bake until golden and slightly browned on the edges, 5 to 6 more minutes. Remove from the oven and serve hot.

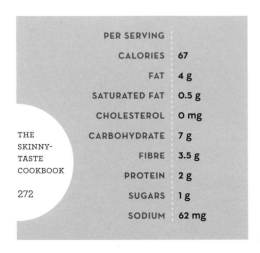

PER SERVING	
CALORIES	67
FAT	4 g
SATURATED FAT	0.5 g
CHOLESTEROL	0 mg
CARBOHYDRATE	7 g
FIBRE	3.5 g
PROTEIN	2 g
SUGARS	1 g
SODIUM	62 mg

Vegetable Fried Brown Rice

SERVES 5

When a craving for Chinese food strikes, I grab my wok and make my own take-away fake-away! I've perfected this healthier version of fried rice made with whole-grain rice and lots of veggies. The key to perfect fried rice is cold, day-old rice, so if I'm cooking rice the night before, I make a double batch of rice. I like to use short-grain brown rice, which stands up to reheating without turning to mush.

2½ tablespoons reduced-salt soy sauce (or tamari* for gluten-free)

1 teaspoon fish sauce (omit for vegetarian)

1 large egg

3 large egg whites

⅛ teaspoon sea salt

Freshly ground black pepper

Cooking spray or oil mister

1 tablespoon sesame oil

½ medium onion, chopped

½ cup (90g) chopped red pepper

6 spring onions, white parts finely chopped and green parts cut into 5mm pieces

3 garlic cloves, crushed

1 teaspoon finely chopped fresh ginger

1 cup (160g) frozen peas and carrots, thawed

3 cups (555g) cooked short-grain brown rice, cold (from 1 cup/220g raw)

Read the label to be sure this product is gluten-free.

In a small bowl, combine the soy sauce and fish sauce (if using) and set aside. In a separate bowl, whisk together the whole egg, egg whites, salt and black pepper to taste.

Heat a large nonstick wok over high heat. Spray with oil, add the eggs and cook until scrambled, about 1 minute. Transfer to a plate.

Let the wok get really hot. Add the oil, then add the onion, pepper and spring onion whites. Cook, stirring, until lightly browned, about 2 minutes. Add the garlic and ginger and cook until fragrant, about 30 seconds. Add the peas and carrots and cook for 3 minutes. Add the cooked brown rice and toss, breaking up any clumps, then spread it over the surface of the wok. Let the rice cook undisturbed for about 2 minutes. Toss well, spread over the wok surface again and let it cook undisturbed for 2 more minutes. Add the cooked egg and soy sauce mixture. Cook 1 minute, add the spring onion greens and cook, stirring, for 30 seconds. Serve hot.

skinny**scoop**

Prep all your vegetables before you start cooking because once the wok gets hot, this rice dish comes together in minutes. I like to use a nonstick wok when I make fried rice because it allows me to use less oil.

PER SERVING	
CALORIES	218
FAT	5 g
SATURATED FAT	1 g
CHOLESTEROL	37 mg
CARBOHYDRATE	36 g
FIBRE	4 g
PROTEIN	8 g
SUGARS	3 g
SODIUM	530 mg

VEGGIE-LICIOUS SIDES

273

Irresistible Vegetable Medley

SERVES 5

What's so irresistible about these vegetables, you may ask? Well, I do a little number on them that makes my family clamour for more. When the vegetables come out of the piping-hot oven, I top them with freshly grated Parmesan, which melts over the vegetables and gives them a wonderfully rich taste. Yum! The best part about roasting vegetables is that although they take a while to cook, the preparation time is pretty much nonexistent.

About 4 heaped cups (350g) broccoli florets

About 4 heaped cups (350g) cauliflower florets

1 large carrot, cut on an angle into 5mm-wide slices

1 small red onion, cut into 8 wedges

6 to 8 large garlic cloves, smashed

3 tablespoons extra-virgin olive oil

½ teaspoon sea salt

Freshly ground black pepper

¼ cup (25g) grated Parmesan cheese

Adjust an oven rack in the lower third of the oven and preheat to 230°C/210°C fan/Gas 8.

Put the broccoli, cauliflower, carrots, onions, and garlic in a 23 × 32cm ceramic or glass baking dish and drizzle with the olive oil. Season with the salt and black pepper to taste and toss well.

Roast, stirring every 10 minutes or so, until the vegetables are tender and browned on the edges, 26 to 30 minutes. Remove the baking dish from the oven and top the vegetables with the Parmesan. Serve hot.

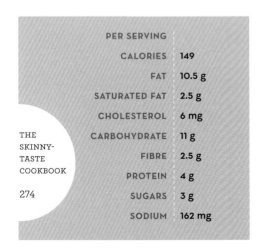

PER SERVING	
CALORIES	149
FAT	10.5 g
SATURATED FAT	2.5 g
CHOLESTEROL	6 mg
CARBOHYDRATE	11 g
FIBRE	2.5 g
PROTEIN	4 g
SUGARS	3 g
SODIUM	162 mg

Tangy Carrot Ribbon Salad

SERES 4

Truth be told, I'm not a huge fan of carrots. I'm always amazed that my toddler can munch on raw carrots all day long. So I find it a bit bewildering that adding a little fresh lemon juice to carrots completely transforms the taste and balances out the sweetness with just the right amount of tang.

3 to 4 carrots (200g), peeled

4 teaspoons extra-virgin olive oil

¼ cup (50ml) fresh lemon juice

¼ teaspoon sea salt

Freshly ground black pepper

Using a vegetable peeler, shave the carrots into thin ribbons.

Put the carrot ribbons in a large bowl and drizzle with the olive oil and lemon juice. Season with the salt and black pepper to taste. Toss well and allow to sit for 10 to 15 minutes before serving. The salad can also be refrigerated in an airtight container for up to 2 days.

FOOD FACTS carrot crush
Carrots are one of those veggies that give you the biggest nutritional bang for one's buck – literally. A cup (150g) gives you all the vitamin A you need for the day.

skinnyscoop

You don't need a fancy tool to shave the carrots into ribbons – all you need is a simple vegetable peeler. If you want to add a little heat to the salad, you can even add a pinch of red chilli flakes.

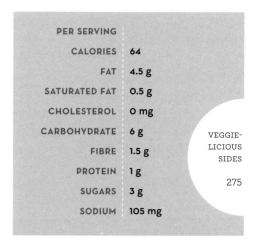

PER SERVING	
CALORIES	64
FAT	4.5 g
SATURATED FAT	0.5 g
CHOLESTEROL	0 mg
CARBOHYDRATE	6 g
FIBRE	1.5 g
PROTEIN	1 g
SUGARS	3 g
SODIUM	105 mg

VEGGIE-LICIOUS SIDES

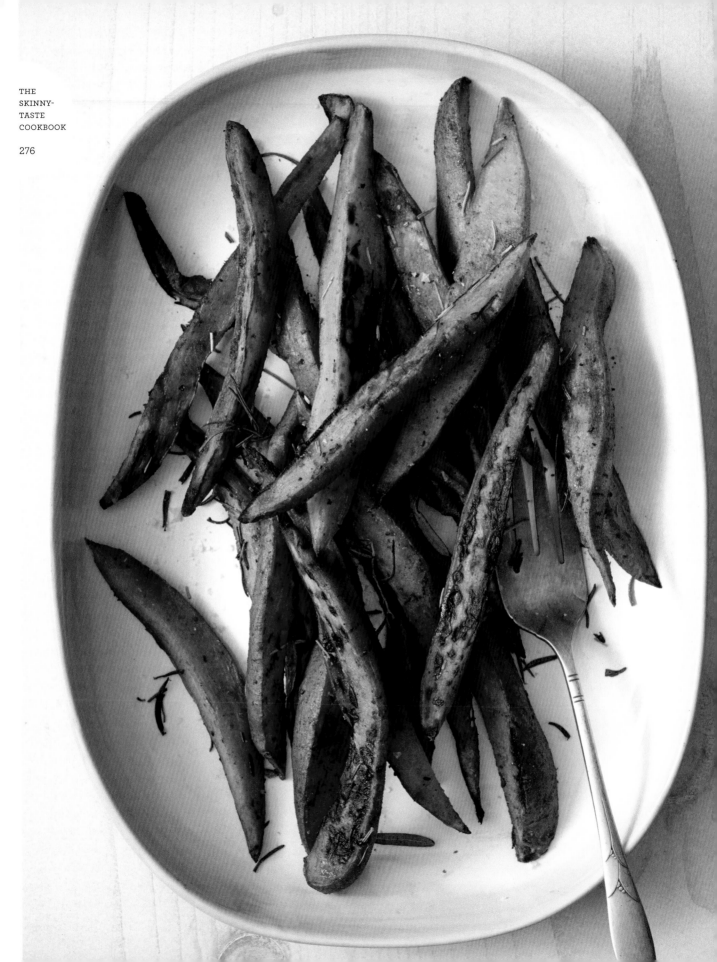

Seasoned Sweet Potato Wedges

MAKES 24 WEDGES · SERVES 4

Sweet and savoury worlds collide with these deliciously seasoned sweet potato wedges.
The seasoning is simple, but when combined with the sweet flavour of the spuds, it's pure harmony.
Roasting the sweet potatoes at a high temperature ensures a soft interior and golden exterior.
No need to fry in any added fat! Leave the skins on for added fibre.

Cooking spray or oil mister

4 medium sweet potatoes
(800g)

4 teaspoons olive oil

1 teaspoon garlic powder

¾ teaspoon sweet paprika

¾ teaspoon dried rosemary

Sea salt

Preheat the oven to 220°C/200°C fan/Gas 7. Lightly spray a
baking sheet with oil.

Halve the sweet potatoes lengthwise, put them cut side down
on a chopping board, and carefully cut each half into 3 equal
lengthwise wedges. You will have 24 wedges.

In a large bowl, toss the sweet potato wedges with the olive oil,
garlic powder, paprika, rosemary and ½ teaspoon salt. Put the
wedges on the prepared baking sheet, flesh side down.

Roast until tender and golden, about 20 minutes, flipping
over once halfway through. Finish with ⅛ teaspoon salt and
serve hot.

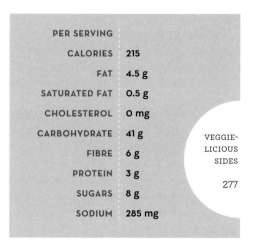

PER SERVING	
CALORIES	215
FAT	4.5 g
SATURATED FAT	0.5 g
CHOLESTEROL	0 mg
CARBOHYDRATE	41 g
FIBRE	6 g
PROTEIN	3 g
SUGARS	8 g
SODIUM	285 mg

VEGGIE-
LICIOUS
SIDES

Lemon-Roasted Asparagus

SERVES 4

I love eating asparagus every which way, but roasting it with a little lemon juice and zest is one of my favourite quick sides. And it goes great with just about everything, from steak to pork to chicken (try it as a side with Chicken Cordon Bleu Meatballs on page 163). I prefer to use thinner spears when roasting asparagus because they're more tender, but if you use thicker spears, simply increase the cooking time. Look for asparagus with compact tips and firm stalks without wrinkles.

450g asparagus, tough ends trimmed

Olive oil spray or oil mister

¼ teaspoon sea salt

Freshly ground black pepper

1 teaspoon grated lemon zest

Wedge of lemon

Preheat the oven to 200°C/180°C fan/Gas 6.

Arrange the asparagus in a roasting pan in a single layer. Spray with olive oil and season with the salt and black pepper. Sprinkle the lemon zest over the asparagus. Roast until crisp-tender, 8 to 10 minutes. Squeeze a little fresh lemon juice on top and serve hot.

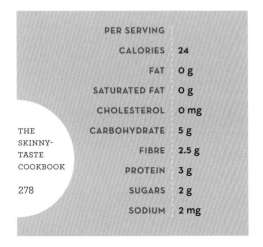

PER SERVING	
CALORIES	24
FAT	0 g
SATURATED FAT	0 g
CHOLESTEROL	0 mg
CARBOHYDRATE	5 g
FIBRE	2.5 g
PROTEIN	3 g
SUGARS	2 g
SODIUM	2 mg

THE SKINNY-TASTE COOKBOOK

Roasted Winter Beetroot and Red Potatoes

SERVES 4

When I was younger, I remember that on occasion my mom would serve jarred pickled beetroot with dinner – blah! I wasn't a fan, and I completely wrote off beetroot until I discovered how great they are roasted. Slowly roasting beetroot turns them into sweets, as all of their natural sugars become concentrated. For this dish, I slice the beetroot and potatoes thinly so that every bite is crispy and browned. This makes a wonderful winter side dish to beef or lamb (try it with the Grilled Lamb Chops with Mint-Yoghurt Sauce on page 202).

Olive oil spray or oil mister

2 medium peeled beetroot (275g), greens and ends trimmed off

450g small red potatoes

2 tablespoons extra-virgin olive oil

¾ teaspoon sea salt, plus more as needed

¼ teaspoon freshly ground black pepper, plus more as needed

Preheat the oven to 220°C/200°C fan/Gas 7. Spray 2 large baking trays with olive oil.

Halve the beetroot lengthwise, put them cut side down on a chopping board and cut crosswise into 5mm-thick slices. Cut the slices in half.

Cut the potatoes into 5mm-thick slices, then cut the slices into quarters. Put the potatoes and beetroot in a bowl and toss with the olive oil. Arrange the vegetables in a single layer on the prepared baking trays. Season with ¾ teaspoon of the salt and ¼ teaspoon of the black pepper and toss well.

Bake until the vegetables are tender and the potatoes are golden, 24 to 28 minutes, flipping over with a spatula halfway through. Season with salt and black pepper to taste and serve hot.

skinnyscoop

The trick to perfectly roasted vegetables every time is to be sure you cut all the vegetables uniformly so everything cooks evenly. Also, don't overcrowd the pan, or they won't crisp.

FOOD FACTS **why beetroot can't be beat**

With nearly 4 grams of fibre, lots of folate and a dose of vitamin C per handful, this root vegetable is a nutritional powerhouse. Its red colour comes from the phytonutrient betalain, which may act as an antioxidant and have some anticancer powers.

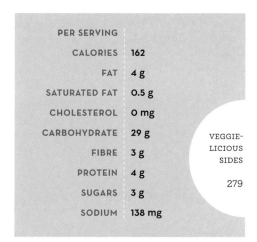

PER SERVING	
CALORIES	162
FAT	4 g
SATURATED FAT	0.5 g
CHOLESTEROL	0 mg
CARBOHYDRATE	29 g
FIBRE	3 g
PROTEIN	4 g
SUGARS	3 g
SODIUM	138 mg

VEGGIE-LICIOUS SIDES

279

Sweet Maple-Roasted Acorn Squash

SERVES 4

I love all things autumn: colourful gourds, cosy sweaters, changing leaves and (of course!) spectacular autumn fruits and veggies. My soul just craves the sweet, buttery taste of this side dish when the weather starts to get cold. I also love how simple it is – in only 5 minutes, you can turn 4 ingredients into a scrumptious side dish. It doesn't get any easier than this.

4 teaspoons coconut oil

2 small acorn squashes, halved lengthwise, seeds scooped out

Sea salt

2 tablespoons pure maple syrup

Preheat the oven to 200°C/180°C fan/Gas 6. Line a baking sheet with baking parchment.

Rub the coconut oil all over the flesh of the squash, then season with a pinch of salt. Put the squash halves cut side up on the prepared baking sheet, then drizzle with the maple syrup.

Bake until you can pierce the flesh with a fork, about 1 hour.

PER SERVING	
CALORIES	151
FAT	4.5 g
SATURATED FAT	4 g
CHOLESTEROL	0 mg
CARBOHYDRATE	29 g
FIBRE	3 g
PROTEIN	2 g
SUGARS	6 g
SODIUM	25 mg

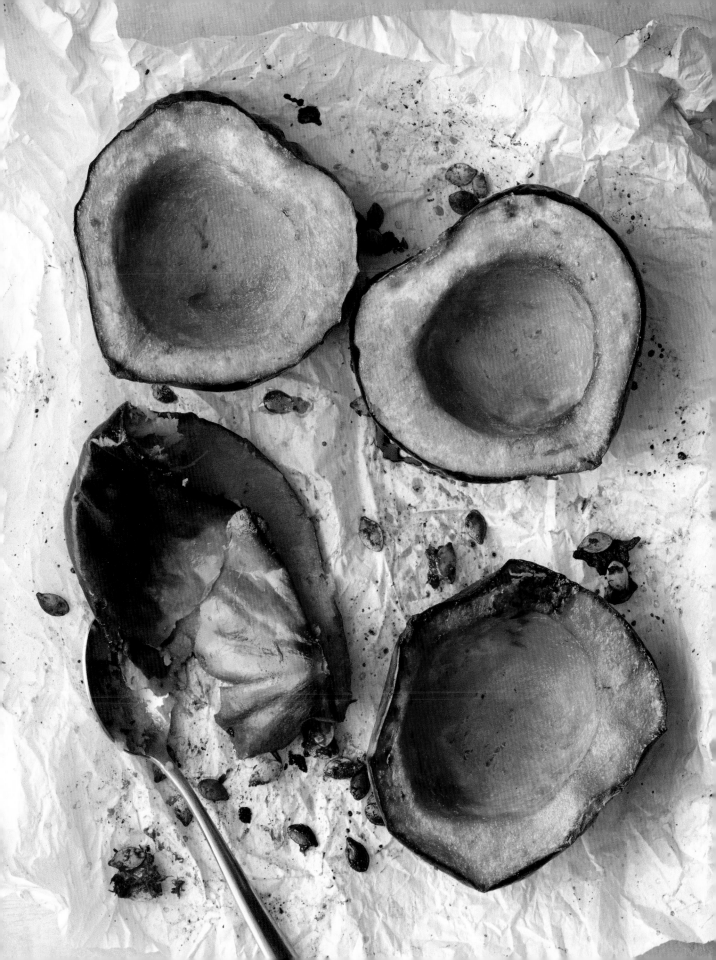

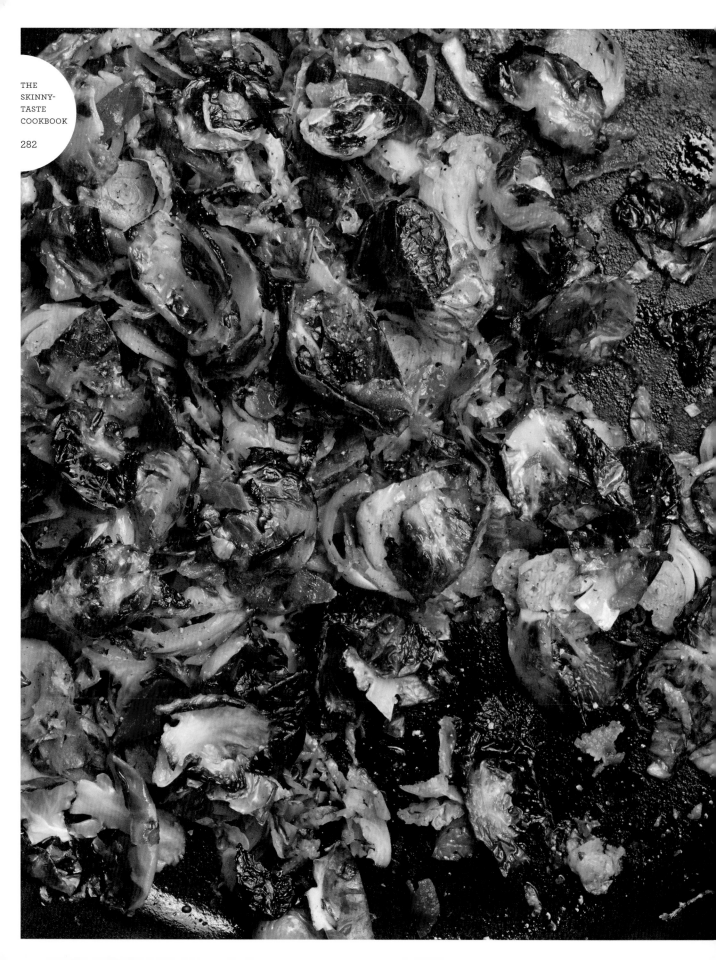

Shredded Brussels Sprouts with Prosciutto

SERVES 4

Don't like Brussels sprouts? Well, this recipe may very well change your mind. In this dish, Brussels sprouts are shredded thin, sautéed until slightly browned and cooked with thin slices of prosciutto and shallots – delish! Shredding the little cabbages makes all the difference, because the veggie can get thoroughly browned and seasoned.

350g Brussels sprouts

2 teaspoons extra-virgin olive oil

¼ cup (30g) finely chopped shallots

2 thin slices prosciutto (25g), chopped

¼ teaspoon sea salt

Freshly ground black pepper

Using a large sharp knife, trim the stems off the Brussels sprouts, then thinly slice the sprouts.

Heat a deep 25cm nonstick frying pan over medium heat. Add the oil and shallots and cook, stirring, 30 to 40 seconds. Add the prosciutto and cook until the shallots are golden, 1 minute. Add the sprouts, season with the salt and black pepper to taste and cook, stirring occasionally, until the sprouts are slightly browned and crisp-tender, about 5 minutes. Cover the frying pan and cook until they begin to wilt, 1 minute. Remove the pan from the heat. Keep covered and allow to sit about 2 minutes to slightly wilt the leaves. Serve hot.

FOOD FACTS **why brussels sprouts deserve a second chance**
There's nothing stinky about sprouts! They're loaded with good-for-you nutrients, including vitamins, minerals and powerful phytonutrients. A cup (100g) contains 3.3 grams of fibre and all your vitamin K needs for the day. It also nearly covers your daily vitamin C and A requirements, all for a mere 38 calories. As a member of the cruciferous vegetable family, Brussels sprouts also offer many of the same benefits of cauliflower and broccoli, including a reduced risk for cancer and other diseases.

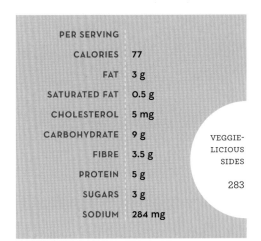

PER SERVING	
CALORIES	77
FAT	3 g
SATURATED FAT	0.5 g
CHOLESTEROL	5 mg
CARBOHYDRATE	9 g
FIBRE	3.5 g
PROTEIN	5 g
SUGARS	3 g
SODIUM	284 mg

VEGGIE-LICIOUS SIDES

Sautéed Rapini with Garlic and Oil

SERVES 4

Rapini (known as broccoli rabe in many parts of the world) is my all-time favourite vegetable. It's one of those vegetables that needs to grow on you, because of its slightly bitter taste. Blanching it before sautéing it with garlic and oil is the secret to mellowing out the bitterness, and it also sets its green colour. Once cooked it can be served as a side or tossed with pasta and sun-dried tomatoes for a quick pasta dish. It's also one of my favourite pizza toppings and is wonderful in a panini with grilled chicken.

1 bunch rapini (about 450g)

2 teaspoons sea salt

1 tablespoon olive oil

5 garlic cloves, thinly sliced

¼ teaspoon crushed red chilli flakes

Trim 4cm off the stems of the rapini, discarding the trimmings, and cut it into 5cm pieces.

Bring a large pot of water and 1 teaspoon of the salt to a boil. Add the rapini and cook until slightly tender and bright green, about 2 minutes. Drain well and set aside.

Heat a large, deep nonstick sauté pan over medium-high heat. Add the olive oil and garlic and cook, stirring, until golden, about 1 minute. Add the rapini, chilli flakes and the remaining 1 teaspoon salt. Cook, stirring, until heated through, 2 to 3 minutes. Serve hot.

FOOD FACTS RAPINI MAKES A NAME FOR ITSELF
This broccoli look-alike is actually a member of the turnip family, but it offers many of the same benefits as broccoli. It's rich in vitamin K and contains a compound called indole-3-carbinol, which has been shown to reduce the risk of cancer in animal studies.

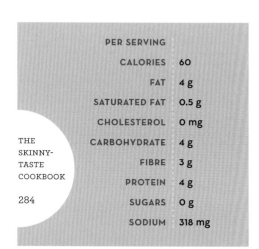

PER SERVING	
CALORIES	60
FAT	4 g
SATURATED FAT	0.5 g
CHOLESTEROL	0 mg
CARBOHYDRATE	4 g
FIBRE	3 g
PROTEIN	4 g
SUGARS	0 g
SODIUM	318 mg

THE SKINNY-TASTE COOKBOOK

Confetti Slaw

SERVES 5

Naturally colourful food is not only beautiful, but it's also healthful. The different colours of foods indicate different phytonutrients and antioxidants, which help protect your body in a variety of ways. Put a multitude of hues on your plate (pictured on page 192) and you could very well colour yourself healthy! And by the way, my kids love this.

4 cups (300g) coleslaw mix

½ cup (40g) thinly sliced red cabbage

½ cup (90g) julienne cut and peeled cucumber

¼ cup (45g) thinly sliced yellow pepper

1½ tablespoons olive oil

1½ tablespoons apple cider vinegar

4 teaspoons fresh lime juice

½ teaspoon sea salt

Freshly ground black pepper

In a large bowl, combine the coleslaw mix, cabbage, cucumber, pepper, olive oil, vinegar and lime juice. Season with the salt and add a pinch of black pepper. Refrigerate for 10 to 15 minutes before serving.

PERFECT PAIRINGS
Serve this side dish with **Slow-Cooker Picadillo (page 193)**, **Buttermilk Oven 'Fried' Chicken (page 151)**, barbecued meats and sandwiches. It makes a perfect crunchy topping for tacos and tostadas, too.

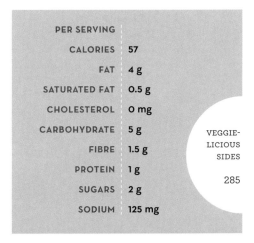

PER SERVING	
CALORIES	57
FAT	4 g
SATURATED FAT	0.5 g
CHOLESTEROL	0 mg
CARBOHYDRATE	5 g
FIBRE	1.5 g
PROTEIN	1 g
SUGARS	2 g
SODIUM	125 mg

VEGGIE-LICIOUS SIDES

285

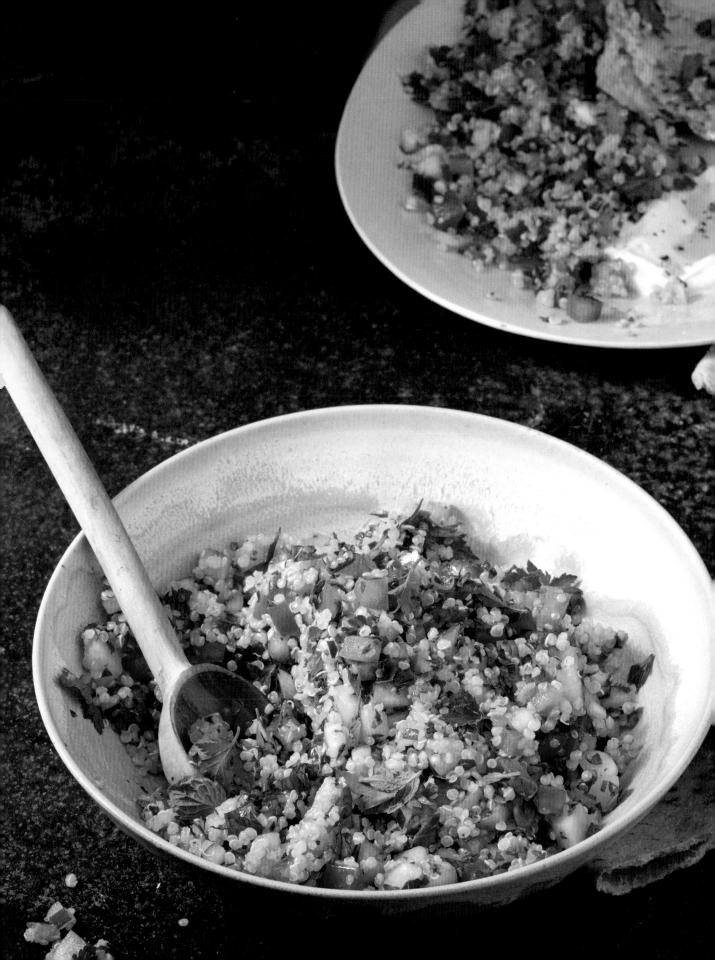

Quinoa Tabbouleh

SERVES 4

Tabbouleh is a wonderful Middle Eastern salad made with lots of chopped herbs, cucumbers, tomatoes, spring onions and bright flavours. It's typically made with bulgur, but I love using quinoa instead because it has a healthy dose of protein.

½ cup (100g) quinoa

Sea salt

1 cup (175g) cucumber, peeled and finely chopped

¾ cup (150g) finely chopped tomatoes

2 tablespoons finely chopped red onion

2 tablespoons sliced spring onions

¼ cup (7g) finely chopped fresh parsley leaves

1½ tablespoons finely chopped fresh mint leaves

½ tablespoon extra-virgin olive oil

1½ tablespoons fresh lemon juice

1 tablespoon red wine vinegar

Rinse the quinoa under running water for about 2 minutes. Cook the quinoa in 1 cup (225ml) of water with ⅛ teaspoon salt according to packet directions. Set aside to cool.

When the quinoa is cool, put it into a large bowl and add the cucumber, tomato, red onion, spring onions, parsley, mint, olive oil, lemon juice and vinegar. Season with the remaining ¼ teaspoon salt and refrigerate until chilled, at least 20 minutes. Serve cold.

PERFECT PAIRING

If I'm grilling in the summer and I want to go with a Mediterranean theme, I make a big bowl of this salad and grill up some skewers, like my **Grilled Lamb Skewers with Harissa Dipping Sauce (page 206),** and serve everything with pitta bread on the side.

PER SERVING	
CALORIES	110
FAT	3 g
SATURATED FAT	0.5 g
CHOLESTEROL	0 mg
CARBOHYDRATE	17 g
FIBRE	2.5 g
PROTEIN	4 g
SUGARS	2 g
SODIUM	95 mg

VEGGIE-LICIOUS SIDES

Summer Giant Couscous

SERVES 5

The first time I tried giant (Israeli or pearl) couscous I instantly fell for it. Although it looks a lot like barley, it's actually small, toasted semolina pasta. Giant couscous is a larger size of the grain that has a wonderful chewiness. This recipe is a fantastic hearty side for grilled chicken or fish, but I also love it as a meal in itself. Although I'm not usually a fan of the taste of wholewheat pasta, I don't mind it at all in this smaller shape. In fact, one way I like to trick fussy vegetable eaters into not picking out the courgette is to dice it so small that it matches the size of the cooked couscous (pictured on page 226).

Sea salt

1 cup (150g) wholewheat giant couscous

½ tablespoon extra-virgin olive oil

3 garlic cloves, crushed

1⅔ cups (210g) diced courgettes, 5mm dice

1 cup (200g) cherry tomatoes, quartered

Freshly ground black pepper

2 tablespoons freshly grated Pecorino Romano cheese

Bring 1¼ cups (300ml) water and ½ teaspoon salt to a boil in a small pot. Add the couscous, cover and simmer for 8 to 10 minutes, or according to the packet directions.

Heat a large frying pan over medium-high heat. Add the oil and garlic and cook, stirring, until golden, 1 to 2 minutes. Add the courgette and tomatoes, season with ¼ teaspoon salt and a pinch of black pepper and cook just until tender, about 2 to 3 minutes. Add the cooked couscous and Romano to the pan and stir to combine; finish with ⅛ teaspoon salt and serve hot.

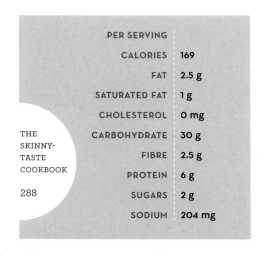

PER SERVING	
CALORIES	169
FAT	2.5 g
SATURATED FAT	1 g
CHOLESTEROL	0 mg
CARBOHYDRATE	30 g
FIBRE	2.5 g
PROTEIN	6 g
SUGARS	2 g
SODIUM	204 mg

Barbecued Mexican Corn Salad

SERVES 5

This vibrant side dish is a staple at backyard parties over the summer, when sweetcorn is at its sweetest. If I'm feeding friends, I make sure to double the recipe so there's enough for everyone. We love the smoky-sweet flavour you get from barbecuing the sweetcorn, which is livened up by the freshly squeezed lime juice and just the right amount of coriander. And, of course, avocado is a must! Heck, I could pile this on a tostada, top it with queso fresco, and call it a meal!

3 medium ears sweetcorn, unhusked, or 1½ cups (225g) thawed frozen sweetcorn kernels

1 cup (200g) chopped tomatoes

¼ cup (40g) chopped red onion

1 jalapeño or other green chilli, finely chopped (optional)

¼ cup (15g) finely chopped fresh coriander

1 small garlic clove, crushed

2 tablespoons fresh lime juice

1 teaspoon olive oil

½ teaspoon ground cumin

Sea salt

Freshly ground black pepper

1 medium avocado, chopped

Preheat the barbecue to medium.

Soak the fresh unhusked sweetcorn in a large bowl of cold water for 30 minutes.

Remove the sweetcorn from the water and shake off any excess. Put the sweetcorn on the barbecue, close the lid and barbecue, turning every 5 minutes, until the kernels are tender when pierced with a paring knife, 20 to 25 minutes. Allow to sit until cool enough to handle.

Increase the heat of the barbecue to high. Carefully remove the husks and silks from the corncobs, put the sweetcorn back on the barbecue and cook, turning, until slightly charred, 2 to 4 minutes. Set aside to cool. When cooled, use a knife to cut the sweetcorn off the cobs.

In a large bowl, combine the barbecued sweetcorn (or thawed frozen sweetcorn), tomatoes, red onion, jalapeño (if using), coriander, garlic, lime juice, olive oil, cumin, ¼ teaspoon salt and black pepper. Refrigerate for at least 20 minutes. Just before serving, toss in the avocado and finish with ⅛ teaspoon salt.

skinny**scoop**

To make this in half the time, you can use thawed frozen sweetcorn kernels instead of fresh grilled sweetcorn.

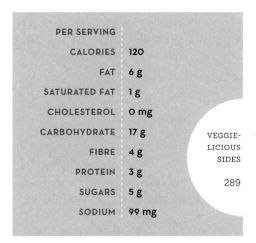

PER SERVING	
CALORIES	120
FAT	6 g
SATURATED FAT	1 g
CHOLESTEROL	0 mg
CARBOHYDRATE	17 g
FIBRE	4 g
PROTEIN	3 g
SUGARS	5 g
SODIUM	99 mg

VEGGIE-LICIOUS SIDES

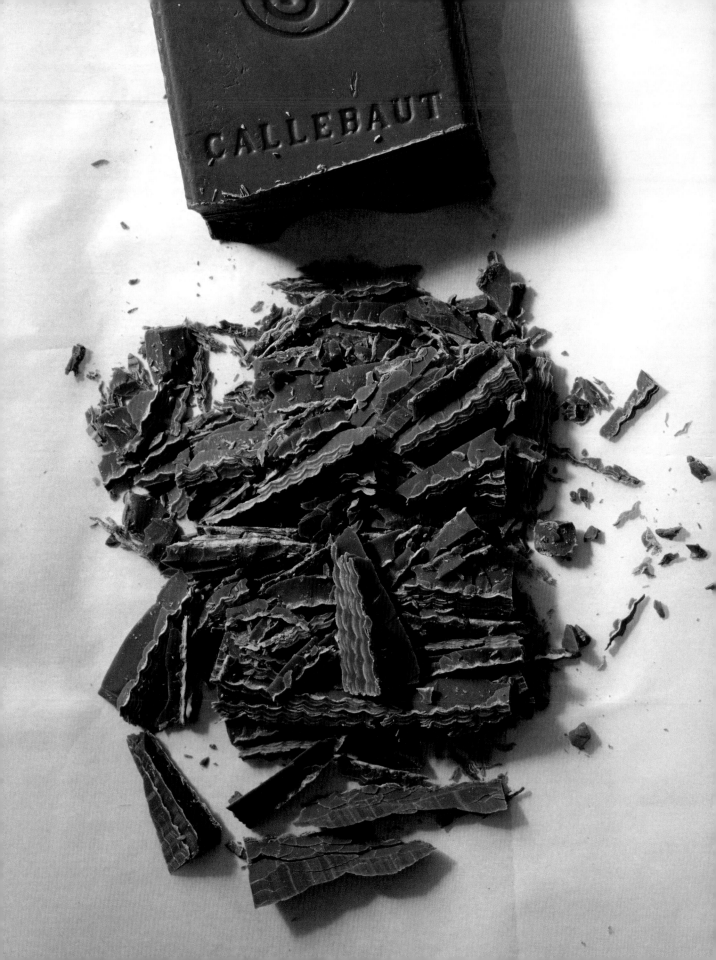

SKINNY SWEET TOOTH

Double Chocolate Chunk Walnut Cookies

MAKES 24 COOKIES

I've done some crazy, unconventional things in baking, but using avocados in place of butter may just be the craziest. Believe it or not, it works! For these chewy cookies made with chunks of chocolate and walnuts in every bite, I use absolutely no butter. They taste too good to be light – and you can't detect the taste of avocados at all. I tested these out on many unsuspecting adults, children and teens, and everyone loved them. Karina, my college-age daughter, was the ultimate test – she's a true chocoholic. She thinks they're pretty awesome!

Cooking spray or oil mister (optional)

½ cup (110g) raw cane sugar

⅓ cup (60g) dark brown sugar

¼ cup (60g) mashed avocado

1 tablespoon unsweetened apple sauce†

1 large egg white

1 teaspoon pure vanilla extract

½ cup (65g) wholemeal flour

⅓ cup (50g) plain flour

⅓ cup (40g) unsweetened cocoa powder

¼ teaspoon bicarbonate of soda

⅛ teaspoon sea salt

⅓ cup (60g) dark chocolate pieces

½ cup (60g) finely chopped walnuts

skinny**scoop**

I love walnuts in my chocolate cookies, but if you have allergies, you can swap the walnuts for more chocolate chunks.

Preheat the oven to 180°C/160°C fan/Gas 4. Line 2 regular baking sheets with silicone baking mats or lightly spray nonstick baking sheets with oil.

In a large bowl, using an electric hand mixer, whisk together the sugars, avocado, apple sauce, egg white and vanilla until the sugar dissolves, about 2 to 3 minutes.

In a separate large bowl, whisk together the flours, cocoa powder, bicarbonate of soda and salt. Fold in the dry ingredients with a spatula in two additions, then fold in the chocolate chunks and walnuts. The dough will be very sticky. Cover the bowl with clingfilm and refrigerate for 15 minutes.

Drop the dough by tablespoonfuls about 2 to 3cm apart onto the prepared baking sheets and smooth the tops.

Bake until almost set, 10 to 12 minutes. Allow to cool for 5 minutes on the sheets, then transfer to wire racks to cool completely.

† If you can't get hold of unsweetened apple sauce, use sweetened as an alternative.

PER SERVING	
CALORIES	152
FAT	5.5 g
SATURATED FAT	1.5 g
CHOLESTEROL	0 mg
CARBOHYDRATE	25 g
FIBRE	2 g
PROTEIN	3 g
SUGARS	15 g
SODIUM	48 mg

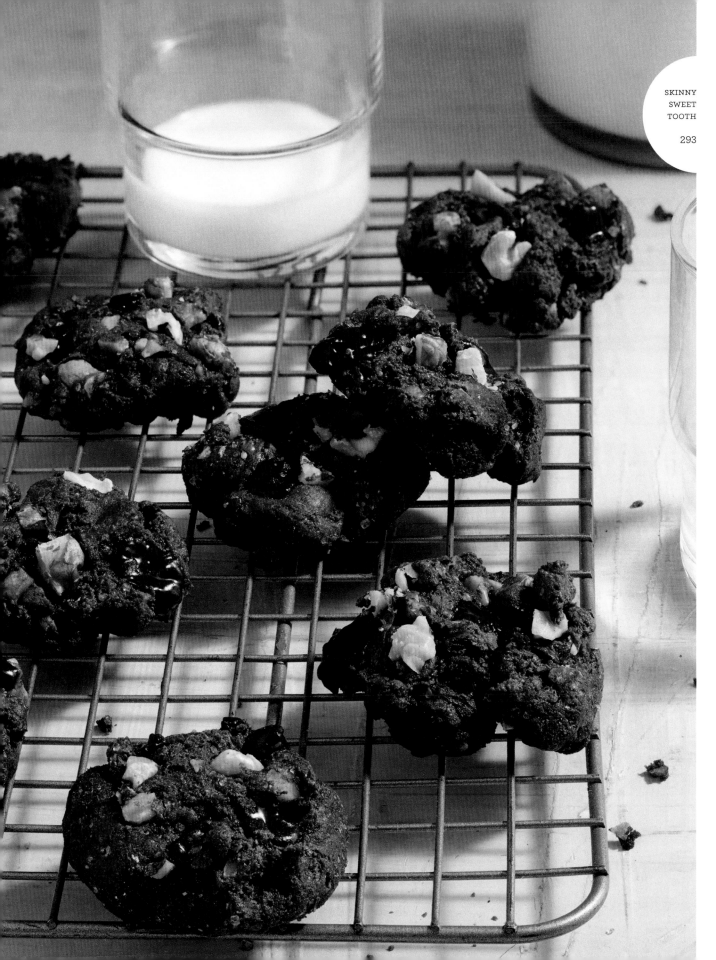

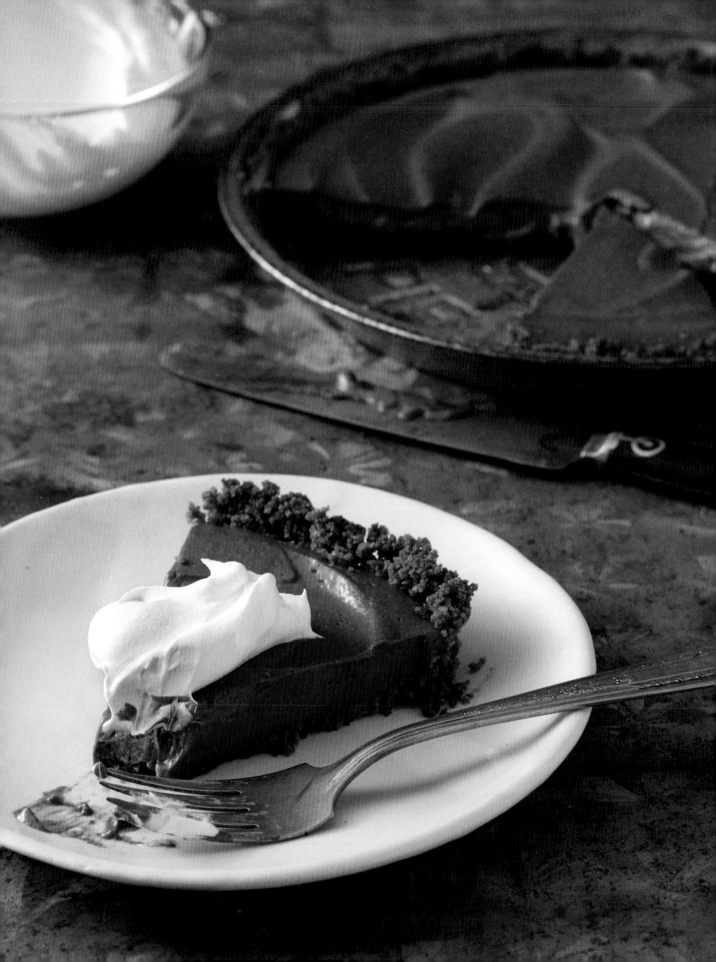

Silky Chocolate Cream Pie

SERVES 8

Chocolate lovers: this dessert is for you! You'll love the rich taste of this decadent, creamy chocolate pie. The secret to keeping it skinny is silken tofu, which has a light texture and a wonderful mouthfeel. Here, it has a puddinglike quality that will fool anyone.

BISCUIT BASE

6 whole reduced-fat graham crackers, crushed†

2 tablespoons raw cane sugar

3 tablespoons cold whipped butter‡

FILLING

350g firm silken tofu

¼ cup (50ml) unsweetened almond milk

2 tablespoons raw cane sugar

140g dark chocolate

For the biscuit base: In a food processor, combine the crushed graham crackers, raw cane sugar and butter. Pulse a few times, then add 1 tablespoon water. Pulse a few more times until it has the texture of coarse bread crumbs. Press the mixture into the bottom and up the sides of a 20cm pie plate or dish. Refrigerate for 30 minutes.

Preheat the oven to 190°C/170°C fan/Gas 5. Bake the biscuit base until the edges are golden, 8 to 10 minutes. Remove from the oven and allow to cool on a wire rack.

For the filling: Lightly mash the silken tofu with a fork and place it in a blender with the almond milk and raw cane sugar. Blend until smooth, about 1 minute.

Place the chocolate in a microwave-safe bowl and microwave on high for 30 seconds. Stir and microwave for another 30 to 40 seconds. Repeat until the chocolate is completely melted. Pour the chocolate into the blender with the tofu and blend for a few seconds until thoroughly combined.

Pour the filling into the cooled biscuit base and refrigerate until set, about 2 hours. Serve chilled and cut into 8 slices.

† If you can't get hold of graham crackers, you can use reduced-fat digestive biscuits instead.

‡ If you can't find whipped butter, you can substitute it with low-fat butter spread.

skinnyscoop

Silken tofu is usually packaged in aseptic boxes that do not require refrigeration. Because of this, it is sometimes sold in a different section of supermarkets or shops than regular tofu, which is packed in water and requires refrigeration. When buying commercial tofu, look for organic, non-GMO brands.

PER SERVING	
CALORIES	219
FAT	10.5 g
SATURATED FAT	5 g
CHOLESTEROL	8 mg
CARBOHYDRATE	30 g
FIBRE	1.5 g
PROTEIN	5 g
SUGARS	19 g
SODIUM	126 mg

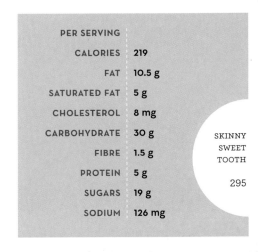

SKINNY
SWEET
TOOTH

295

Coconut Panna Cotta with Fresh Raspberries

SERVES 6

This is one of my favourite desserts in the whole cookbook. Traditionally, panna cotta is made with double cream and milk, but with a little bit of tinkering, it can easily be adapted to work with just about any type of milk. I'm coconut-obsessed, so I like to make this dairy-free version with a combination of tinned light coconut milk and coconut milk drink, usually found in the refrigerated section of the supermarket.

¾ cup (175ml) unsweetened coconut milk drink

3½ teaspoons (12g) gelatine powder

2 cups (450ml) tinned light coconut milk

¼ cup (90g) honey

Sea salt

1½ cups (185g) raspberries

1 tablespoon grated lime zest (optional)

skinny**scoop**

Panna cotta is the perfect dessert to make when you have dinner guests. The reason: it needs to be made at least 4 hours in advance to set (it stays chilled in the refrigerator until ready to serve), which leaves you free to mingle with company instead of fussing in the kitchen. It can also be made a day or two ahead.

Pour the coconut milk drink into a medium heavy-based saucepan. Sprinkle the gelatine over the milk and allow to stand until the gelatine softens, about 10 minutes. Meanwhile, fill a large bowl with ice water.

Turn the heat under the saucepan to medium and whisk the gelatine until it has dissolved, but don't let the milk boil, about 3 minutes. Whisk in the light coconut milk, honey and a pinch of salt. Cook, whisking, until the mixture is hot, but do not let it boil, 4 to 5 minutes. Transfer the milk to a clean, medium metal bowl. Put the bowl in the prepared ice bath and allow to cool, stirring slowly so no bubbles form, until the mixture begins to thicken, about 12 minutes.

Ladle the mixture into each of the small dessert bowls or sundae or other glasses. Cover each with clingfilm and refrigerate until firm, 4 to 6 hours or overnight.

To serve, remove the clingfilm and spoon the fresh berries over the panna cotta along with lime zest (if using).

PER SERVING	
CALORIES	152
FAT	7.5 g
SATURATED FAT	4 g
CHOLESTEROL	0 mg
CARBOHYDRATE	19 g
FIBRE	2 g
PROTEIN	2 g
SUGARS	13 g
SODIUM	29 mg

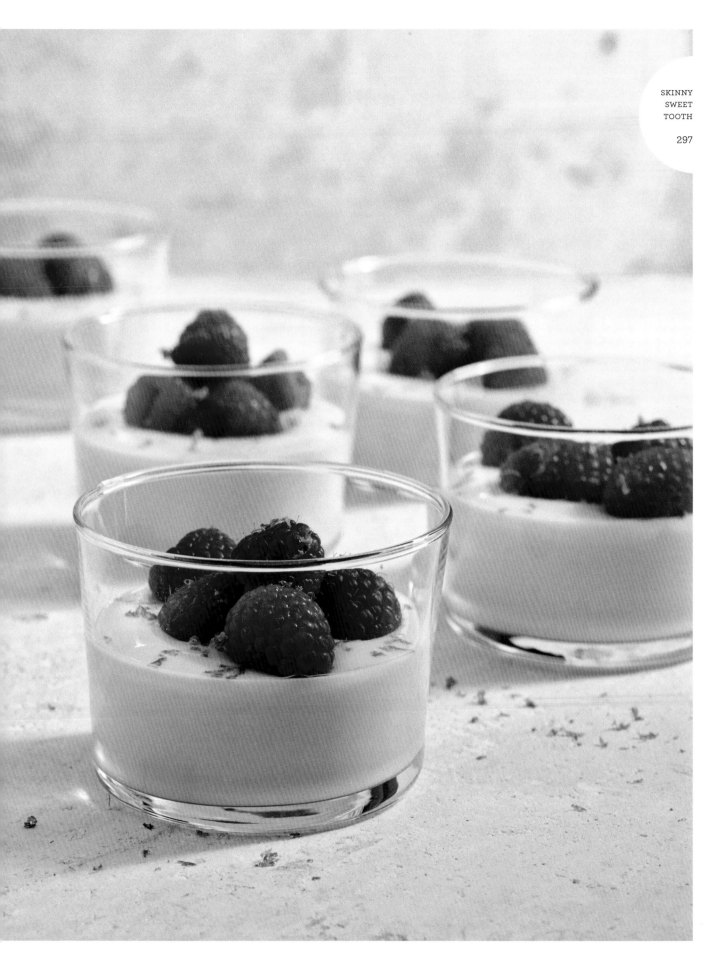

Warm Apple-Pear Crumble

SERVES 8

There's nothing better to me than a warm dessert on a chilly autumn evening. I'm all about hot desserts with cold toppings – a dab of fat-free frozen yoghurt on top of something warm and sweet is enough to make me swoon. With this nutrient-packed dessert, you'll score an impressive 3 grams of filling fibre and 2 grams of satiating protein all for less than 200 calories. Goodbye, guilt!

Cooking spray or oil mister

FILLING

2½ cups (565g) peeled, sliced pears

2½ cups (300g) peeled, sliced Gala apples

¼ cup (90g) honey

1 tablespoon fresh lemon juice

1 tablespoon plain flour

½ teaspoon ground cinnamon

TOPPING

¾ cup (75g) rolled oats

¼ cup packed (55g) light brown sugar

¼ cup (30g) chopped walnuts

1 tablespoon plain flour

¼ teaspoon sea salt

3 tablespoons virgin coconut oil

skinny**scoop**

Coconut oil is a great substitute for lard, butter, margarine or vegetable oil. If you're not a fan of the taste of coconut, use expeller-pressed coconut oil, which has a neutral flavour, rather than cold-pressed, which tastes more like coconut

Preheat the oven to 160°C/140°C fan/Gas 3. Lightly spray a 23 x 23cm baking dish with oil.

For the filling: In a large bowl, combine the pears, apples, honey, lemon juice, flour and cinnamon. Pour the mixture into the prepared baking dish.

For the topping: In a separate bowl, combine the oats, brown sugar, walnuts, flour, salt and coconut oil. Sprinkle the topping evenly over the filling.

Bake until browned and bubbling, 55 minutes to 1 hour. Serve warm.

PER SERVING	
CALORIES	199
FAT	8 g
SATURATED FAT	4.5 g
CHOLESTEROL	0 mg
CARBOHYDRATE	32 g
FIBRE	3 g
PROTEIN	2 g
SUGARS	21 g
SODIUM	75 mg

Baked Bananas Foster à la Mode

SERVES 4

We go *bananas* for this simple, slimmed-down dessert in my home. It's the perfect treat whenever you have ripe bananas sitting on your counter just begging to be used. And guess what? By baking them in the oven with just a little brown sugar, cinnamon and vanilla, the bananas taste decadent with zero guilt. And bananas are available year-round, so you can make this any time you need a last-minute dessert.

2 ripe medium bananas, sliced into 1cm rounds

⅛ teaspoon ground cinnamon

1½ tablespoons light brown sugar

1 teaspoon pure vanilla extract

2 cups (400g) low-fat vanilla frozen yoghurt

Preheat oven to 200°C/180°C fan/Gas 6.

Arrange the bananas in a 23 x 23cm oven-safe dish and sprinkle them with cinnamon and brown sugar. Drizzle the vanilla extract over the bananas, wrap tightly with foil and bake 10 to 12 minutes, or until the bananas are soft.

To serve, scoop ½ cup (80g) frozen yoghurt into each dessert bowl. Divide the bananas among the bowls and spoon the sauce that accumulates in the bottom of the baking dish over each. Serve immediately.

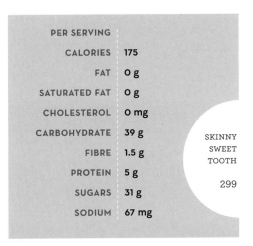

PER SERVING	
CALORIES	175
FAT	0 g
SATURATED FAT	0 g
CHOLESTEROL	0 mg
CARBOHYDRATE	39 g
FIBRE	1.5 g
PROTEIN	5 g
SUGARS	31 g
SODIUM	67 mg

SKINNY
SWEET
TOOTH

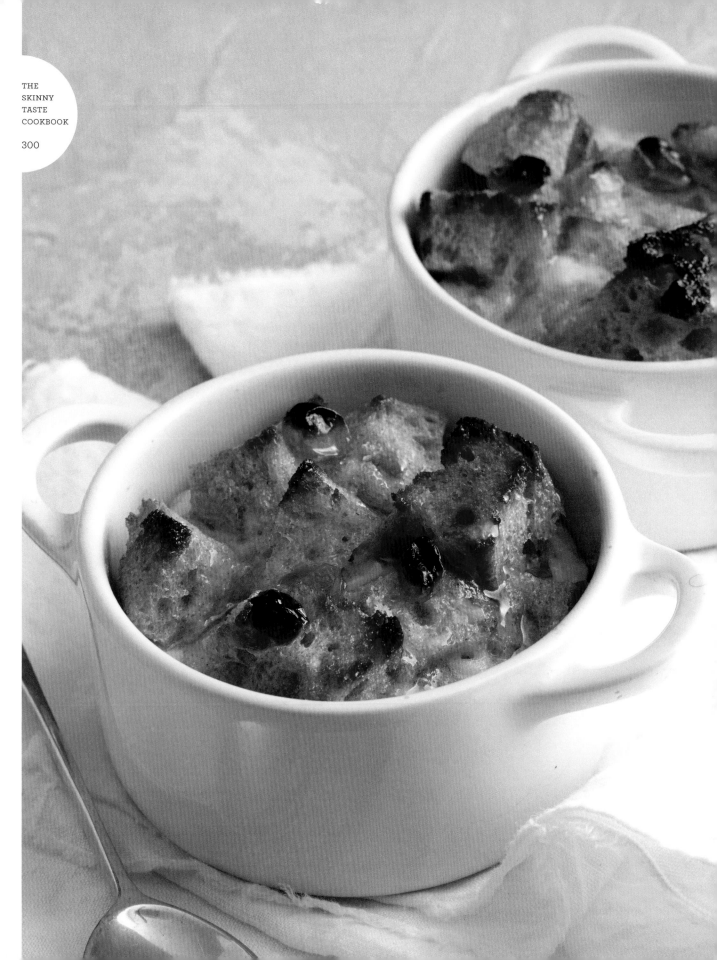

Almost Sinful Maple-Raisin Bread Pudding

SERVES 4

I've always found bread pudding pretty hard to resist, especially when it's still warm from the oven and topped with a touch of whipped cream. But how do you make a dessert that's based on bread and eggs a little less sinful? I swapped the white bread for wholemeal French bread, swapped the cream for skimmed milk and cut back on the eggs. To sweeten it, I like to go natural, using pure maple syrup and raisins instead of refined sugar. But most importantly, I keep portions in check by baking them in individual ramekins, so I don't 'accidentally' have more than my share.

2 cups (60g) wholemeal French bread, crusts removed, cut into 1cm cubes

1 cup (225ml) skimmed milk

¼ cup (50ml) pure maple syrup

2½ teaspoons pure vanilla extract

2 large eggs

⅓ cup (40g) raisins

Cooking spray or oil mister

Preheat the oven to 180°C/160°C fan/Gas 4.

Arrange the bread cubes in a single layer on a baking sheet. Bake until golden, 5 to 6 minutes, stirring halfway through the cooking time. Allow to cool.

In a medium bowl, whisk together the milk, 3 tablespoons of the maple syrup, vanilla and eggs. Stir in the raisins. Fold in the toasted bread cubes. Cover and refrigerate for at least 30 minutes or up to 4 hours.

Preheat the oven to 160°C/140°C fan/Gas 3. Spray 4 (140g) ramekins with oil.

Divide the bread mixture equally among the prepared ramekins. Put the ramekins in a 20 × 20cm baking tin and add 2 to 3cm hot water to the pan.

Bake until set, 45 to 50 minutes. Drizzle with the remaining tablespoon of maple syrup. Serve warm.

PERFECT PAIRINGS
For a little extra indulgence, I like to serve these with either a little fat-free frozen yoghurt or light whipped topping.

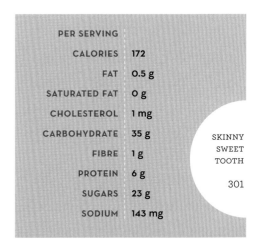

PER SERVING	
CALORIES	172
FAT	0.5 g
SATURATED FAT	0 g
CHOLESTEROL	1 mg
CARBOHYDRATE	35 g
FIBRE	1 g
PROTEIN	6 g
SUGARS	23 g
SODIUM	143 mg

SKINNY SWEET TOOTH

Piña Colada Chia Pudding

SERVES 4

Each spoonful of this healthy pudding offers a little taste of paradise. Chia pudding is one of my favourite guiltless desserts, because it's low in calories and is super easy because there's no cooking involved. Chia seeds are the perfect 'pudding' ingredient because they absorb any liquid you combine them with and expand to eight or nine times their weight. They end up with a nice texture that's similar to tapioca. Because the seeds have no flavour, they take on the taste of whatever liquid they absorb, like these delicious piña colada-inspired ingredients.

1 cup (225ml) tinned light coconut milk

1 cup (225ml) unsweetened coconut milk drink

1½ cups (240g) chopped fresh pineapple

¼ cup (40g) chia seeds

3 tablespoons sweetened desiccated coconut

10 drops liquid stevia (or your favourite sweetener)

In a large bowl or container with a lid, combine the coconut milk, coconut milk drink, pineapple, chia seeds, desiccated coconut and stevia. Cover, shake well and allow to sit for 15 minutes. Shake again and refrigerate for 4 to 6 hours, or up to overnight. The pudding will keep in the refrigerator for up to 3 days.

Divide among 4 dessert bowls.

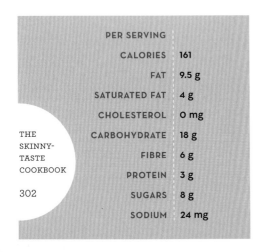

PER SERVING	
CALORIES	161
FAT	9.5 g
SATURATED FAT	4 g
CHOLESTEROL	0 mg
CARBOHYDRATE	18 g
FIBRE	6 g
PROTEIN	3 g
SUGARS	8 g
SODIUM	24 mg

Delightful Poached Pears with Yoghurt

SERVES 4

My cousin Katia shared this recipe with me, and it's something she learned from her mom. It's a naturally light dessert option, but we played around with the original recipe to cut back on sugar – without losing any of the sweetness – by cooking the pears in a sweeter wine combined with pear juice and pomegranate juice. The results were just lovely, and the yoghurt adds a creamy finish that complements the sweet pears perfectly.

PEARS

2 peeled ripe pears

1½ cups (350ml) Pink Moscato wine

1 cup (225ml) pear juice

¼ cup (50ml) pomegranate juice

½ tablespoon vanilla extract

2 tablespoons raw cane sugar

1cm piece fresh ginger, peeled and halved

2 cinnamon sticks

3 (5cm) strips orange zest

¾ cup (185g) fat-free vanilla Greek yoghurt

For the pears: Halve the pears lengthwise, leaving the stems on, and remove the core and seeds. Put the pears, wine, pear juice, pomegranate juice, vanilla, sugar, ginger, cinnamon sticks and orange zest in a medium saucepan, with the cut sides of the pears facing up. Bring to a boil, reduce the heat to medium-low, cover and simmer until the pears are soft but not falling apart, 30 to 40 minutes (or longer depending on the ripeness of the pears), carefully flipping the pears over halfway through.

Using a slotted spoon, transfer the pears to a 23 × 23cm baking dish, reserving the liquid in the saucepan, and discard the cinnamon sticks. Increase the heat under the saucepan to medium-high, bring to a boil and cook until the liquid has reduced by half, about 5 minutes. Pour the liquid over the pears and allow to cool for 20 minutes. Cover and refrigerate until chilled, about 1 hour or overnight.

To serve, place a pear half, cut side up, on each plate and drizzle each with the sauce and 3 tablespoons of yoghurt.

PER SERVING	
CALORIES	230
FAT	0 g
SATURATED FAT	0 g
CHOLESTEROL	3 mg
CARBOHYDRATE	41 g
FIBRE	3 g
PROTEIN	4 g
SUGARS	30 g
SODIUM	27 mg

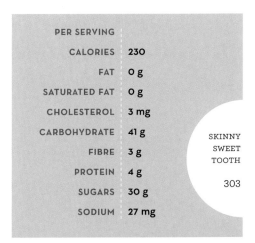

SKINNY
SWEET
TOOTH

303

Summer Berry Cobbler

SERVES 6

Because cobbler is a favourite of mine, I've been playing around with this recipe for years. Traditional cobbler toppings are usually made with so much butter, but I've been able to cut down substantially by using sweet whipped butter. I use ramekins here for automatic portion control.

FILLING

½ cup (110g) raw cane sugar

1½ tablespoons cornflour

Ground cinnamon

Sea salt

1½ cups (185g) raspberries

1½ cups (185g) blackberries

1½ cups (225g) strawberries, cored and sliced

½ teaspoon grated lemon zest

1 tablespoon fresh lemon juice

TOPPING

¼ cup (35g) wholemeal flour

¼ cup (30g) plain flour

2 tablespoons raw cane sugar

½ teaspoon baking powder

¼ teaspoon bicarbonate of soda

Sea salt

2 tablespoons cold unsalted whipped butter, cut into small pieces†

⅓ cup (75ml) buttermilk

1 tablespoon rapeseed oil

2 teaspoons sugar

Preheat the oven to 190°C/170°C fan/Gas 5.

For the filling: In a large bowl, whisk together the raw cane sugar, cornflour and a pinch each of cinnamon and salt. Add the berries and gently mix to coat. Add the lemon zest and juice and divide the filling among 6 (225g) ramekins. Put the ramekins on a baking tray and bake until the berries are hot and bubbling at the edges, 22 to 24 minutes.

For the topping: In a bowl, whisk together the flours, raw cane sugar, baking powder, bicarbonate of soda and a pinch of salt. Cut in the butter using a pastry cutter or 2 knives until the butter pieces are the size of small pebbles. In a small bowl, combine the buttermilk and oil. Add to the dry ingredients and stir until just moistened.

Carefully remove the ramekins from the oven and increase the oven temperature to 200°C/180°C fan/Gas 6. Spoon about 2 tablespoons of topping over the berries. Sprinkle with sugar. Bake until the berries are bubbling and the topping is golden and cooked through, 15 to 18 minutes. Remove from the oven and allow to cool for 15 to 20 minutes before serving.

† If you can't find whipped butter, you can substitute it with low-fat butter spread.

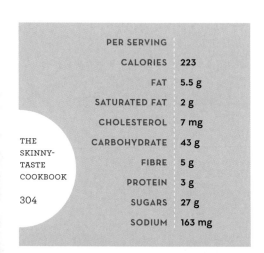

PER SERVING	
CALORIES	223
FAT	5.5 g
SATURATED FAT	2 g
CHOLESTEROL	7 mg
CARBOHYDRATE	43 g
FIBRE	5 g
PROTEIN	3 g
SUGARS	27 g
SODIUM	163 mg

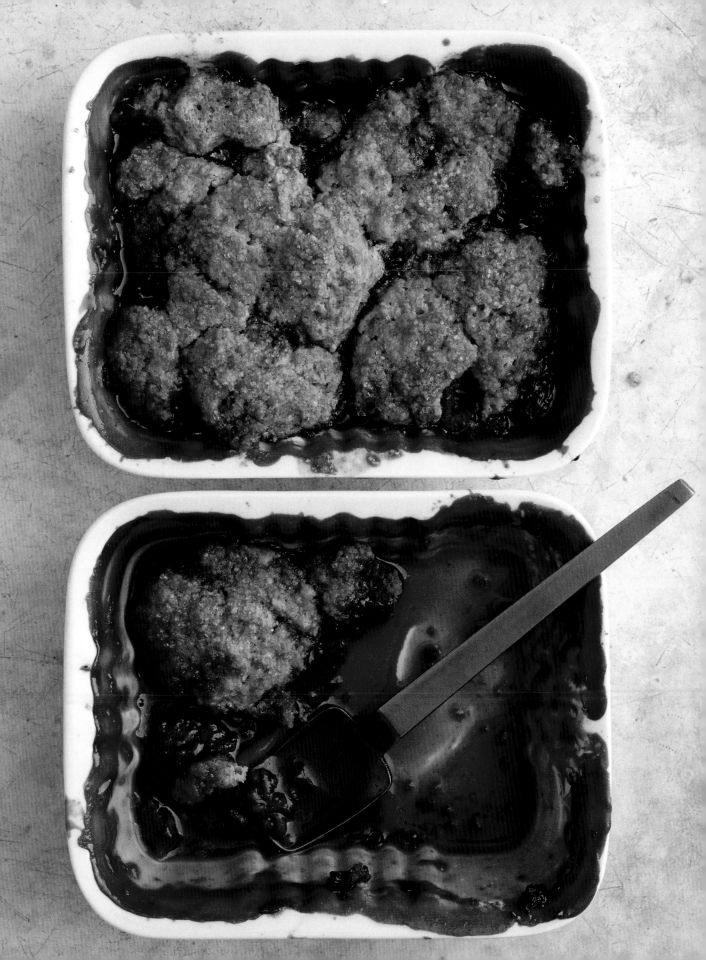

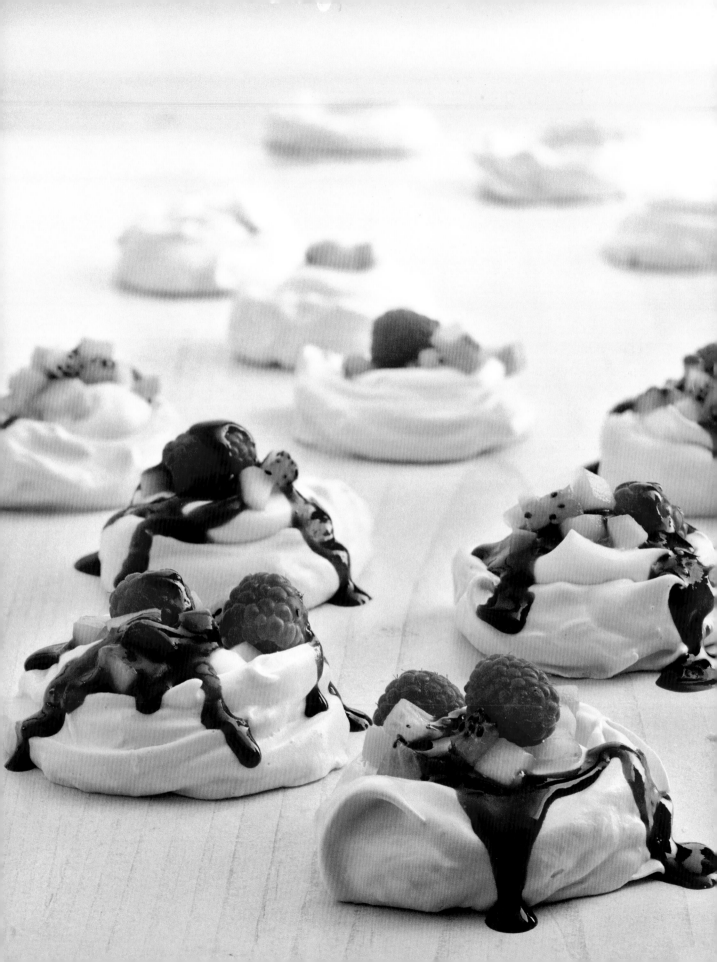

Mini Pavlovas with Fresh Fruit

SERVES 9

These sweet meringues are a great dessert if you're having company or want to bring something sweet to a party. Since they're nothing more than whipped egg whites, sugar, cornflour and vanilla topped with fresh fruit, they're naturally fat-free. But I do like to top them with a little fresh cream, so I came up with this delicious lighter alternative to full-fat whipped cream by whipping up only half of the cream, then folding in fat-free Greek yoghurt. It works beautifully and the yoghurt gives it a little extra tang.

MERINGUES

2 large egg whites, at room temperature

½ teaspoon pure vanilla extract

1 teaspoon cornflour

⅛ teaspoon sea salt

6 tablespoons sugar

FRUIT TOPPING

1¼ cups (155g) raspberries

2 tablespoons sugar

1 teaspoon fresh lemon juice

10 tablespoons finely chopped mango

2 small kiwifruits, finely chopped

LIGHTER WHIPPED CREAM

1 tablespoon sugar

¼ cup (50ml) well-chilled whipping cream

¼ teaspoon pure vanilla extract

¼ cup (60g) fat-free Greek yoghurt

Adjust the rack in the centre of the oven and preheat to its lowest temperature. Line a large baking tray with baking parchment.

For the meringues: In the bowl of a stand mixer fitted with the whisk, beat the egg whites, vanilla, cornflour and salt at medium speed until foamy, 1 to 2 minutes. Increase the speed to medium-high and beat until the egg whites are soft and billowy, 2 to 3 minutes. Slowly add the sugar, 1 tablespoon at a time, beating until thick and glossy peaks form, 3 to 4 minutes.

Using a spatula, scoop 9 generous mounds of meringue onto the prepared baking tray and use the spatula to make an indent in the centre of each (like a bowl).

(recipe continues)

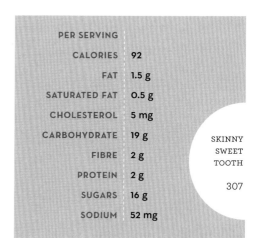

PER SERVING	
CALORIES	92
FAT	1.5 g
SATURATED FAT	0.5 g
CHOLESTEROL	5 mg
CARBOHYDRATE	19 g
FIBRE	2 g
PROTEIN	2 g
SUGARS	16 g
SODIUM	52 mg

SKINNY
SWEET
TOOTH

307

Bake until firm on the outside and smooth, about 1 hour 30 minutes. Turn off the oven and leave the meringues in the oven with the door closed until they are hard and dry, about 3 hours. Carefully remove the meringues from the paper. Immediately store them in an airtight container.

For the fruit topping: In a small saucepan, combine ¾ cup (90g) of the raspberries, the sugar and lemon juice. Bring to a boil over medium heat and cook, stirring, for 2 minutes. Remove the pan from the heat and allow to sit for about 10 minutes. Strain the mixture through a fine-mesh sieve into a bowl, using a spoon to press on the raspberries; discard the seeds. Refrigerate until ready to serve.

In a small bowl, combine the remaining raspberries with the mango and the kiwifruits.

For the lighter whipped cream: Put a metal bowl and the beaters of a hand mixer into the freezer for 10 to 15 minutes.

Remove the bowl and beaters from the freezer. Put the sugar, cream and vanilla into the bowl and beat with a hand mixer just until the cream reaches stiff peaks, 2 to 3 minutes. Fold in the yoghurt.

Assemble the pavlovas by spooning 1 tablespoon light whipped cream into each meringue shell. Top each with 1 tablespoon of the fresh fruit and 2 teaspoons raspberry sauce. Serve immediately.

Frozen Dark Chocolate-Almond Bananas

SERVES 4

I eat a banana just about every day, sometimes in my smoothie or oatmeal, other times as a quick snack on the go. But my favourite way to enjoy this potassium-filled pick, particularly in the summer when I need a chocolate fix, is frozen on a stick, dipped in dark chocolate and sprinkled with chopped almonds. It's a guiltless frozen treat!

1 large ripe banana

4 ice lolly sticks

225g dark chocolate*

1 teaspoon rapeseed oil

3 tablespoons coarsely chopped dry-roasted almonds

*Read the label to be sure this product is gluten-free.

Line a baking sheet with greaseproof paper.

Halve the banana lengthwise, then cut in half crosswise. Insert an ice lolly stick into each piece of banana and lay them on the prepared baking sheet. Freeze until completely frozen, at least 1 hour.

In a microwave-safe mug or bowl, combine the chocolate and oil. Melt the chocolate in the microwave on high, 30 seconds at a time, stirring until the chocolate is melted. Dip the bananas one at a time into the chocolate, scraping off the excess from the flat part of the banana, and put them on the baking sheet. Working quickly, before the chocolate sets, sprinkle the bananas with the chopped almonds. Put the bananas back into the freezer until the chocolate is hard, about 1 hour. Keep frozen until ready to serve.

Note: In order to coat the bananas with chocolate, you'll need to start with 225g, but only 50g will adhere to the bananas. The nutritional information accounts for 50g of chocolate.

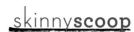

Don't let those browning bananas on your counter go to waste! They are perfect for this sweet treat!

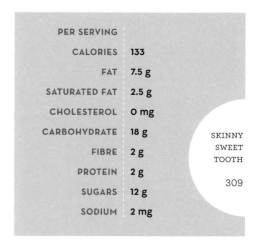

PER SERVING	
CALORIES	133
FAT	7.5 g
SATURATED FAT	2.5 g
CHOLESTEROL	0 mg
CARBOHYDRATE	18 g
FIBRE	2 g
PROTEIN	2 g
SUGARS	12 g
SODIUM	2 mg

SKINNY
SWEET
TOOTH

Watermelon Lime Granita

SERVES 4

Eating a sweet, juicy watermelon on a hot summer's day is hard to beat – but this Italian-ice-like dessert comes pretty darn close! And it's made with just three ingredients. Trust me, you'll want to make this all summer long! A granita is made by scraping frozen ice crystals as they form in the freezer. You don't need to own any fancy appliances or equipment – all you need is a blender, a metal baking pan, a freezer and a fork!

4 cups (600g) chopped seedless watermelon

Juice of 1 lime

2 tablespoons sugar

In a blender, combine the chopped watermelon, lime juice and sugar. Blend until smooth. Pour the purée into a 23 × 23cm metal baking tin. Cover with clingfilm and freeze for about 1½ hours. Using a fork, scrape the surface and mix it up. Return the pan to the freezer until almost set, about 2 hours. Using a fork, scrape the granita into chunky snowlike ice crystals. Freeze and repeat the scraping process until the entire mixture is frozen and shaved, 1 more hour.

Store, covered in clingfilm, until ready to serve. To serve, spoon into 4 small glass bowls.

skinny**scoop**

For the sweetest results, always buy a whole, fresh watermelon instead of one that has already been cut. Look for a firm, symmetrical watermelon that's free of any bruises, cuts or dents. The watermelon should be heavy for its size, and the underside of the watermelon should have a creamy yellow spot from where it sat on the ground and ripened in the sun. If it doesn't have that, it was picked too early and won't be as sweet.

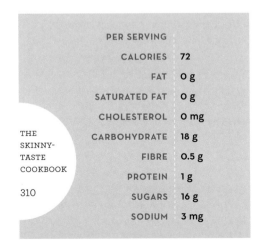

PER SERVING	
CALORIES	72
FAT	0 g
SATURATED FAT	0 g
CHOLESTEROL	0 mg
CARBOHYDRATE	18 g
FIBRE	0.5 g
PROTEIN	1 g
SUGARS	16 g
SODIUM	3 mg

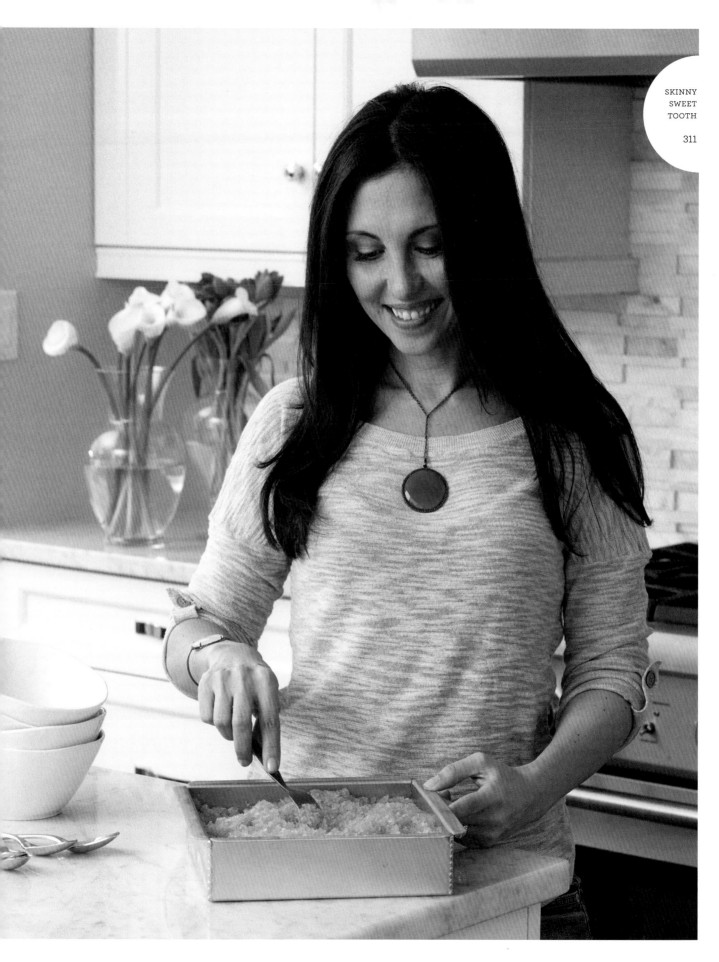

Sweet Plum Custard

SERVES 4

I love the taste and rustic simplicity of this French-inspired dessert. The sweet plums sink into the batter, like purple crescent moons. The batter puffs up while it bakes in the oven and then collapses into a soft custard that's lightly dusted with icing sugar just before eating. Use really ripe plums when you make these – they should be practically falling out of their skins. Other stone fruits, such as peaches or apricots, can be substituted, or try ripe pears in the autumn.

Cooking spray or oil mister

1⅓ cups (235g) halved, stoned plums, cut into 5mm-thick wedges (about 4)

¼ cup (55g) raw cane sugar

2 tablespoons cornflour

Sea salt

2 large eggs, at room temperature

½ cup (120ml) skimmed milk

1 teaspoon pure vanilla extract

Icing sugar, for dusting

Preheat the oven to 190°C/170°C fan/Gas 5. Lightly spray 4 (170g) shallow gratin dishes with oil.

Place the gratin dishes on a baking sheet and arrange the plums in each gratin dish in a single layer.

In a large bowl, whisk together the raw cane sugar, cornflour and a pinch of salt. Add the eggs, milk and vanilla and whisk until smooth. Pour the egg and milk mixture over the plums.

Bake until lightly golden and a toothpick inserted into the centre comes out clean, about 30 minutes. Transfer the gratin dishes to a wire rack and allow to cool until warm.

When ready to serve, dust with icing sugar. Serve warm.

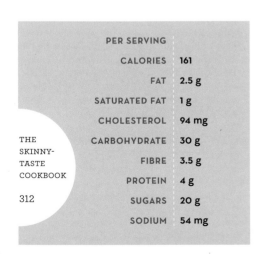

PER SERVING	
CALORIES	161
FAT	2.5 g
SATURATED FAT	1 g
CHOLESTEROL	94 mg
CARBOHYDRATE	30 g
FIBRE	3.5 g
PROTEIN	4 g
SUGARS	20 g
SODIUM	54 mg

Matcha Milkshake

SERVES 2

I love the taste of matcha, a traditional Japanese green tea powder. It has a complex, rich flavour that's unique and easily dissolves in any liquid (no need to boil water). Matcha offers the same health benefits as green tea leaves, plus it has two amino acids (theophylline and L-theanine) that have both an energizing and calming effect – maybe this explains why Buddhist monks have been drinking matcha for centuries!

1 cup (200g) low-fat vanilla frozen yoghurt

1 cup (225ml) sweetened vanilla almond milk

4 teaspoons matcha powder

4 to 5 ice cubes

In a blender, combine the frozen yoghurt, almond milk, matcha powder and ice cubes and blend until smooth. Divide between 2 glasses.

skinnyscoop

After opening, matcha should be refrigerated or kept in the freezer in an airtight container.

FOOD FACTS magnificent matcha

Green tea is famous for its health-promoting properties, many of which stem from one powerful antioxidant called epigallocatechin-3-gallate (EGCG). Matcha green tea, a powder made from ground tea leaves, has triple the EGCG found in traditionally steeped green teas. It also boasts the amino acids theophylline and L-theanine, which improve focus, reduce stress and contribute to an energy boost.

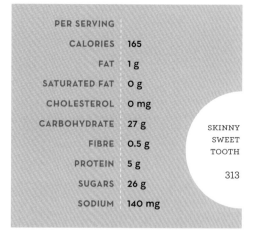

PER SERVING	
CALORIES	165
FAT	1 g
SATURATED FAT	0 g
CHOLESTEROL	0 mg
CARBOHYDRATE	27 g
FIBRE	0.5 g
PROTEIN	5 g
SUGARS	26 g
SODIUM	140 mg

SKINNY
SWEET
TOOTH

ACKNOWLEDGEMENTS

Mom and Dad, we sat to eat together as a family every night; you're my inspiration and I am forever thankful for you both. My brother, Ivan, I can't imagine my life without you. To my loving and supportive husband, and my two favourite girls, Karina and Madison – thank you for being my official taste-testers; your honesty only made the recipes better. I love you!

A huge thank-you to Heather K. Jones, R.D., for all the time you poured into this book; your positive attitude lifted me up on those nights when I let self-doubt creep into my head; I couldn't have partnered with a better person and a true friend. To my aunt Ligia, thank you for your meticulous recipe testing and dedication. My editor, Ashley Phillips; you are sweet, brilliant and talented. Thank you for guiding me through the process.

To the amazing photography team who inspired me every day on set: photographer Penny De Los Santos, who taught me that photos should always tell a story; Simon Andrews, thank you for your flawless food styling and for the invaluable lessons learned; Kaitlyn DuRoss, your positive energy and love of prop styling was contagious. Jay Kim, Stephanie Mungia, Barret Washburne, Idan Bitton – I couldn't have been in better hands. To the vendors who loaned their props: ABC Home, abchome.com; CLAM LAB ceramics, Brooklyn, NY, clamlab.com; Young In the Mountains, Boulder CO, younginthemountains.com; MONDAYS ceramics, Brooklyn, NY, mondaysprojects.com; and Looks Like White ceramics, Montreal Quebec, lookslikewhite.com. Thanks to Aloft Studios for making us feel at home.

To my girlfriends who came through for me when I needed them most, I love you all so very much: Denise H, Katia, Raquel, Doreen, Denise P, Kim, Gabbie, Nicole and Julia – I am forever grateful for our friendship. My uncle and cousins, Rene, Nina and Camila, who tasted most of these recipes in this book more than once. Jimmy and Maureen, neighbours extraordinaire who also doubled as taste-testers. Susan Hanover Designs, for letting me use your fabulous kitchen and wear your stunning jewellery. To Tara, for styling me, and Jacqueline Shepherd Makeup for making me pretty.

A special thank-you to Donna Fennessy, for polishing my writing. And Heather's nutrition team – Caroline Kaufman, M.S., R.D., Danielle Hazard, Juhie Bhatia, B.Sc., M.S. – as well as her nutrition interns: Hayley Morgan, Ryan Locke, Stephanie L. Leong, Kendall Wright and Nicole Karetov.

And, of course, this book would not have been possible without my wonderful agent, Janis Donnaud, and the entire team at Clarkson Potter.

Last, a giant THANK-YOU to all my *Skinnytaste*, Facebook, Twitter, Pinterest and Instagram fans who took part in naming the book, and helping me choose this winning cover design.

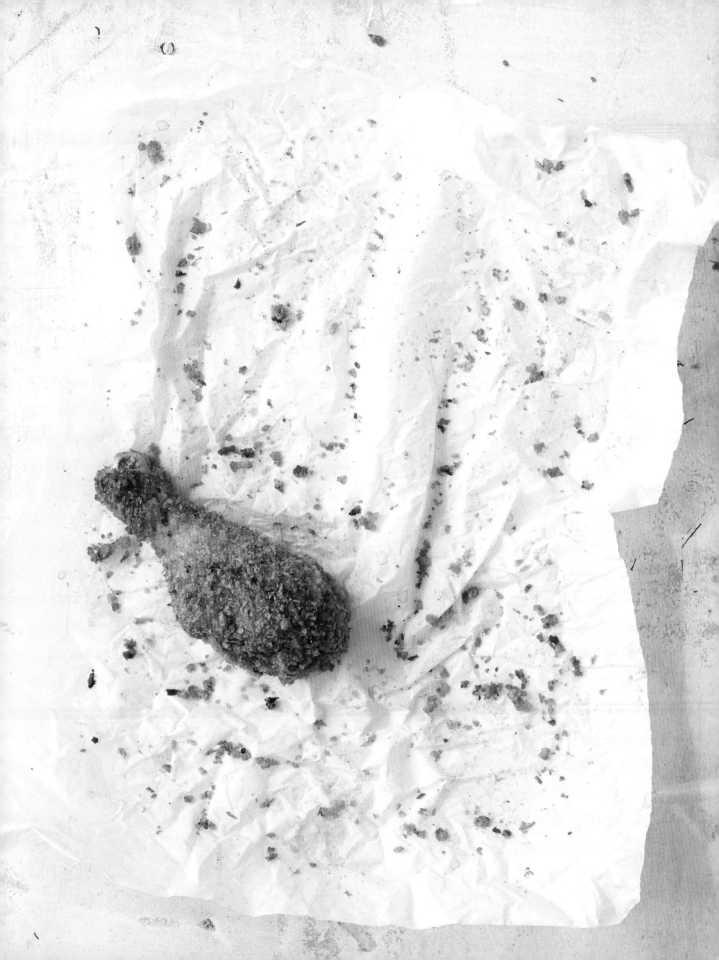

INDEX